TO MRS. MARIE ST. RAVN

Very best wishes
Thanks for all you
withhend

Alex Robin
April '86.

D0275198

Liver Disorders in Childhood

POSTGRADUATE PAEDIATRICS SERIES

under the General Editorship of

JOHN APLEY
CBE, MD, BS, FRCP

Emeritus Consultant Paediatrician,
United Bristol Hospitals

Liver Disorders in Childhood

ALEX P. MOWAT

MB, ChB, FRCP, DCH, DObst RCOG

Consultant Paediatrician
King's College Hospital, Bethlem Royal Hospital
and Maudsley Hospital, London

BUTTERWORTHS
London - Boston
Sydney - Wellington - Durban - Toronto

United Kingdom London	**Butterworth & Co (Publishers) Ltd** 88 Kingsway, WC2B 6AB
Australia Sydney	**Butterworths Pty Ltd** 586 Pacific Highway, Chatswood, NSW 2067 Also at Melbourne, Brisbane, Adelaide and Perth
Canada Toronto	**Butterworth & Co (Canada) Ltd** 2265 Midland Avenue, Scarborough, Ontario, M1P 4S1
New Zealand Wellington	**Butterworths of New Zealand Ltd** T & W Young Building, 77–85 Customhouse Quay, 1, CPO Box 472
South Africa Durban	**Butterworth & Co (South Africa) Ltd** 152–154 Gale Street
USA Boston	**Butterworth (Publishers) Inc** 19 Cummings Park, Woburn, Massachusetts 01801

All rights reserved. No part of this publication may be reproduced or transmitted in any form or by any means, including photocopying and recording, without the written permission of the copyright holder, application for which should be addressed to the Publishers. Such written permission must also be obtained before any part of this publication is stored in a retrieval system of any nature.

This book is sold subject to the Standard Conditions of Sale of Net Books and may not be re-sold in the UK below the net price given by the Publishers in their current price list.

First published 1979

© Butterworth & Co (Publishers) Ltd, 1979

ISBN 0 407 00163 8

British Library Cataloguing in Publication Data

Mowat, Alex P
   Liver disorders in childhood. – (Postgraduate paediatrics series).
   1. Liver – Diseases 2. Children – Diseases
   I. Title II. Series
   618.9′23′62   RJ456.L5   78–40690

   ISBN 0–407–00163–8

Typeset by Scribe Design, Chatham, Kent
Printed and bound at William Clowes & Sons Limited, Beccles and London

To
Ann, Neil and Adrian

Editor's Foreword

It is noteworthy that this book is the work of a paediatrician, not of a physician for adults who would be writing about children as a sideline. Knowledge and experience of liver disorders in childhood have been accumulating so rapidly that there has been an indisputable need for a comprehensive volume bringing them into the paediatric ambit. It had to be done and now it has been done, fully and well. This is the first book on the subject, so far as I know, and by a single author. That itself is a matter for congratulation, for now readers (and their patients) can reap the benefit of one man's balance and perspective.

Dr Mowat offers experience and expertise that have accrued largely from his work in a teaching hospital which has a highly reputed unit for liver disorders adjacent to and working closely with a paediatric department. Help and advice for children with liver disorders are sought by paediatricians from far afield. The patients enjoy a triple advantage. They benefit from extensive, pooled know-how. They share out-patient clinics and centralized and highly specialized support services for investigation, treatment and research. Yet they are cared for – and thought about – by staff with paediatric training and habits. The patients are not just 'liver problems' but sick children.

Because Dr Mowat is a paediatrician the presentation is based on a clinical approach. The main focus is on day-to-day practical problems of diagnosis and management; but he discusses controversial topics and research developments, too, with the non-specialist reader in mind. It was illuminating for me to find so much reasoned argument based on anatomy, physiology and metabolism, and to be able to follow it through even though my somewhat dusty souvenirs of these subjects only vaguely resemble the crystal-sparkling items that he offers. The mystery that has surrounded liver disorders is being cleared away as new knowledge is collated, tested and made available. Nowhere is this more welcome than in paediatrics. I hope that from this book many children all over the world will benefit.

John Apley

Preface

This book aims to provide a comprehensive and up-to-date account of disorders of the liver and biliary system in childhood. The main justification for writing such a book at this time is the need to synthesize for the clinician the many important developments in diagnosis, categorization and treatment of liver disease in childhood which have occurred in the last two decades. The developments considered range through new knowledge of the mechanisms of physiological jaundice; the controversy of jaundice associated with breast feeding; surgery for extrahepatic biliary atresia; the role of hepatitis B virus infection in chronic liver disease; presymptomatic diagnosis of Wilson's disease; liver transplantation to surgical treatment of metabolic disorders such as glycogen storage disease. Throughout, important aspects in diagnosis and management are stressed from the viewpoint of the paediatrician. The value and limitations of investigative procedures, both old and new, are critically discussed.

The secondary aim is to summarize recent research developments and to indicate some of the outstanding clinical problems and areas in which research is urgently required. The book incorporates advances in knowledge of hepatocyte and bile duct cell structure and function derived from electronmicroscopic and biochemical studies, where these contribute to our understanding of the pathogenesis of liver disease.

Information gleaned from studies in genetic disorders which lead to liver damage have also been included since these give important insights both into liver function and mechanisms of liver damage. Such advances in knowledge are important to the clinician and clinical research worker trying to understand and modify the many metabolic disturbances which can occur secondarily to liver damage or bile duct obstruction.

Recent developments in the understanding of disordered immune mechanisms associated with liver disease suggest that these are important not only because of their role as diagnostic indicators but because of their putative role in pathogenesis. Evidence relating the outcome of liver disease to the interaction between the many cell types within the liver and the cells of the reticulo-endothelial system is also scrutinized.

This book has been written primarily for clinicians, especially paediatricians, paediatric surgeons and gastroenterologists; but it is hoped that it will be of value also to pathologists, biochemists and laboratory research workers concerned with understanding aspects of hepatic function and elucidating pathogenic mechanisms.

I wish to acknowledge my indebtedness to all my many teachers, especially Dr G.A. Levvy, Professor Ross G. Mitchell and Dr Irwin M. Arias who gave me so much help in developing my interest in liver disease.

This work would not have been possible without the help and encouragement of many colleagues at King's College Hospital. I am particularly grateful to Professor C. Eric Stroud, Dr Roger Williams, Dr Adrian L.W.F. Eddleston and Mr. Edward R. Howard for their help in providing an academic environment in which to pursue clinical research in liver disease.

My thanks are due to the many past and present fellow students in the Department of Child Health and the Liver Unit for contributing to my continuing education by stimulating discussion.

Dr K. Cottrall, Dr D.I. Johnston, Dr V.C. Larcher, Mr. D.J. Manthorpe, Dr G. Mieli, Dr A. Nicholson, Dr C.A. Porter, Dr B.I. Portmann, Dr H.T. Psacharopoulos, Dr A.L. Smith and Dr M.S. Tanner, co-workers in the last seven years, have contributed much information which has modified my understanding of conditions considered in this book.

Clinical photographs were the work of Mr. Blewitt and his staff of the Photographic Dept. King's College Hospital. Dr Mieli, Dr Portmann and Dr W.G.P. Mair provided photomicrographs.

Dr Heather Nunnerley performed many of the radiographic procedures shown, and provided the radiographs.

I would like to thank the Editors of the *Archives of Disease in Childhood, Tohoku Journal of Experimental Medicine, Journal of Clinical Investigations* and Churchill Livingstone, Publishers, for permission to include illustrations and tables from their works.

Many colleagues have invited me to see patients under their care and advised me on their subsequent progress. These patients and their parents provided the stimulus which has seen this book to completion, assisted by the tactful, succinct and helpful guidance of Dr John Apley.

The complete manuscript was typed by Mrs. Pamela Golding, while continuing her duties as a secretary in the Department of Child Health, King's College Hospital. Without her the book would not have been completed.

I am greatly indebted to my wife and children for their patient support and understanding during the gestation of this book.

Alex P. Mowat

Contents

CHAPTER 1

Anatomy and Physiology of the Liver

Clinical assessment of liver

Inspection Where hepatomegaly is massive, or where there are large nodules on the surface of the liver, this may be evident on inspection.

Palpation and percussion The lower edge of the liver should be palpated just lateral to the right rectus muscle. In the newborn and in the first four months of life, the liver edge may be palpable up to 2 cm below the costal margin without indicating hepatomegaly. In older children, it is rarely more than 1 cm below the costal margin, except in deep inspiration. It may be normally palpable in the mid-line 3 or 4 cm below the base of the xiphisternum.

If the liver is palpable at a lower level, one cannot immediately conclude that the liver is enlarged until the position of the upper border has been determined by percussion. It should be at the level of the fifth or sixth rib in the right mid-axillary line, at about the seventh intercostal space in the mid-axillary line, and at the ninth rib posteriorly. There is some doubt as to whether light percussion is more informative than heavy percussion for this purpose. I favour the former, but it is probably more important for a clinician to use a consistent method and interpret the results with some allowance for the effect of subcutaneous fat, oedema, and the state of the lungs. Emphysema displaces downwards the upper limits of hepatic dullness. The left lobe extends from the mid-line out as far as the left mid-clavicular line.

A Reidel's lobe is a downward tongue-like projection from the right lobe of the liver. It may extend as far as the right iliac crest.

Percussion is of value in detecting a reduction in the size of the liver. In cirrhosis the area of hepatic dullness will have a lower upper border than normal and dullness will stop well above the edge of the rib cage.

Very large livers are associated with storage disorders, disorders of the reticulo-endothelial system, such as leukaemia, gross fatty change, malignant disease and congestive cardiac failure. Rapid changes in size occur in congestive cardiac failure and in bile duct obstruction.

Some information on the nature of the liver disease may be inferred from the consistency of the edge of the liver and from its surface. The normal edge is soft, fairly sharp, and is not tender. Livers swollen because of congestive cardiac failure, or acute hepatocyte infiltration are firm, have somewhat rounded edges, smooth surfaces and are tender if the swelling is acute. In cirrhosis the liver is hard and has an irregular surface and edge. The liver is pulsatile in tricuspid incompetence.

Auscultation Auscultation is of value in detecting increased hepatic blood flow in vascular lesions such as tumours and haemangiomata. It has also been used to try to assess the position of the lower border of the liver. A stethescope may be placed on the xiphisternum and the abdomen scratched lightly in a transverse direction, advancing the line of the scratch cephalad in the right mid-clavicular line. If the edge of the liver is below the costal margin a change in intensity and quality of the auscultated sound is noted as the edge is crossed. In general, this technique has little to add to palpation, but it may be helpful when the liver is large but soft; for example, in glycogen storage disease.

Where serial recordings of liver size are desirable, the most consistent is that obtained by palpating the edge of the liver in the right midclavicular line recording the distance below the rib cage at which the edge is palpable. An alternative method is to determine the upper limit of hepatic dullness in the mid-clavicular line and to record the distance between this point and the palpated edge of the liver in the midclavicular line. Where the latter technique has been compared with isotope scintiscans, considerable discrepancies have been found.

Spleen

The spleen can be palpated from 1 to 2 cm below the left costal margin during the first few weeks of life. The tip is often palpable in well infants and young children. It is very commonly enlarged during generalized infections. Gentle palpation starting from the right iliac fossa and moving towards the left costal margin is the best technique. The spleen is a very superficial organ, and the edge is very distinct. The splenic notch is very rarely palpable. On percussion the dullness extends up beyond the costal margin. Careful palpation and percussion detects the vast majority of spleens which have been shown to be enlarged by scintiscanning. The scintiscan is particularly valuable in the presence of ascites.

ANATOMY OF THE LIVER

The liver is essentially a mass of cells permeated by a complex but ordered system of channels carrying its blood supply and bile. Electronmicroscopic examination of hepatocytes shows an equally complex arrangement of channels connecting intracellular organelles. In this chapter emphasis will be given to the structural arrangements which ensure that each hepatocyte is in intimate contact with the blood flowing through the liver, facilitating transport of materials into and out of the hepatocyte, and at the same time facilitating secretion of bile.

Gross structure

The liver is a continuous, uniform organ adopting a shape enforced on it by body cavities, other intraperitoneal structures and vascular forces; the positive pressure from the portal vein and the hepatic artery and the often negative pressure in the hepatic veins. The conventional division into right and left lobes does not coincide with the intrahepatic branching of vessels and ducts. Some knowledge of the normal distribution of these structures is necessary to understand some of the pathological consequences of disease within the liver or in the portal venous system.

Portal vein branches

Since the hepatic artery and bile ducts follow the portal vein and its branches these will be described. The portal vein, which is formed by the junction of the superior mesenteric vein and the splenic vein, is directed towards the right lobe as it approaches the portahepatis. It branches into a short right trunk and a longer left trunk. The intrahepatic branches are subject to minor variations but a 'typical' pattern can be described. The right branch gives rise to a lateral branch directed to the right upper lobe, an inferior branch supplying the area to the right of the gallbladder and a large central branch supplying the anterosuperior portion of the liver. From the left trunk, superior, intermediate and inferior branches supply the lateral aspects of the left lobe and branches run also to the caudate and quadrate lobes (*Figure 1.1*). Anastomoses between the branches of the right and left portal vein branches are unusual. Each terminal branch has a sharply defined territory, the smaller branches having the characteristic of 'end-arteries'. The portal vein 'territories' are shared by branches of the hepatic artery and tributaries of the hepatic duct which accompany the veins.

Hepatic artery The hepatic artery and its intrahepatic branches are much less constant. In 55 per cent of individuals the main hepatic artery arises as a single trunk from the coeliac artery but in the

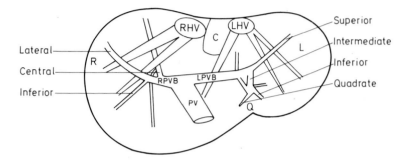

Figure 1.1. Diagrammatic representation of portal blood distribution to the right (R), left (L), quadrate (Q), and caudate (C) lobes of the liver, and the main right (RHV) and left (LHV) hepatic veins

remainder two or three main arteries arise from the coeliac, superior mesenteric, gastro-duodenal, left or right gastric arteries, or even direct from the aorta.

Within the liver the artery or its branches follow the appropriate branches of the portal vein. Sometimes two anastomosing arteries may accompany one vein, but the terminal branches are end-arteries supplying independently a circumscribed volume of liver. There are no intrahepatic communications between the right and left hepatic arteries.

Hepatic vein tributaries

The hepatic vein tributaries have sharply defined areas of drainage which do not relate directly to the portal vein end-branch or hepatic end-artery territory, yet they do interdigitate with these to give uniform drainage of the liver. On both a microscopic and a macroscopic scale, portal vein and hepatic veins run as nearly perpendicular to one another as is geometrically possible. There are three main hepatic veins: the right hepatic vein drains the right upper lobe, the middle vein drains an area supplied by both the right and left portal veins, and the left vein the left lobe. Other fairly constant veins drain the posterior cranial parts of both lobes, the inferior part of the right lobe, and a number lead from the caudate lobe. These hepatic veins are straight and follow a radial course to the inferior vena cava. The branches of the portal vein weave between these vessels, the convexity of their course being directed to the diaphragm and to the anterior and lateral body walls.

Portal tract

The portal vein and hepatic artery branches, bile ducts, lymph vessels and nerves are surrounded by a coat of connective tissue continuous with the external capsule of the liver. This connective tissue, referred to as the 'limiting plate', bounds the portal canal or tract. This is sometimes described as the portal *triad* because it contains the portal vein radical, the hepatic artery and the bile duct, as the three most prominent structures within it.

From the portal triads, portal venous blood and the hepatic artery branches pass through the limiting plate, through channels which are controlled by a sphincter. These channels discharge into a specialized network of capillaries termed 'sinusoids'.

Sinusoids

Sinusoids carry the blood to the hepatocytes, which are polyhedral cells arranged as plates or sheets one cell in thickness. Up to the age of two years many sheets, having many lacunae, are two cells in thickness. The sinusoids form a three-dimensional network of vessels within these lacunae. They are separated from the hepatocytes by the space of Disse. This perisinusoidal space contains argyrophilic reticulum fibres which have the electronmicroscopic characteristics or collagen. They are arranged in thick fibres which run parallel to sinusoids and fine ones which seem to bind them together. The microvilli of the hepatocyte cell membrane project into the space of Disse. The sinusoids are lined by specialized *endothelial* cells, the sides of which do not adhere to one another but overlap loosely. They have holes in their cytoplasm through which large molecules can pass. A second type of cell is the specialized endothelial cell usually given the eponym *Kupffer cell*. These are cells which are actively engaged in phagocytosis, their number increasing when an antigen load coming to the liver increases. The Kupffer cells are also thought to have the ability to bulge into the lumen of the sinusoid and perhaps control sinusoidal blood flow. A third type of cell in the wall of the sinusoid is the so-called 'fat cell' or *Ito cell*, which are thought to have a role in fibrogenesis, they may produce the collagen found in the space of Disse and also participate in collagen deposition in disease. It is believed that the fluid in the space of Disse drains to the periportal space from which it passes through the limiting plate into lymphatics within the portal triads (*Figure 1.2* to *1.5*).

Hepatic development

Much of our current knowledge of the development of the liver and its functions has been derived from animal work or very abnormal situations in the human fetus. Extrapolation of these findings to the intact human fetus may lead to erroneous conclusions.

The liver is formed at an early stage in embryonic life from an invagination of the foregut into the mesoderm of the septum transversum. Both bile ducts and hepatocytes are derived from endoderm. The mesoderm forms the marrow elements, endothelial cells, Kupffer cells, fibrous tissue and blood vessels. By the 10 mm stage all branches of the portal and hepatic veins are evident. Umbilical venous blood from the placenta is largely deviated from the liver via the ductus venosus to the inferior vena cava. The remainder of the umbilical vein blood passes via the portal vein through the liver, rejoining the circulation via the hepatic veins. At this stage, the right and left hepatic lobes are of equal size, but the portal venous drainage to the left lobe is less satisfactory than that to the right, causing a relative retardation

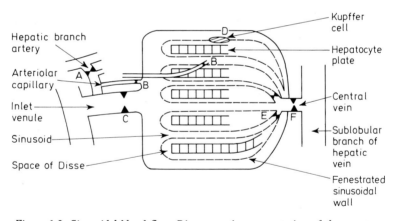

Figure 1.2. Sinusoidal blood flow. Diagrammatic representation of the structure of sinusoids showing at points indicated (A,B,C,D,E and F) the sites of possible sphincters (⚡ *) involved in controlling blood flow through the hepatic sinusoids. Sphincters are present on the arterioles of capillaries, tiny arteries entering the liver substance, on the inlet venule draining the portal vein, on the sinusoids themselves (D) at the exits from the sinusoids (E) and in the central vein branch. The Kupffer cell may also have a sphincteric effect*

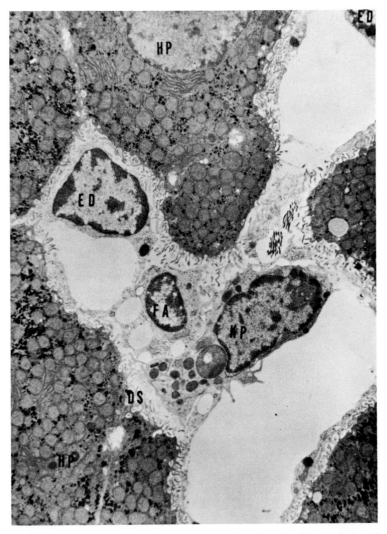

Figure 1.3. A survey picture of the sinusoid of rat liver fixed by perfusion. A Kupffer cell (KP). an endothelial cell (ED); a fat storage cell (FA); a hepatocyte (HP); the space of Disse (DS). The Kupffer cell has small nucleo-cytoplasmic ratio, many cytoplasmic projections, ample cytoplasm containing many lysosomes with various size and density. An endothelial cell is characterized by large nucleo-cytoplasmic ratio, the smooth cell surface, attenuated cytoplasmic processes forming the large part of the sinusoidal wall and well developed vacuolar apparatus. There is a paucity in lysosomes (× 6,800, reduced to ninetenths in reproduction). (Reproduced by courtesy of the Editor of the Tohoku Journal of Experimental Medicine)

of growth of the left lobe prior to birth. The ductus venosus probably closes soon after birth. By 10–20 days of age closure is complete.

By late gestation the morphological characteristics of liver cells are similar to those in the adult. Liver cells are arranged in plates which are two cells in thickness, which presumably limits the effectiveness of transfer of materials into and out of the hepatocytes. By the age of two years the majority of plates have become one cell in thickness, but it is not until the age of five years that all plates are composed of single hepatocytes.

PHYSIOLOGY OF THE LIVER

Hepatocellular activities

The liver plays a major role in metabolism, maintaining within narrow limits the supply of carbohydrates, proteins and lipids to other tissues, in spite of wide variations in dietary intake and in metabolic demands.

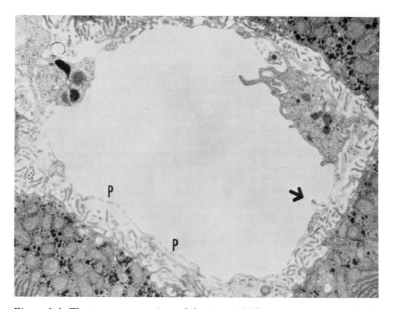

Figure 1.4. The transverse section of the sinusoid. There are many pores in the attenuated process of the endothelial cell (P). The size of the pores is almost about 0.1μ. A microvillus of the hepatocyte penetrates the sinusoidal wall through the pore (arrow) (× 10,200, reduced to seven-tenths in reproduction). (Reproduced by courtesy of the Editor of the Tohoku Journal of Experimental Medicine)

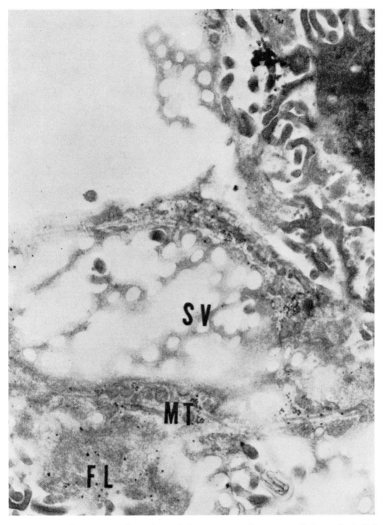

Figure 1.5. The tangential section of the attenuated process of the endothelial cell. The pores are round or oval in shape creating the sieve plate-like structure (SV). Fine filaments (FL) and microtubules (MT) can be seen in the cytoplasm around the pores (× 20,900, reduced to nine-tenths in reproduction). (Reproduced by courtesy of the Editor of the Tohoku Journal of Experimental Medicine)

The liver is involved in the chemical transformation of many endogenous and exogenous substances, thereby vastly changing their metabolic, therapeutic or toxic effects. It has a major role in bilirubin excretion. By bile formation it contributes to digestion and absorption. It serves as a store for carbohydrates in the form of glycogen, and also for the fat-soluble vitamins, A, D, E and K and vitamin B_{12}.

During much of childhood the liver has considerable reserve capacity for these functions. A temporary hepatic inefficiency is a feature of the newborn, most marked in infants born prematurely.

In fetal life many enzymes concerned with various homeostatic functions of the liver show negligible activity, possibly because many of the functions of the liver are at this time performed by the placenta and maternal tissues. It is thought that changes in the function of the liver in the perinatal period are mediated by intrahepatic and extra-hepatic vascular changes, together with extensively studied, but only partially understood, changes in enzymatic activity. Many of the enzymatic studies on which current knowledge is based have been carried out in experimental animals, often using artificial substrates for the enzyme.

Each of the main physiological roles of the liver are considered below, together with those changes during development which may be of clinical or pathological relevance.

Carbohydrate metabolism

Monosaccharides, glucose, galactose and fructose absorbed from the intestinal tract are avidly taken up by the liver, where they may be utilized for immediately required energy, being incorporated in the citric acid cycle, or they may be used to form glycogen. Hepatic glycogen is an invaluable source of carbohydrate which prevents hypoglycaemia by releasing glucose to other tissues during fasting. Muscle glycogen does not release glucose into the general circulation.

Large amounts of glycogen appear in the liver towards the end of gestation. These stores are lower in the premature or light-for-gestational age infant. Glycogen is rapidly mobilized immediately following birth; hypoglycaemia may occur at this stage. It is thought that this arises because of ineffective gluconeogenesis which does not replenish hepatic glycogen.

Lipids: steroids: bile salts

Neutral fats absorbed from the small intestine are oxidized within the liver into glycerol and free fatty acids. Fatty acids may be further oxidized to acetyl CoA which enters Krebs' tricarbonylic acid cycle. Glycerol may be utilized to form other triglycerides or degraded via acetyl CoA. Phospholipids sphingolipids and steroids may all be synthesized within the liver.

The liver has an important role in the metabolism of glucocorticoids and mineralocorticoids. The main step is usually production of an inactive metabolite which is then conjugated to either glucuronic acid or sulphate which can then be excreted by the kidney.

Cholesterol is synthesized in the liver, intestinal mucosa, adrenal cortex and arterial walls. It is excreted in the bile as a neutral steroid. As well as providing the basic structure for steroid hormones, cholesterol is the precursor of bile salts. These are synthesized only within the liver. The liver also has a key role in conjugating free bile acids arriving in the portal blood. These are rapidly conjugated with glycine or taurine, prior to biliary secretion.

Serum bile acid and cholesterol concentrations are lower in the newborn infant than in older children or in adults. Bile acid synthesis is reduced. The bile acid pool, when corrected for surface area, is less in the neonate than in the adult. As a result, bile acid secretion is low although there is no defect in bile acid transport. Malabsorption of fats results. These physiological defects are not seen in infants who have been born to mothers who have received dexamethazone to prevent hyaline membrane disease. Presumably this agent induces metabolic pathways involved in bile acid formation.

Protein and aminoacid metabolism

Aminoacids absorbed from the intestine are rapidly taken up by the liver. There they are deaminated, transaminated, or utilized in protein synthesis. Ammonia produced by the deamination of aminoacids is rapidly converted to urea.

Most of the proteins in plasma, other than the immunoglobulins, are synthesized by the rough endoplasmic reticulum of the hepatocytes. Quantitatively, albumin is the most important of these, but haptoglobin, transferrin, caeruloplasmin, C reactive protein, alpha-1 antitrypsin, alpha-2 globulin, and alpha and beta lipoprotein are also formed in the liver.

The other important proteins are those involved in clotting mechanisms. Fibrinogen, prothrombin and Factors V, VII, IX, X and to some extent, Factor VIII, are formed within the liver. Factors II, VII, IX and X are dependent on the presence of vitamin K for their synthesis. Inhibitors of the coagulation system, notably anti-thrombin -3 and components of the fibrinolytic system, for example, plasminogen, are also synthesized within hepatocytes.

Protein synthesis is very active in fetal life and in the newborn period. The main serum protein in fetal life is alpha-fetoprotein. It first appears in the serum at six weeks gestation, rising to a peak concentration of 300 mg/dl at 13 weeks gestation and then declining linearly to around 7 mg/dl in cord blood. By the age of six weeks the concentration has fallen to less than 25 μg/litre. Albumin synthesis starts at approximately three to four months gestation, the serum concentration is at the adult value by birth. Low levels are commonly found in prematurely born infants. Proteins involved in coagulation are frequently of low concentration around the time of delivery but increase to normal levels within a few days. Caeruloplasmin is low at birth and reaches its highest concentration at about the age of three months, thereafter falling slowly to the adult level by the age of two years. There is thus no uniformity in the time course of changes in homeostasis of different proteins. Alpha-fetoprotein production is prolonged in neonatal obstructive liver diseases; it is also produced by 40–50 per cent of hepatocellular tumours.

Although aminoacids except cystine are in higher concentrations in fetal blood than in the adult, the enzymes involved in metabolism or degradation of aminoacids are at low activity around the time of birth. The elevated phenylalanine levels frequently found in premature infants is attributed to a deficiency of enzymes involved in this degradation. Premature infants given high protein intake may be unable to metabolize this and have dangerously elevated serum aminoacid concentrations as a result.

Drug metabolism

The metabolism of drugs within the liver occurs in two stages in most instances. The first step is a biochemical transformation resulting in demethylation, oxidation or reduction. This is followed by conjugation to sulphate or glucuronide which renders the compound more water-soluble, making it more readily excreted in the urine or bile. Continuous administration of drugs such as phenobarbitone, phenytoin or rifampicin, which are metabolized by the endoplasmic reticulum, has the effect of increasing the concentration and activity of enzymes involved in drug metabolism. This process, known as 'enzyme induction', is a non-specific process. One drug may induce an increased metabolism of other drugs or endogenous substances such as steroids. It may affect other processes, for example, the rate of catabolism of vitamin D. Patients treated with phenobarbitone have increased vitamin D requirements due to enzyme induction.

In the first two–four weeks of life, drug metabolism is frequently very different from that in the adult because of differences in the binding of drugs by serum proteins, inefficient renal function, as well as by differences in hepatic metabolism. The metabolic handicaps in drug handling in the newborn are very similar to those found in bilirubin excretion. As a result, both the pharmacological action of drugs and their half-life is often very different in the newborn period. It is generally necessary to give low doses less frequently.

Reticulo-endothelial function

In fetal life, the liver is an important site of haematopoiesis, activity being maximal at seven months gestation. Beyond the age of six weeks this is normally confined to the bone marrow, but in the presence of haemolytic anaemia, or where the bone marrow space has been destroyed, the reticulo-endothelial cells of the liver are again found to be involved in haem formation.

Kupffer cells are phagocytic and have an important function in removing a variety of bacterial products, such as endotoxin, and other antigens which have been absorbed into the portal blood. The Kupffer cells may have an important role in conjunction with the rest of the reticulo-endothelial system in producing antibodies.

HEPATIC ULTRASTRUCTURE AND FUNCTION

Electronmicroscopy coupled with advances in histochemistry, at a subcellular level, has permitted exciting advances in the correlation of structure and function within the hepatocytes. Histochemical studies, although they have been used to demonstrate only a few enzymes, are important since they have provided a correlation between cell morphology and the results of biochemical studies which have exploited classical cell fractionation techniques. These histochemical studies allow speculation about function of the structures seen with the electronmicroscope.

The hepatocyte is permeated by a continuous complex tubular network from which only the mitochondria are excluded. The major structures within the hepatocytes – organelles – will be described and their function considered.

Plasma membrane The plasma membrane of the hepatocyte is a complex and active tissue, possibly conferring on the liver cell many of its unique properties of selective hepatic uptake of chemicals and their biliary excretion. The sinusoidal aspects of the cell are bounded by long, often tortuous villi, which stain actively with such enzymes as alkaline phosphatase and nucleosidase-monophosphatase. In the cytoplasm immediately adjacent to the membrane, are numerous vesicles which probably participate in the transport of proteins and lipids into the hepatocyte. Cholesterol, albumin, fibrinogen and other proteins are secreted into the circulation via this membrane.

The other main area of specialization on the hepatocyte cell membrane is the bile canalicular surface. It is bound by slender villi up to 0.5 mμ in length which stain strongly for nucleoside triphosphate and monophosphatases and diphosphatases. This enzyme localization suggests that an active transport mechanism is involved in bile secretion. The bile canaliculi are lined by such specialized areas of cell membrane on opposing liver cells. The third area of specialization of the plasma membrane is the so-called 'junctional' complex, a reinforced adherent area of plasma membrane bounding the bile canaliculi and effectively separating the lumen of the canaliculi from the sinusoids. The lateral or intrahepatic plasma membranes are relatively simple, being interrupted with occasional interdigitations, but they do have microvilli.

Endoplasmic reticulum Endoplasmic reticulum is a complex system of membranous cysterna traversing the cytoplasm and closely associated, if not continuous with, all other organelles except the mitochondria. Its functions are thought to include synthesis and transport of proteins, lipids and mucopolysaccharides. Two types are recognized: a smooth endoplasmic reticulum, and a rough endoplasmic reticulum which has attached to it many ribosomes (*vide infra*).

Nucleus The nucleus is the principal site for the regulation of hereditary characteristics. The nuclear envelope consists of an outer ribosome-studded membrane and an inner smooth membrane. The membranes fuse in parts called 'membrane pores'. Continuity between the outer nuclear membrane and the endoplasmic reticulum has been reported in many cell types.

A nuclear cytoplasmic pathway has been demonstrated in some types of cells. The nucleus has many fibrillary desoxyribonucleic acid and granular components containing ribonucleic acid precursors. It has an important role in ribosomal ribonucleic acid biosynthesis. Euchromatin, representing active parts of the genome, or complete gene complement, is seen as dense fibres in isolated chromatin fractions.

Mitochondria The main function of these organelles is in oxidative phosphorylation and in the storage of energy as adenosine triphosphate. Mitochondria are closely related to the endoplasmic reticulum but are most dense in the perinuclear and sub-sinusoidal zones. They have a characteristic appearance, being delineated by a smooth outer membrane which is separated by a small space from the inner membrane. It is convoluted with prominent, fine projections into the matrix of the mitochondrion. On the inner membrane, numerous club-shaped particles can be seen. Each base part is thought to represent an electron transport system, while the head of the club represents molecules of ATP-ase. Within the matrix, granules containing calcium and phosphorus may be seen. The mitochondria also contain both desoxyribonucleic acid and ribonucleic acid. They thus have a complete mechanism for the transport of genetic material, although the exact relationship of this mechanism to the nuclear genetic material is unclear.

Ultrastructural histochemical techniques show that the enzymes cytochrome, B5 and monoamine oxidases are localized to the outer layers of the mitochondrial membrane, while enzymes of the respiratory chain are on the inner membrane.

Mitochondria are sensitive indicators of cell damage. Swelling, bizarre shape, and the development of crystal-like material in the matrix has been described in a variety of hepatic disorders.

Golgi apparatus The Golgi apparatus is a complex arrangement of vesicles and sacules, often stacked in a parallel fashion near the bile canaliculi. Adjacent to the Golgi apparatus is a distinct system of smooth membrane tubules from which lysosomes may arise. The Golgi apparatus is involved in the addition of carbohydrates moities to polysaccharides, glycoproteins and glycolipid proteins. It may be involved in the coupling of lipids with protein and in their 'packaging' prior to secretion from the hepatocytes.

Lysosomes Lysosomes are a morphologically heterogeneous group of organelles found throughout the hepatocyte. They may contain other organelles in various states of degeneration, haemosiderin granules or ferritin particles and lipofuscin. Whether they function entirely as intracellular scavengers has not been resolved. They contain more than 30 acid hydrolysases which are capable of degrading a wide range of biological compounds if activated.

Perioxisomes These round organelles of 0.4—0.8 mμ contain enzymes involved in oxygen transport. They are often found in close association with glycogen and may possibly be involved in gluconeogenesis as well as in oxygen transport.

Microtubules Microtubules are smooth membrane tubules found throughout the hepatocyte. They are less prominent in the liver cells than in many other cells. The main role is thought to be in intracellular transport, but this has yet to be fully defined.

Ribosomes and their actions

Ribosomes are complex structures intimately involved in the synthesis of proteins and lipids. They may be found in the cytoplasm, singly or in clusters or polyribosomes in association with messenger ribonucleic acid (mRNA). Most commonly they are attached to the endoplasmic reticulum as polyribosomes.

Each ribosome consists of two parts. The larger is attached to the endoplasmic reticulum in such a way that material synthesized passes directly from it into the cisternae of the endoplasmic reticulum. The protein and ribosomal ribonucleic acid (RNA) content of the two parts of the ribosome differ.

Some of the complex functional relationship between these cell structures is illustrated by considering the formation of ribosomes and their role in polypeptide synthesis. The initial step is formation of ribosomal proteins in the cytoplasm. These proteins move to the nucleus where they combine with a special form of RNA, ribosomal RNA, to form ribosomes. These migrate into the cytoplasm, some becoming attached to the endoplasmic reticulum. Before they can form polypeptides, they combine with mRNA.

Messenger RNA has a key role in the expression of gene actions. Nuclear desoxyribonucleic acid (DNA) acts as a template for the single strand of mRNA. The base sequence of one DNA strand is mirrored by the mRNA sequence. Three sequential nucleotide bases on DNA or mRNA are necessary to code for any particular aminoacid. mRNA migrates from the nucleus to the cytoplasm, where it becomes associated with ribosomes. The mRNA–ribosomal complex incorporates appropriate aminoacid in the correct sequence for the protein structure by a process termed 'translation'. A third form of RNA, transport RNA (tRNA), is involved in the process of translation. By means of specific aminoacyl synthetases, tRNA becomes attached to aminoacid in the cytoplasm. The sequence of three bases on tRNA then 'reads' the base sequence on mRNA and when the appropriate bases are exposed inserts the aminoacid in the correct position in the polypeptide chain.

For protein synthesis to occur, the other requirements include a pool of 20 common aminoacids, a minimum of 20 specific aminoacyl synthetases, adenosine triphosphate and guanidine triphosphate as energy sources. The specificity of the synthetase enzyme is critical.

An ordered complex then forms of ribosome, mRNA and aminoacyl, tRNA (*Figure 1.6*). As each specific aminoacyl tRNA inserts its aminoacid into peptide, the ribosome moves along the mRNA exposing new codons. When the ribosome reaches the other end the polypeptide is released and the mRNA and the ribosome become dissociated. In the meantime, other ribosomes become attached to the mRNA. Factors

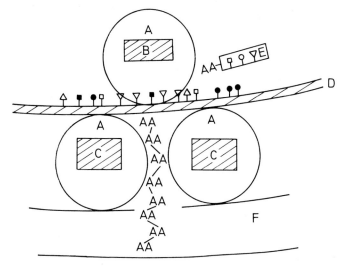

Figure 1.6. Diagrammatic representation of polypeptide synthesis by ribosomes: (A) represents ribosomes; (B) and (C) represent the two forms of ribosomal RNA; (D) is messenger RNA; (E) is transport RNA; (AA) indicate aminoacids; and (F) is the cisterna of the endoplasmic reticulum

which control the initiation of protein synthesis and the release of the polypeptide chain, are as yet unknown. In spite of the complexity of this process it is believed that up to ten aminoacids may be polymerized by a ribosome in one second.

BIBLIOGRAPHY AND REFERENCES

Hepatic anatomy
Elias, H. and Sherrick, J.C. (1969). *Morphology of the Liver.* London: Academic Press
Grisham, J.W., Nopanitaya, W. and Compagno, J. (1976). Scanning, electronmicroscopy of the liver: a review of methods and results. In *Progress in Liver Diseases,* Vol. 5, p. 1. Ed. by Popper, H. and Schaffner, F. New York: Grune and Stratton
Ma, M.H., Goldfisher, S. and Biempica, L. (1972). Morphology of the normal liver cell. In *Progress in Liver Diseases*, Vol. 4, p. 1. Ed. by Popper, H. and Schaffner, F. New York: Grune and Stratton
Ogawa, K., Minase, T., Enomoto, K. and Onoe, T. (1973). Ultrastructure of fenestrated cells in the sinusoidal wall of rat liver after perfusion fixation. *Tohoku J. exp. Med.* **110**, 89.
Wisse, E. (1972). An ultrastructural characterisation of the endothelial cell in the rat liver sinusoid. *J. Ultrastruct. Res.* **38**, 528

Liver size

Holder, L.E., Striefe, J. and Padical, E.M. (1975). Liver size determination in paediatrics using sonographic and scintigraphic techniques. *Radiology* **117**, 349

Smith, A.L., Mowat, A.P. and Williams, R. (1977). Hepatic scintigraphy in the management of infants and children with liver disease. *Archs Dis. Childh.* **52,** 633

Sullivan, S., Krasner, N. and Williams, R. (1976). The clinical estimation of liver size: a comparison of techniques and analysis of the source of error. *Br. med. J.* **2,** 1042

Younoszai, M.K. and Mueller, S. (1975). Clinical assessment of liver size in normal children. *Clin. Pediat. Philad.* **14,** 378

Physiology of the liver

Mowat, A.P. (1976). Development of liver function. In *Topics in Paediatric Gastroenterology*, p. 51. Ed. by Dodge, J.A. London: Pitman Medical

Stein, L.B. and Arias, I.M. (1976). Physiology of the liver. In *Gastroenterology*, 3rd ed. Vol.III, p. 40. Ed. by Boccus, H.L. Philadelphia: Saunders

Watkins, J.B. and Perman, J.A. (1977). Bile acid metabolism in infants and children. *Clin Gastroenterol.* **6,** 201

Ribosomal function

Weisman, S.M. and Brawerman, G. (1974). Gene structure and function. In *Duncan's Diseases of Metabolism*, 7th ed. p. 1. Ed. by Bondy, H. and Rosenberg, L.M. Philadelphia: Saunders

CHAPTER 2

Anatomy and Physiology of the Biliary Tract

ANATOMY AND PHYSIOLOGY

Anatomy and ultrastructure

Gross anatomy of the extrahepatic biliary system is shown in *Figure 2.1*. The biliary tract, however, is not an inert tube but is lined by cells which play an important part in controlling bile secretion. It is pertinent, therefore, to consider details of the microstructure of the cells lining the biliary tract and to emphasize that throughout its length the surface area is increased by the presence of microvilli while its role in secretion and perhaps absorption of bile is emphasized by its profuse blood supply.

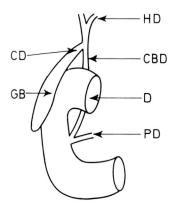

Figure 2.1. Diagrammatic representation of a normal extrahepatic biliary tree showing the hepatic duct (HD), common bile duct (CBD), gallbladder (GB), cystic duct (CD), duodenum (D), and pancreatic duct (PD)

Bile is formed in the *bile canaliculi*, which are channels of uniform diameter between two or three adjoining liver cells. The walls of bile canaliculi are specialized segments of the cell wall bearing regularly shaped cylindrical microvilli which jut into the lumen of the canaliculi. Along the margin of the grooves which form the bile canaliculi the

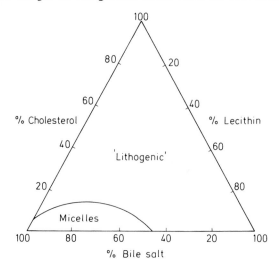

Figure 2.2. Phase-diagram showing the influence of bile salt phospholipid and cholesterol concentration on the formation of micelles in aqueous solution at 37°C. Micelles are formed only if the relative concentrations are such that when plotted on a triangular co-ordinate the point of intersection falls within the micellar area. Concentrations falling outwith this area produce crystals or liquid crystals. Bile behaves like this model and although the exact critical micellar concentrations have not been finally agreed, it has become customary to assess the degree of cholesterol saturation of bile by plotting its composition using such triangular co-ordinates. If the concentrations fall outwith the micellar phase, bile is considered lithogenic. (Reproduced from The physico-chemical basis of gallstone formation in man, by Admirand and Small, by courtesy of the Editor of the Journal of Clinical Investigation)

hepatocytes are attached to one another by so-called 'tight junctions' which form continuous bands along the entire length of the canalicular network.

From the canaliculi bile flows into fine ductules with a diameter less than that of a liver cell and lined by a simple squamous epithelium.

These epithelial cells are smaller than hepatocytes, have a clear cyto-plasm, fewer mitochondria, but have up to 70 widely spaced microvilli on their epithelial surface. These ductules join ducts of ever-increasing calibre which form plexuses around portal vein branches as they carry bile towards the portahepatis. Larger channels are formed which drain into the major right and left hepatic ducts before emerging from the

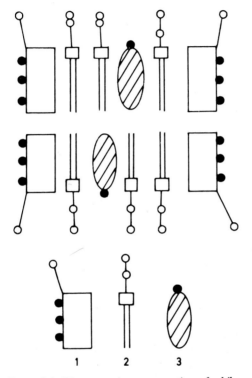

Figure 2.3. Diagrammatic representation of a bile salt micelle. Polar groups are shown as open circles, closed circles indicate less polar but charged groups. 1 represents bile acid; 2, phospholipid; and 3, the cholesterol

right and left lobes of the liver at the portahepatis to form the common hepatic duct. The lining cells of these larger ducts become more cylin-drical but still bear many microvilli. Another feature of these major tributaries of the common hepatic duct are two diametrically opposed rows of glands which produce both serous and mucus secretions. These glands lie outwith the ducts but open into them. Simpler, smaller, but less frequent glands are seen outwith the common bile duct. The common bile duct has a columnar epithelium with prominent micro-villi. The mucosa is often arranged in longitudinal oblique folds or rugae with a highly vascular lamina propria. A few thin smooth muscle fibres are found in the connective tissues surrounding the duct. The common hepatic duct is joined by the cystic duct from the gallbladder to form the common bile duct, which terminates at the choledocho-duodenal junction uniting with the main pancreatic duct in a *complex ampulla* which opens on to a papilla on the mediodorsal aspect of the second part of the duodenum. A sphincter is found at the lower end of the common bile duct with another within the ampulla and its papilla. The ampulla has a complex arrangement of valve-like structures with smooth muscle and mucus-producing glands which may assist in the mixing of bile and pancreatic juices.

The *gallbladder* is a pear-shaped bag, the broad end of which is directed anteriorly towards the abdominal wall. The body extends into a narrow neck continuing into the cystic duct. The mucosa of the gallbladder is markedly increased in area by its prominent highly vascular rugae or interconnecting ridges. It, too, is lined by columnar epithelium bearing long, fine microvilli. The folds of the gallbladder continue into the cystic duct forming a spiral valve.

The wall of the gallbladder consists of muscular elastic fibres without definite layers except in the neck and fundus where the muscle is particularly prominent. The gallbladder receives its blood supply from the cystic artery, usually a branch of the hepatic artery, which follows a tortuous course.

Physiology of bile formation

Bile secretion is a complex process involving at least three steps: (a) uptake or synthesis of substances by the liver or bile duct cell; (b) transport of these across the cell membrane; and (c) excretion of water, organic and inorganic material into the bile canaliculi.

Great difficulties exist in performing quantitative studies of biliary secretion, particularly in man, but qualitative studies determining the constituents of bile and their concentrations have been possible. Collections usually involve having a T tube in the common bile duct, which implies that the circumstances studied are more likely to be pathological than physiological; or by duodenal intubation, in which substantial amounts of bile may be lost. Endoscopic cannulation of the ampulla of Vater and the common bile duct may give additional in-formation and obviate the problem of loss of bile but has too many complications to be used as a physiological investigation. Unfortunately, there are substantial differences from species to species in bile constituents and in bile flow. Thus, the results of animal studies cannot be applied to man. Nevertheless, by using techniques comparable to those used in determining glomerular filtration rate, in which the biliary clearance of inert solutes such as erythritol is determined, and by the use of methods validated *in vitro* and *in vivo* in the experimental animal, a tentative assessment of bile flow and the factors controlling it in man may be made.

Bile acid dependent secretion of bile

A linear relationship exists between the excretion of bile acid, bile flow, and electrolyte output in bile in man and many other species. Factors controlling bile acid metabolism are thus important in consideration of the control of bile flow.

Bile salts are synthesized in the liver from cholesterol. They are excreted in bile in concentrations which are approximately 5,000 times greater than that in serum — an enormous concentration gradient. Before secretion, bile salts are conjugated with the aminoacids glycine or taurine and passed into the canaliculi on a carrier-mediated active transport system. Only a small amount of the total bile salts excreted at any one time is newly synthesized, the remainder having already undergone an enterohepatic circulation. They will have been concentrated and stored in the gallbladder to be released in high concentration into the duodenum when food is taken.

Digestion and enterohepatic circulation of bile salts In the upper small intestine bile salts play a crucial role in digestion and absorption of lipids. The exact mechanism of their action in this regard is still not clear but they do aid in the formation of micelles and accelerate the uptake of both fatty acid and monoglyceride by the small bowel mucosa. They activate pancreatic lipase and may have a role in the release of enterokinase and enteric hormones. They are also necessary for the absorption of fat-soluble vitamins A, D, E and K, as well as calcium. The bile salts themselves are not absorbed in the upper small bowel but pass into the ileum where they are absorbed by an active transport system ideally adapted for taurine and glycine conjugates of bile acids but also efficient at absorbing unconjugated bile acids.

This whole process is so efficient that the total bile salt pool (2–4 g in the adult) may be excreted and reabsorbed twice in any meal with only 3 per cent of the total pool being lost in the faeces.

Cholesterol metabolism and bile salts The metabolism of bile salts and cholesterol are closely related in a variety of ways; as follows.

(1) Bile salt excretion probably accounts for 40 per cent of cholesterol turnover.

(2) Absorbed bile salts exert a negative feedback control on their own synthesis (that is, the more absorbed, the less new bile salts are formed) and thus influence cholesterol degradation.

(3) Bile salts control the synthesis of cholesterol both in the liver and in the intestine.

(4) Bile salts promote the secretion of insoluble cholesterol and maintain it in micellar solution in bile.

Just how bile salts play a part in controlling bile flow is uncertain. It is generally believed that the mechanism is increased water and electrolyte secretion in response to the bile acids themselves by osmotic filtration, but this is probably induced by associated ions since the bile salts in bile are usually in micellar form which has low osmotic activity.

Bile acid independent component of bile flow

In a number of species bile flow independent of bile acid secretion has been demonstrated to occur in many studies. Secretion is produced by hepatocytes. It is reduced by agents which inhibit the enzyme sodium potassium ATPase and is thus thought to be produced by active sodium transport across the bile canaliculi. In the dog both phenobarbitone and hydrocortisone increase this component of bile flow. Agents such as glycogen, which increase cyclic AMP, also increase this component of bile flow.

Specific pathways of secretion into bile

At least three further distinct and independent pathways of hepatocyte secretion into bile have been identified for the following classes of substances: (a) organic anions such as bilirubin glucuronide; (b) organic cations; and (c) neutral substances, for example, cardiac glycosides.

In general, compounds excreted in the bile in concentrations much higher than in plasma increase bile flow, but others such as bilirubin do not influence bile flow, while yet others, such as lithocholic acid, bromsulphthalein and radio-opaque dyes, may be cholestatic, that is, they may reduce bile flow.

Studies using isolated segments of bile ducts and *in vivo* experiments, confirm the contribution of these structures to bile flow. This function appears to be under the control of the hormone secretin, which increases bile flow causing a characteristic change in its composition with increased bicarbonate concentration, a rise in pH and a fall in bile salt concentration.

Role of the gallbladder

In the fasting state, bile produced in the liver is diverted into the gallbladder, the sphincteral body at the lower end of the common bile duct being closed. In the gallbladder there is active reabsorption of sodium bicarbonate and water by means of a neutral anion–cation pump which causes a ten-fold increase in the concentration of non-absorbable organic compounds.

Within 30 minutes of eating, there is a sharp increase in bile acid concentration of the duodenum due to contraction of the gallbladder and relaxation of the sphincter of Oddi, brought about by the action of cholecystokinin. If the gallbladder is removed, is non-functioning due to disease, or is inert as in coeliac disease, the sharp rise in duodenal concentration of bile does not occur and enteric absorption of fats may be impaired.

BIBLIOGRAPHY

Biava, C.G. (1964). Studies on cholestasis; a re-evaluation of the fine structure of normal human bile canaliculi. *Lab.Invest.* 13, 840

Elias, H. and Sherrick, J.C. (1969). In *Morphology of the Liver*. New York and London: Academic Press

Erlinger, S. (1972). Physiology of bile flow. In *Progress in Liver Diseases*, Vol. 4, p.63 Ed. by Popper, H. and Schaffner, F. New York and London: Grune and Stratton

Heaton, K.W. (1972). The enterohepatic circulation. The life-cycle of bile salts. In *Bile Salts in Health and Disease*, p. 58. Edinburgh and London: Churchill Livingstone

Ma, M.H., Goldfisher, S. and Biempica, L. (1972). Morphology of the normal liver cell. In *Progress in Liver Diseases*, Vol. 4, p. 1, Ed. by Popper, H. and Schaffner, F. New York and London: Grune and Stratton

Prandi, D., Erlinger, S., Glasinovic, J.C. and Dumont, M. (1965) Canalicular bile production in man. *Eur. J. clin.Invest.* 5, 1

CHAPTER 3

Unconjugated Hyperbilirubinaemia

JAUNDICE

Jaundice, a yellow discoloration of sclera, skin and other tissues caused by the accumulation of bilirubin, is an important sign of disease or functional disorder affecting the hepatic, biliary or haematological systems. It appears in children and in adults when the serum bilirubin concentration exceeds 2 mg/dl (34 μmol/litre), but in neonates it is rarely noticeable below a concentration of 5 mg/dl (85 μmol/litre). Except in the newborn, the total serum bilirubin is less than 1.5 mg/dl (25 μmol/litre) with less than 0.5 mg/dl (7 μmol/litre) in the direct reacting or conjugated form. In all these groups investigation of the causes of jaundice is simplified if it is classified into unconjugated or conjugated hyperbilirubinaemia.

Unconjugated hyperbilirubinaemia is characterized clinically by jaundice without bile in the urine and biochemically by a raised total serum bilirubin with less than 15 per cent bilirubin in the direct reacting form. It may be physiological in the newborn. It is frequently due to haematological causes; rarely, it is due to genetic or familial functional disorders considered in this chapter. Very high concentrations of unconjugated bilirubin cause brain damage.

Conjugated hyperbilirubinaemia is characterized clinically by jaundice with bile in the urine. The stools may be pale brown or even chalky white in colour. The total serum bilirubin is raised and more than 15 per cent of the bilirubin is in the direct reacting form. It is always pathological.

Bilirubin metabolism

Bilirubin is an orange organic anion with a molecular weight of 584, exclusively derived from haem of haemoglobin in senescent red blood cells or from other tissue haem proteins such as the enzyme cytochrome P450. It is produced largely in the reticulo-endothelial system of the spleen, liver and bone marrow. Haem is first converted to biliverdin by the rate limiting microsomal enzyme haemoxygenase, which produces equimolar amounts of carbon monoxide and biliverdin. Biliverdin is changed to bilirubin by the action of the abundant biliverdin reductase enzyme. Bilirubin has a limited aqueous solubility at physiological pH. It is carried from the reticulo-endothelial system to the liver in the circulation firmly bound to serum albumin. Within the liver an ill-understood but very efficient mechanism dissociates bilirubin from albumin and the bilirubin passes into the hepatocyte. What determines hepatic selectivity of bilirubin uptake is not clear, nor is the process of uptake understood; recent research, however, has shown that this process requires no energy but is saturable, suggesting that it may be one of facilitative diffusion.

Within the hepatocyte bilirubin is transported to the endoplasmic reticulum, possibly being carried by cytoplasmic proteins with a high affinity for bilirubin, such as ligandin or Z protein. In the endoplasmic reticulum an enzymatic process converts bilirubin to a water-soluble form, largely bilirubin diglucuronide but as recent studies have shown also to the monoglucuronide and possibly also forming conjugates with glucose, xylose and sulphate. In man it would seem that glucuronide is the major conjugate. The exact enzymatic process involved in these conversions is probably complex, and as yet the enzymes involved have not been purified or characterized. A surprising new finding is that bilirubin monoglucuronide is formed in the endoplasmic reticulum but is subsequently converted to bilirubin diglucuronide and bilirubin by an enzyme in the liver cell membrane. The bilirubin conjugates are excreted into the biliary system by an energy-dependent process. The bilirubin is then carried in the bile to the bowel where it is converted to stercobilin and excreted in the stool. There is little or no enteric reabsorption.

GENETIC ABNORMALITIES IN BILIRUBIN METABOLISM

Crigler–Najjar syndrome (Type 1)

In 1952, Crigler and Najjar described a syndrome of severe persistent unconjugated hyperbilirubinaemia, without haemolysis or evidence of hepatic disease, usually complicated by the early onset of kernicterus and, frequently, death in the first year of life. The condition is inherited in an automosal recessive fashion. There is complete absence of the enzyme bilirubin uridine diphosphate glucuronyl transferase (bilirubin UDPGTase) in the liver. Heterozygotes are phenotypically normal with normal serum bilirubins but may have impaired glucuronidation of other substrates.

Clinical features

Jaundice appears soon after birth, the bilirubin rapidly rising to 20mg/
dl (340 μmol/litre), is poorly controlled by phototherapy in the
first few days and exchange transfusion is usually necessary. Only with
continuous phototherapy is it possible to keep the serum bilirubin
below 340 μmol/litre. Investigations fail to show haemolysis or other
aggravating factors of neonatal jaundice but a history of parental
consanguinity and instances of similar severe icterus in other family
members may be found. Without continuous phototherapy kernicterus
will ensue and death is frequent in the first year of life. In a few
instances, however, kernicterus does not appear until the late 'teens.

Diagnosis

A provisional diagnosis may be made on the basis of the clinical
features in the absence of other causes of hyperbilirubinaemia. Confirmation requires percutaneous liver biopsy. There is no histological
abnormality. Bilirubin UDPGTase activity is absent.

Treatment

The only effective treatment is phototherapy which presumably must
be continued for life. It will be necessary to administer this for periods
of up to 15 hours per day to keep the bilirubin in a safe range. The
simultaneous administration of cholestyramine by mouth may diminish
the duration of phototherapy.

Crigler—Najjar (Type 2)

This variant of the Crigler—Najjar syndrome is characterized by less
severe non-haemolytic unconjugated hyperbilirubinaemia, the bilirubin concentration being in the range of 5—20 mg/dl (100—350 μmol/
litre). The inheritance is autosomal dominant with variable expres-
sivity. There is defective but not absent UDPGTase activity. Some
conjugated bilirubin may be found in bile.

Clinical features

Jaundice may start in the first year of life but may be delayed until childhood or even early adult life; its severity varies from time to time. A past family history of similar jaundice may be obtained. Hyperbilirubinaemia in relatives may be shown chemically. Brain damage is infrequent.

Diagnosis

A provisional diagnosis may be made if there is no other evidence of liver disease and there is a positive family history of unconjugated hyperbilirubinaemia. Confirmation requires the demonstration of normal hepatic pathology and deficient activity of UDPGTase.

Treatment

The bilirubin falls to normal levels in two to four weeks when enzyme-inducing agents such as phenobarbitone are given in a dose of 1–5 mg/kg bodyweight each evening.

Gilbert's syndrome

Definition

Mild, chronic, variable, unconjugated hyperbilirubinaemia with serum bilirubin levels of around 2 mg/dl (40 μmol/litre) without significant haemolysis or abnormality of liver function are the characteristic features of this condition.

Family studies suggest an autosomal recessive mode of inheritance. The pathogenesis is undetermined but there is impaired hepatic uptake of bilirubin and deficient UDPGTase activity. Fifty per cent of cases have slightly reduced red blood cell survival.

Clinical features

There is a mild fluctuating jaundice often accompanied by unexplained vague symptoms such as upper abdominal discomfort, lethargy and general malaise. Intercurrent infection and exertion may exacerbate the jaundice. Recent research has shown that fasting – particularly if lipid is withdrawn from the diet – causes aggravation of the jaundice to a greater extent than seen in jaundice due to chronic liver disease or haemolytic states. Intravenous nicotinic acid in a dose of 50 mg in the adult also causes a sharp increase in serum bilirubin levels. Such an injection and fasting have been used clinically to support the diagnosis. Males are more commonly affected than females. The age of onset is difficult to determine but most cases come to light at around the age of ten years but there is frequently much delay in diagnosis.

Diagnosis

Diagnosis should be restricted to patients who have no past history of liver disease, who show no abnormality on clinical examination, except icterus, who have normal haematological studies and liver function tests including normal serum bile acids but do have a persistent documented mild hyperbilirubinaemia. The liver histology should be shown to be normal. The main conditions to be considered in differential diagnosis are compensated haemolytic states, the post-viral hepatitis syndrome, shunt hyperbilirubinaemia and the Crigler–Najjar syndrome Type 2.

Treatment

The disorder is benign. If the jaundice is distressing the patient it may be cleared by the administration of phenobarbitone in a dose of 6–10 mg/kg of bodyweight given each evening in gradually increasing doses. Surprisingly, this therapy often causes diminution of other symptoms.

NEONATAL UNCONJUGATED HYPERBILIRUBINAEMIA

Introduction

Of all the liver disorders, unconjugated hyperbilirubinaemia in the newborn infant is by far the most frequent, and because it can cause brain damage is by far the greatest cause of anxiety, primarily in the paediatrician but secondarily in the mother. The appearance of jaundice has two beneficial effects, namely, the earlier diagnosis of disorders such as septicaemia, haemolysis or galactosaemia which cause jaundice and which require specific treatment; measures are taken to prevent kernicterus (irreversible brain damage due to staining of the brain by bilirubin). A great deal of research effort has gone into factors controlling the production and excretion of bilirubin. Unfortunately, in the study of neonatal jaundice much research has been done on experimental animals which do not suffer from physiologic jaundice.

Frequently, substances more easily measured than bilirubin have been used in *in vitro* work. Extrapolation of the results of such work to bilirubin metabolism in the newborn infant has caused a great deal of confusion. Since, in most circumstances, bilirubin does neither harm nor good, the results of such studies may be of more importance for the information they provide about the metabolism of other organic anions, of greater physiological or pharmacological importance, which share the same metabolic pathways as bilirubin.

PHYSIOLOGIC JAUNDICE OF THE NEWBORN

Physiologic jaundice of the newborn is a transient benign icterus which occurs during the first week of life in otherwise healthy newborn infants. Clinically detectable jaundice becomes present after the age of 24 hours and rises to a maximum level of 6 mg/dl (100 μmol/litre) on the second to fourth days of life returning to normal by the seventh day. In premature infants levels of between 12–15 mg/dl (200–240 μmol/litre) are commonly reached on the fifth to seventh days of life and return to normal by the fourteenth day.

Pathogenesis

It is now considered likely that there is no single cause of physiologic jaundice in the neonate but that it results from the complex inter-action of factors which cause: (a) increased bilirubin production; (b) impaired hepatic uptake and excretion of bilirubin; and (c) enteric reabsorption of bilirubin. In the individual infant all the factors in-fluencing bilirubin metabolism can rarely be rigorously investigated. Statistical associations between the parameters that can reasonably be measured only point at aspects which require further study. Much of the laboratory research into this condition has been done with experimental animals which do not have physiologic jaundice adding to interpretative difficulties when the results are applied to man.

Studies of possibly greater significance in understanding the condition in man are those performed in the Rhesus monkey which does have a physiologic jaundice, albeit a biphasic one. The serum bilirubin increases from less than 1 mg/dl (17 μmol/litre) to 4.5 mg/dl (76 μmol/litre) in the first 24 hours of life (phase 1), falling to 2 mg/dl (42 μmol/litre) on the second, third and fourth day (phase 2) returning to 0.1 mg/dl (less than 2 μmol/litre) on the fifth day. By effusion studies on this animal it has been shown that bilirubin formation is at five times the adult value in the first 18 days of life, activity of the enzyme bilirubin UDPGTase is almost zero at birth but very rapidly reaches high levels in the first 24 hours, attaining adult levels by the third day. Hepatic uptake which is at only 30 per cent of the adult value at birth rises more slowly, reaching adult levels only on the fifth day. It is thus considered that the rapid rise of bilirubin in phase 1 is due to deficient bilirubin conjugation, but that the impaired hepatic uptake may be a major factor in phase 2. The cause of the impaired hepatic uptake has still to be identified but the virtual absence of ligandin within the hepatocyte at birth but reaching adult levels during the first week of life may possibly be related. By cannulating the bile duct and interrupting the passage of bile into the bowel it has been shown that absorption of bilirubin from the bowel adds considerably to the load of bilirubin which has to be excreted in this age group.

In the *human infant* there is good evidence of increased bilirubin production from reduced red blood cell survival shown experimentally both by the use of radioactively labelled glycine incorporated in haemoglobin and also from studies of the production of carbon monoxide, released from haem. Both techniques give the red blood cell life of approximately 90 days in the newborn as compared with 120 days in the adult. There is, in addition, increased bilirubin production from non-haemoglobin sources giving a total bilirubin production of approximately 8.5 ± 2.3 mg/kg of bodyweight per day (145 ± 39 μmol/kg per day) in infants compared with 3.6 mg/kg of bodyweight per day (75 μmol/kg per day) in the adult.

Lower ligandin levels have been demonstrated in human neonatal livers. The role of the possible deficient activity of the enzyme bilirubin UDPGTase is yet to be established. In the early study of this enzyme activity done on human biopsy material the time course of development was totally different from that seen in physiologic jaundice, adult levels not being reached until the seventieth day. It should be noted, however, that methylumbelliferone was used as a substrate rather than bilirubin. There is at present no direct evidence to implicate ineffective hepatic perfusion or diminished transport across the hepatocellular membranes as a factor in physiologic jaundice.

PATHOLOGICAL NEONATAL UNCONJUGATED HYPERBILIRUBINAEMIA

Pathological neonatal unconjugated hyperbilirubinaemia indicates that a disease process or processes may be present aggravating or accentuating physiological neonatal unconjugated hyperbilirubinaemia, and in clinical practice is considered to exist when serum bilirubin concentration exceeds that found in normal healthy infants. In addition any degree of clinical jaundice in the first 24 hours of life is pathological. In full-term infants bilirubin concentrations should not exceed 12 mg/dl (200 μmol/litre) on the second to fourth day and should have returned to normal by the eighth day. In prematurely born infants the peak concentration may not occur until the fifth to seventh day but should be less than 15 mg/dl (255 μmol/litre) and return to normal by the fourteenth day. Any deviation from this pattern is abnormal and is indicative of possible underlying disease. An infant with such jaundice must be urgently investigated to identify treatable conditions such as septicaemia or galactosaemia and measures to prevent kernicterus have to be considered.

Causes of pathological neonatal jaundice

The many factors which may contribute to hyperbilirubinaemia in the newborn are listed in *Tables 3.1, 3.2* and *3.3*. It would be inappropriate in a textbook such as this to consider these in detail. The conditions listed in *Table 3.1* require active treatment, and priority in investigation must be to exclude these. Those listed in *Table 3.2* are important to

TABLE 3.1
Causes of Neonatal Unconjugated Hyperbilirubinaemia which Require
Urgent Identification and Treatment

Haemolytic disorders, for example, blood group incompatibility, defects of red blood cell membranes, red blood cell enzyme deficiencies, ingestion of haemolytic agents infections.
Increase red blood cell mass, for example, placental transfusion, twin-to-twin transfusion, infant of diabetic mother, late clamping of the cord.

Hypoxia	Fructosaemia
Hypoglycaemia	Administration of drugs competing
Hypothyroidism	with bilirubin for hepatic excretion
Dehydration	Meconium retention
Galactosaemia	High intestinal obstruction

TABLE 3.2
Established Causes of Neonatal Hyperbilirubinaemia

Prematurity	Excessive bruising
Infant of diabetic mother	Down's syndrome
Breast milk jaundice of late onset	Transient familial neonatal
Gilbert's syndrome	hyperbilirubinaemia

TABLE 3.3

Factors Possibly Implicated in Aggravating Physiologic Jaundice

Male sex – summer birth	Previous use of oral contraceptives
Previous use of oral contraceptives with breast feeding	Progestogen therapy
	Breast feeding
Prolonged labour	Antipartum haemorrhage
Family history of hyperbilirubinaemia	Vitamin E deficiency

TABLE 3.4

Laboratory Investigations in Unconjugated Hyperbilirubinaemia
in the Newborn

Serial determination of total and direct serum bilirubin
Haemoglobin and reticulocyte determination
Red blood cell morphology
Blood group of mother and child
Direct Coomb's test in saline and albumin on infant's red blood cells
Maternal antibodies and haemolysins
Urine microscopy and culture
Urine analysis for reproducing substances
Blood culture and other appropriate bacteriological investigations
Specific enzyme test for abnormality of red blood cells
Serum thyroxine and T.S.H. concentration

appreciate since they may save the child much unnecessary investigation. The conditions listed in *Table 3.3* are some of those in which a statistical correlation has been shown although the mechanism of action is far from clear.

Iatrogenic factors in hyperbilirubinaemia

The changing incidence of neonatal jaundice from time to time, and particularly the increased incidence in the United Kingdom and North America over the last ten years of idiopathic hyperbilirubinaemia, has led to the suggestion that changes in obstetrical or neonatal practice may be important factors in this increased incidence. A statistically greater incidence of hyperbilirubinaemia has been demonstrated with operative delivery, most marked with ventouse extraction, rotation and extraction with Keilland's forceps and less with breech extraction, manual rotation and caesarean section. The possible implication of infusion of oxytocin in aggravating jaundice causes much controversy as to whether this is a drug effect or reflects hepatic immaturity in an infant born before spontaneous onset of labour. An increased incidence of hyperbilirubinaemia follows its use in accelerating labour which starts spontaneously, and the effect is dose-related. A direct pharmacological action seems possible.

An important and frequently overlooked fact in assessing causes of hyperbilirubinaemia is the effect of delay in clamping the umbilical cord. Recent research by Seigel *et al.* (1972) in premature infants showed that only 6 per cent developed serum bilirubins of greater than 15 mg/dl (235 μmol/litre) if the cord was clamped immediately following birth as opposed to 35 per cent if the cord was clamped at 5 minutes. The difference was due to the increased red blood cell mass following delayed clamping of the cord. An important post-natal factor which is also frequently overlooked, although it is easily observed and recorded, is how long the infant takes to clear meconium from the bowel. This is important since the gut at birth contains an average 360 μmol of bilirubin (greater than 300 mg) and if none is passed in 12–15 hours

TABLE 3.5

Maternally Administered Drugs and Serum Bilirubin Concentrations in the Newborn Infant

Drugs causing a reduction in serum bilirubin concentration	*Drugs causing an increase in serum bilirubin concentration*	*Drugs having no effect on serum bilirubin concentration*
Narcotic agents	Diazepam	Phenothiazine derivatives
Barbiturates	Oxytocin	General anaesthetics
Aspirin		Local anaesthetics
Chloral hydrate		Sulphadimidine
Reserpine		Ampicillin
Sodium phenytoin		Penicillin
Alcohol		

a 15 per cent incidence of hyperbilirubinaemia (bilirubin greater than 15 mg/dl) (240 μmol/litre) is seen in healthy full-term infants. Drugs administered during pregnancy, in labour, or in the neonatal period may also affect bilirubin metabolism adversely. Most important are those causing depressed respiration with hypoxia and its sequellae. In *Table 3.5* the effect on serum bilirubin in the newborn infant of drugs given to the mother is listed. It is important to appreciate, however, that these effects are often minimal and of no clinical significance; they are included to illustrate how difficult it is in this field to associate a particular event with subsequent bilirubin metabolism.

Breast milk jaundice

During the first week of life jaundice may be observed more commonly in breast-fed infants than in bottle-fed infants. The reasons for this are not clear but possibly result from the combination of handicaps in bilirubin handling causing physiologic jaundice, aggravated by low calorie intake, steroids in breast milk, possibly in inhibition of bilirubin excretion by fatty acids in breast milk and contentiously by some action of prostaglandins. In most instances jaundice disappears within two weeks of birth.

A rarer form of jaundice associated with breast feeding is that in which the serum bilirubin concentration rises to between 15 and 20 mg/dl (255–360 µmol/litre) in the second or third week of life in infants who are otherwise entirely well. Such jaundice may persist for as long as four months. If breast feeding is discontinued, however, the jaundice will resolve spontaneously within six days and, surprisingly, may not recur if breast feeding is recommenced.

The *aetiology* of the syndrome is not known. Seventy-five per cent of siblings of affected infants are similarly affected. Breast milk from the mothers of affected infants can be shown to competitively inhibit gucuronide formation *in vitro*. Recent research into the mechanism of this has concentrated on two factors in the breast milk. The first of these is 3 alpha–20 beta pregnanediol, an isomer of a natural steroid found in breast milk. It was implicated because *in vitro* it is a powerful inhibitor of glucuronide formation by preparations from guinea-pig liver microsomes. It has been found in a few instances in breast milk of mothers of affected infants. When given to two infants it did cause a rise in serum bilirubin. It is not found in every case, however, nor does it cause *in vitro* inhibition of bilirubin glucuronide formation by human liver slices, its role is therefore as yet uncertain.

The implication of second factor free fatty acids, powerful inhibitors of bilirubin conjugation *in vitro*, has already been challenged by recent research work. The concentration of free fatty acids in stored breast milk has been shown to be related to the concentration and activity of the enzyme lipoprotein lipase. Unfortunately, if breast milk is stored without first being heated to 56°C this enzyme remains active and increasing amounts of free fatty acids are released. It has now been shown that the concentration of this enzyme and of free fatty acids in the breast milk of mothers whose infants have not become jaundiced is as high as that found in the breast milk of mothers whose infants have become jaundiced.

Clinical aspects

As has already been stated, these children are entirely well. It is important, however, to consider hypothyroidism in differential diagnosis. Kernicterus has not complicated this condition but it is my practice to recommend that breast feeding be stopped for a period of 24–48 hours if the serum bilirubin levels are greater than 17 mg/dl (290 μmol/ litre). If the jaundice is less than this the mother should be encouraged to continue breast feeding.

Transient familial hyperbilirubinaemia

Infants with this condition are also well but develop jaundice in the first few days of life which persists into the second or third week. The mothers are apparently healthy but all their children develop jaundice. It is thought to be caused by an unidentified inhibitor of bilirubin glucuronide formation which can be recovered from the serum of the mothers and of their infants.

CONTROL OF HYPERBILIRUBINAEMIA

Identification and specific treatment of the causes of hyperbilirubinaemia in *Table 3.1*, minimizing the effects listed in *Table 3.2*, and the prevention of kernicterus are the objectives in management. Prevention by good antenatal care, followed by an atraumatic delivery of a mature infant and an appropriate environment in the newborn period with an adequate intake of both fluid and calories, is paramount. It would be inappropriate to consider in detail all that is implied by the above. Laboratory investigations required for diagnosis and treatment are listed in *Table 3.4*. Some comments on the relative place of exchange transfusions, phototherapy and phenobarbitone – the major specific measures in controlling hyperbilirubinaemia – are appropriate.

Kernicterus is a disorder in which death or permanent neurological damage follows the deposition of unconjugated bilirubin in the brain. It occurs when the serum concentration of unconjugated bilirubin exceeds the capacity of the serum proteins to bind bilirubin, and unconjugated bilirubin diffuses into the brain. It is not possible to measure unbound bilirubin. The accurate estimation of the reserve capacity of serum proteins to bind bilirubin may provide a more precise indication of the risk of kernicterus than serum bilirubin concentration itself. This, however, has only been demonstrated using the salycilate saturation index which is technically difficult and only available in a limited number of laboratories. Many other methods which are considered to measure *in vitro* bilirubin binding by albumin have not, as yet, been shown to provide a better guide to the risk of kernicterus than the unconjugated serum bilirubin concentration.

In full term infants a serum bilirubin concentration of greater than 20 mg/dl (340 μmol/litre) or more is associated with a significant risk of kernicterus. Acidosis, asphyxia, hypo-albuminaemia, prematurity, and the administration of drugs which compete with bilirubin for albumin binding may cause kernicterus to occur at lower serum bilirubin concentrations. A wide range of endogenous anions such as haematin, bile acids and fatty acids compete with bilirubin for albumin binding.

Exchange transfusion

When the serum bilirubin level exceeds 20 mg/dl (340 μmol/litre) in full-term infants, or is greater than 15 mg/dl (250 μmol/litre) in premature infants, immediate exchange transfusion is indicated. In infants with haemolytic disorders a rise of serum bilirubin of greater than 0.5 mg/dl per hour (8.5 μmol/litre per hour) usually indicates that bilirubin will accumulate more rapidly than it can be excreted and exchange transfusion will be necessary. In the exchange transfusion twice the calculated blood volume is replaced by compatible whole blood. This is by far the most effective method of immediately controlling hyperbilirubinaemia.

Phototherapy

In newborn infants hyperbilirubinaemia may be prevented and controlled by exposing the jaundiced infant to artificial light which provides a radiant flux of between 4 and 6 μW/m² per nm. The light should be of a wavelength between 400 and 500 nm but is perhaps most effective near 450 nm. However, white light is to be preferred since observation of the patient is easier. Photo degradation of bilirubin occurs predominantly in the exposed skin but a well documented effect is the excretion in the bile of bilirubin which reacts chemically like unconjugated bilirubin. It is not known whether this results from an action of the phototherapy on the hepatocyte or biliary system or from photobiochemical transformation of the bilirubin in skin. The *in vivo* photo degradation products remain ill-characterized. *In vitro* the photochemical derivatives of bilirubin are less toxic to microsomal function than bilirubin.

Side-effects A number of side-effects have been recognized as complications of phototherapy. The most important is an increase by two or three-fold in the insensible water loss which may lead to dehydration and thereby aggravate hyperbilirubinaemia. It is important to replace this water loss by an increased water intake. Loose stools are frequently reported but when detailed control observations are made the evidence for diarrhoea or increased bowel motility with such phototherapy is less clear. In patients with liver disease, acute haemolysis and an unusual bronzing of the skin has been reported. It is important to protect the eyes because of the possibility of retinal damage. To date no permanent abnormality has been detected in human infants treated with phototherapy, but because of the immense biological effects of light on the neuro-endocrine system it would seem prudent to limit the use of phototherapy to infants who have been shown to require it. Although it is postulated that neonatal hyper-bilirubinaemia may cause a continuum of brain damage extending from kernicterus to minor intellectual impairment, this has never been confirmed in careful studies. It has yet to be shown that the widespread use of phototherapy in the prevention and control of non-haemolytic jaundice in low-birth-weight infants is in the patient's best interest. It is particularly disastrous where phototherapy is used without first excluding treatable conditions such as meningitis. Phototherapy is the only means of controlling the hyperbilirubinaemia in Crigler–Najjar Type 1.

Phenobarbitone

Carefully controlled studies have shown that phenobarbitone, particularly if given to the mother for some days before delivery of the infant, is effective in both premature and full-term infants in controlling neonatal hyperbilirubinaemia even when due to haemolysis. The mode of action of phenobarbitone in man has not been determined. Animal studies suggest that the drug stimulates hepatic uptake, conjugation and excretion of bilirubin as well as increasing the bile salt dependent component of bile flow. Since the effect of phenobarbitone on reducing serum bilirubin is not apparent until 48 hours after commencing therapy, it is of little value in the treatment of established hyperbili-rubinaemia. It should be remembered that phenobarbitone has been shown to influence many other metabolic systems including hormones, clotting factors, vitamins and drugs in addition to changing the inter-cellular ratios of reduced and oxidized forms of NAD(H) and NADP(H). Routine use of phenobarbitone in the management of hyperbiliru-binaemia is therefore to be discouraged.

It has to be recognized, however, that many infants are born in conditions where optimum highly technical perinatal care is not possible. In these circumstances the small risk of complications with relatively simple measures, particularly phototherapy, may be discounted if they give an increased chance of survival without brain damage.

JAUNDICE IN LATER INFANCY AND CHILDHOOD

Unconjugated hyperbilirubinaemia with normal coloured stools and urine is likely to be due to haemolytic disorders, Gilbert's disease, primary shunt hyperbilirubinaemia, or the Crigler–Najjar syndrome. Biochemically it is characterized by an elevated unconjugated bilirubin usually to levels of less than 6 mg/dl (100μmol/litre). The serum conjugated bilirubin, alkaline phosphatase, transaminase, albumin and globulin will be normal. In haemolytic disorders the serum haptoglobulins will be diminished. The total haemoglobin is low with a reticulocyte count greater than 2 per cent of the total red cell count: frequently it is as high as 20 per cent.

If anaemia is severe this may cause hepatocellular dysfunction with an elevation in the conjugated bilirubin. This may also occur if haemolytic anaemia is due to infection, or complicates the haemolytic uraemic syndrome. It may be found also in haemolytic anaemia complicating Wilson's disease.

BIBLIOGRAPHY

Arias, I.M., Gartner, L.M., Cohen, M., Ben Ezzer, J. and Levi, A.J. (1969). Chronic non-haemolytic unconjugated hyperbilirubinaemia with glucuronyl transferase deficiency. *Am.J.Med.* 47, 395

Arias, I.M. (1976). Extracellular and intracellular transport of bilirubin. In *Liver Diseases in Infancy and Childhood*, p. 1. Ed. by Berenberg, S.R. The Hague: Martinus Nijhoff Medical Division

Crigler, J.F. and Najjar, V.A. (1952). Congenital familial non-haemolytic jaundice with kernicterus. *Pediatrics* 10, 169

Gartner, L.M., Lee, K-S., Vaisman, S., Lane, D. and Zarafu, I. (1977). Development of bilirubin transport and metabolism in the newborn rhesus monkey. *J.Pediat.* 90, 513

Maisels, M.J. (1972). Bilirubin: on understanding and influencing its metabolism in the newborn infant. *Pediat. Clins N. Am.* 19, 447

Mowat, A.P. (1976). Obstetric causes of neonatal jaundice. In *The Management of Labour*, p. 257. Ed. by Brudenell *et al.* London: Royal College of Obstetricians and Gynaecologists

Odell, G.B. (1976). Neonatal jaundice. In *Progress in Liver Diseases*, p. 457. Vol.V. Ed. by Popper, H. and Schaffner, F. New York: Grune and Stratton

Odievre, M. (1976). Breast feeding and neonatal hyperbilirubinaemia. In *Liver Diseases in Infancy and Childhood*, p. 34. Ed. by Berenberg, S.R. The Hague: Martinus Nijhoff Medical Division

Ostrow, J.D. (1972). Photochemical and biochemical basis of the treatment of neonatal jaundice. In *Progress in Liver Diseases*, Vol IV, p. 447. Ed. by Popper H. and Schaffner, F. New York: Grune and Stratton

Seigel, S. *et al.* (1972). Placental transfusion and hyperbilirubinaemia in the premature. *Paediatrics* **46**, 406

Vaisman, S.L. and Gartner, L.M. (1975). Pharmacologic treatment of neonatal hyperbilirubinaemia. *Clins Perineonatal.* **2**, 37

CHAPTER 4

Conjugated Hyperbilirubinaemia

Conjugated hyperbilirubinaemia is always pathological, in contradistinction to unconjugated hyperbilirubinaemia which may be physiological in infancy. It most commonly arises from inflammatory intrahepatic causes or from lesions of the biliary tree (*Table 4.1*), giving rise to a hepatitis syndrome with clinical and biochemical features which are difficult to distinguish. Its causes are legion (*Table 4.1*). Urgent investigation is necessary to identify causes for which there are specific effective treatments and to exclude surgically correctable lesions. In addition, it is important to recognize genetically determined causes even if no treatment is available, since this may indicate the likely prognosis in the individual case, and is essential if the family are to be advised of the risks of recurrence in subsequent pregnancies. Very rarely, conjugated hyperbilirubinaemia may be caused by a specific genetically determined abnormality in the excretion of bilirubin glucuronide.

CONJUGATED HYPERBILIRUBINAEMIA DUE TO INHERITED DISORDERS IN BILIRUBIN GLUCURONIDE TRANSPORT

The Dubin—Johnson syndrome

Definition

This familial disorder is characterized by chronic benign conjugated hyperbilirubinaemia, and the deposition of melanin-like pigment in the liver. The exact mode of inheritance is uncertain but recent research suggests autosomal recessive rather than dominant as was previously considered likely. There is no mechanical bile duct obstruction.

Pathological features

The exact pathogenesis is undetermined. There is deficient hepatic excretion of cholecystographic agents, Bromsulfophthalein Sodium, methylene blue and indocyanine green, but bile salts are excreted normally. Jaundice is exacerbated by trauma, surgery, pregnancy, oral contraceptives and anabolic steroids. There is no pruritis. The

TABLE 4.1
Causes of Conjugated Hyperbilirubinaemia in Infancy

Structural defects

                Bile duct abnormalities

                            Biliary atresia
                            Spontaneous perforation
                              of bile duct
                            Choledochal cyst
                            Bile duct stenosis
                            Biliary hypoplasia
                              syndromes
                            Choledocholithiasis
                            Cholangiolitis
                Polycystic disease
                Vascular lesions

                            Veno-occlusive disease
                            Poor perfusion syndromes
                            Haemangioendothelioma
                            Lymphatic defects
                Chromosomal abnormalities
Metabolic defects
Infections
Post-haemolytic disorders
Toxic or deficiency disorders
                Intravenous nutrition
                Drugs
Familial syndromes
Neonatal hepatic necrosis
Idiopathic

precise nature of the pigment which gives the liver its characteristic greenish-black appearance is controversial. It is found predominantly in the central lobular region as fine granules or globules associated with lysosomes. It has melanin-like properties and may be derived from noradrenaline or adrenaline (*Figure 4.1*).

Clinical features

The apparent age of onset of jaundice is from birth to 40 years. It is often intermittent but rising to levels as high as 300 μmol/litre (17 mg/dl) with between 25 and 75 per cent of the bilirubin conjugated. There are no other features of liver disease but vague upper abdominal pain and nausea may occur. There is no hepatomegaly and standard

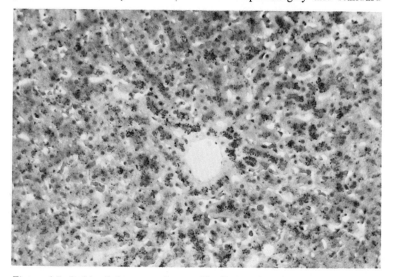

Figure 4.1. Dubin–Johnson syndrome. The liver architecture is normal. There are dark granules in the hepatocytes, particularly around the central vein. Cholestasis is not seen. There is no cellular infiltrate or fibrosis. (Percutaneous biopsy: haematoxylin and eosin; × 100, reduced to seven-eights in reproduction)

tests of liver function are normal. Oral cholecystography fails to reveal the gallbladder. Bromsulfophthalein Sodium retention in the serum at 45 minutes is generally between 10 and 20 per cent but higher concentrations may be found at 120 minutes. There is a reversal of the normal coproporphyrin/coproporphyrin isomer ratio in the urine. Liver biopsy shows the characteristic histology but this may not be apparent in early infancy.

No treatment is required for this benign disorder. Drugs aggravating the jaundice should clearly be avoided.

The rotor syndrome

This is a rare benign familial disorder with predominantly conjugated hyperbilirubinaemia, similar to the Dubin—Johnson syndrome but without pigment deposition in the hepatocytes. The exact mode of inheritance is uncertain. In some families both the Dubin—Johnson syndrome and the rotor syndrome have been described.

Clinical features

There is lifelong mild conjugated hyperbilirubinaemia with bilirubin levels of around 80—100 μmol/litre (4—5 mg/dl) with 85 per cent of the bilirubin conjugated. There are no clinical abnormalities, liver function tests are normal except for increased Bromsulfophthalein Sodium retention in the serum at levels of around 35 per cent at 45 minutes after injection. No rise occurs in the Bromsulfophthalein Sodium concentration at 120 minutes. Cholecystography is normal, and the liver biopsy is often normal.

Prognosis is excellent, no treatment is required.

HEPATITIS SYNDROMES IN INFANCY

Clinical features and laboratory findings (Figures 4.1—4.4)

The vast majority of patients present with jaundice, usually in the first four weeks of life, but with a small number presenting at five to eight weeks of life and a few as late as four months. Very rarely, jaundice may not be observed and the patient presents with malabsorption. Conjugated hyperbilirubinaemia is accompanied by dark bile-containing urine, and in many instances by clay-coloured stools. Hepatomegaly is usual, splenomegaly occurs in approximately 50 per cent of cases and a smaller percentage fail to thrive. A mild haemolytic anaemia is commonly found. Standard tests of liver function show elevation of the serum aspartate aminotransferase to levels of between one and a half and six times the normal, with similar elevations of the alkaline phosphatase. The prothrombin time may be prolonged and the serum albumin low.

Pathological features

On liver biopsy there is conspicuous cholestasis with bile staining within the hepatocytes and occasionally within bile canaliculi and bile ductules. Hepatocytes show to a variable degree multinucleated giant cell transformation. Hepatocellular necrosis is less readily seen in an

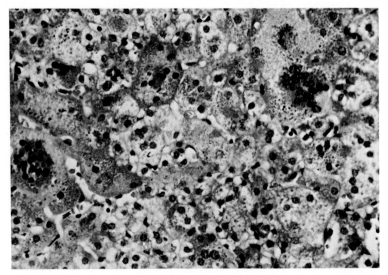

Figure 4.2. Hepatitis in infancy. Hepatic parenchyma showing great variability of hepatocyte size with many giant cells. Two multinucleated cells are seen. The normal lobular pattern cannot be distinguished. There is slight cellular infiltrate. (Percutaneous liver biopsy: haematoxylin and eosin; × 250, reduced to seven-eighths in reproduction)

Figure 4.3. Child aged 6 months with alpha-1 antitrypsin phenotype PiZ. There is marked hepatomegaly, splenomegaly, and an everted umbilicus. The child demonstrated marked pruritus. Jaundice had been present since the third day of life. By the age of 3 weeks the stools were acholic and the urine dark. There was marked hepatomegaly, splenomegaly but no ascites. Laboratory investigations showed features of severe cholestasis with Rose Bengal faecal excretion of < 5 per cent in 72 hours. Jaundice persisted until the age of 5½ months. Routine tests of liver function remained abnormal. By the age of 11 months ascites was evident and there was marked failure to thrive. The infant died of cirrhosis at the age of 17 months.

Figure 4.4. Infant aged 2 weeks with conjugated hyperbilirubinaemia, purpura and abdominal distension due to ascites. The birth weight was 2.3kg at 39 weeks gestation. No cause for the liver disease was identified. Steroids were started at 5 days after birth because of persistent purpura with thrombocytopaenia, the platelet count being less than 10,000 and the prothrombin time prolonged by 110 seconds. The bleeding diathesis settled over the course of 2 weeks. Steroids were continued when liver function tests remained abnormal and a percutaneous liver biopsy showed features consistent with chronic aggressive hepatitis. Steroids were eventually stopped at the age of 2 years when liver function tests had been normal for 12 months. A repeat liver biopsy 12 months later showed slight fibrosis but no evidence of hepatitis. Although the outcome was satisfactory in this case, there is no evidence that steroids affect the course of hepatocellular disease in this age group

acute hepatitis in the adult but evidence of hepatocellular loss is frequently demonstrated by crowding of reticulum fibres with appropriate stains. Conspicuous but diffuse acute and chronic inflammatory cell infiltrate is seen in the hepatic parenchyma as well as in the portal tracts. Clumps of haemopoietic cells are seen in the parenchyma.

The portal tracts are often widened with cellular infiltration, conspicuous bile duct proliferation and increased fibrosis. Such changes may be seen irrespective of whether the disease affects primarily the hepatic parenchyma, the portal tracts, the major intrahepatic bile

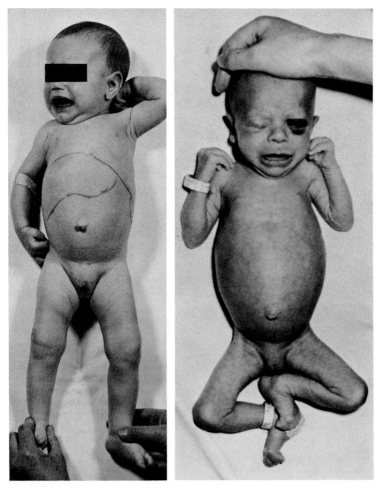

Figure 4.3   *Figure 4.4*

ducts, or the extrahepatic bile ducts. It should be noted that giant cell transformation occurs in extrahepatic biliary atresia, in hepatitis of known cause, as well as in the familial and idiopathic varieties.

The term 'giant cell hepatitis' thus has little to recommend it. It should be appreciated that there may be differences in the appearance in the two lobes, fibrosis being much more prominent in the left. Where there is obstruction of the extrahepatic bile ducts, it is extremely rare in this age group to see dilatation of proximal extrahepatic ducts or dilatation of the intrahepatic bile ducts. It should be appreciated that patients with marked hepatitis may have negligible bile flow and the extrahepatic bile ducts may be very narrow and the lumen difficult to identify.

Three aspects of these histological changes have been the subject of much recent research since they are unique to this age group and are particularly important from the point of view of prognosis.

Giant cell transformation The exact nature of giant cell transformation of hepatocytes, producing multi-nucleated balloon cells with pale cytoplasm and variably stained nuclei, is still a mystery, but it is generally held that this is a non-specific response to injury, particularly occurring in intrauterine life or in the first 24 months of extrauterine life. While the increased number of nuclei suggest a regenerative process, the electronmicroscopic appearances suggest degeneration. When serial biopsies have been done, it has been concluded that these cells have a short life span. They may represent a relapse to a more primitive level of functioning since the degree of elevation of serum alpha-fetoprotein found in such patients may be related to the degree of giant cell change seen on liver biopsy. Both phenomena, however, could represent an unrelated response to injury. The causes of giant cell transformation are not clear, but in the experimental animal it has been shown that endotoxin from *Escherichia coli* can produce such changes.

Bile duct proliferation The second distinct histological change is marked ductular proliferation seen particularly in biliary atresia but also in infants with genetic deficiency of the serum protein alpha-1 antitrypsin and in idiopathic disease. It is uncertain whether these distorted angulated bile ductules arise by cholangiocyte proliferation or are derived from hepatocytes by direct transformation, or even from peri-lobular cells which are incompletely differentiated into hepatocytes or cholangiocytes in this age group. Experimentally, bile duct ligation, hepatocellular injury (for example, by aflatoxin), and abnormalities of bile salt metabolism, are all associated with bile duct proliferation.

Fibroblastic activity There is always associated fibroblastic activity almost as if these abnormal bile ductules provided a template on which collagen is deposited. The factors which control the abnormal deposition of collagen in many instances of hepatitis in infancy are not known. In various forms of liver disease, abnormalities of collagen metabolism have been observed. These include an increased number of fibroblasts, increased proline concentration, an increased activity of the enzyme prolyl-hydroxylase, increased transfer of collagen from the fibroblasts to the extracellular tissue and, paradoxically, increased collagenase activity. It is the outcome of these interactions which determines whether liver disease will be reversible or cirrhosis inevitable.

Aetiological factors

Some specific causes of hepatobiliary disease in infancy are considered below. The aetiology of much of hepatobiliary disease in this age group is, however, poorly understood. Consideration must be given not only to the possible environmental and genetic factors indicated in *Table 4.2*, which independently or in unison may cause symptomatic liver disease, but also to the interaction between the cell types within the liver, namely, hepatocytes, bile duct epithelial cells, sinusoidal endothelial cells, Kupffer cells and Ito cells which appears to maintain the reticulum framework and control the deposition and removal of collagen. An injury to any one of these cell types may disturb the functions of the other. The outcome, be it a fulminant, dramatic disturbance of liver function, acute disease followed by complete resolution or progressive liver disease may depend not only on the interaction of these five cell types but also on their interaction with migrant polymorphonuclear leucocytes, lymphocytes and macrophages. Research into the causes of liver disease in this age group must therefore not be limited to hepatocytotrophic viruses or hepatocyte toxins, but include factors affecting the other cells within the liver and elements of the reticulo-endothelial system.

Complications

Complications arise when the hepatocellular disease is severe or where cholestasis with diminished bile flow is complete or prolonged. Problems arise from retention of bile salts, cholesterol from malabsorption of fat and fat-soluble vitamins, portal hypertension, cirrhosis and hepatocellular failure (*Table 4.3*).

TABLE 4.2
Possible Aetiological Factors in Cryptogenic Hepatobiliary
Disease in Infancy

Causes	Timing	Mechanisms	Examples
genetic and/or environmental	Antenatal	Infections	Bacterial toxins Unidentified viruses
		+ or −	
		Toxins	Drugs in pregnancy or labour, sedatives, antihistamines, milk additives, DDT in maternal fat stores, intravenous fat
	Perinatal	+ or −	
		Immunological factors	Mother–infant incompatibility Absorption of polypeptides Transient immuno-deficiency Abnormalities of cell-mediated immunity
		+ or −	
	Postnatal	Perinatal handicaps	Transient depressed enzymatic activity Impaired hepatic perfusion during post-natal vascular changes Excessive demand due to haemolysis especially in severe haemolytic disease Perinatal hypoxia Stress of initiation of intrahepatic circulation

TABLE 4.3

Patho-physiological Consequences of Prolonged Cholestasis

Abnormality	Effect
Diminished bile salt excretion	Pruritus and malabsorption
Hypercholesterolaemia	Xanthelasma
Diminished fat absorption	Steatorrhoea, loose offensive stools, growth retardation
Calcium and magnesium deficiency	
Deficiency of fat-soluble vitamins, namely:	
Vitamin K	Hypoprothrombinaemia
Vitamin D	Rickets
Vitamin A	Night blindness
Vitamin E	Haemolytic anaemia
Cirrhosis	
Portal hypertension	
Hepatocellular failure	Fluid retention, encephalopathy, hypo-prothrombinaemia unresponsive to Vitamin K
Increased susceptibility to infection	

Diagnosis

The differential diagnosis of conjugated hyperbilirubinaemia or the hepatitis syndrome in infancy requires consideration of all the disorders listed in *Table 4.1*. These are considered in detail elsewhere in this Chapter. The priority in diagnosis must be the immediate detection of medically treatable infections, namely, bacterial, syphilis or toxoplasmosis, and of metabolic disorders for which effective dietary treatment is available. Galactosaemia is frequently associated with septicaemia, and is not invariably accompanied by galactosuria. Urgent consideration must be given to excluding the surgically correctable disorders, spontaneous perforation of the bile duct (page 339) and choledochal cyst (page 332). Precise identification of the other causes may influence management of the individual case and may yield information of prognostic value or with genetic implications. The important distinction between idiopathic hepatitis and extrahepatic biliary atresia is considered with this latter topic (*see* Chapter 5).

Course and prognosis

The course and prognosis is determined by the underlying cause and the effectiveness of therapy. Where liver disease is caused by systemic infection it is frequently of short duration and the prognosis is determined by the extent of injury to other vital organs such as the brain or the heart.

Where the syndrome has arisen from an intrahepatic cause, complete resolution may occur. Liver disease is associated with genetic metabolic abnormalities, it is commonly progressive, but in both alpha-1 antitrypsin deficiency and cystic fibrosis, an asymptomatic period may occur before cirrhosis and its complications appear.

Where the disease is cryptogenic, the prognosis is variable. In most reported series, between 10 and 33 per cent of those with cryptogenic disease die of progressive liver failure early in infancy, and an estimated 5–20 per cent may develop progressive liver disease, leading ultimately to cirrhosis.

GENETICALLY DETERMINED METABOLIC DISORDERS

Of the metabolic disorders causing the neonatal hepatitis syndrome (*Table 4.4*), *galactosaemia, fructosaemia* and *tyrosinaemia* must be excluded since specific treatment is effective in the former two and may be helpful in the third. Galactosaemia or fructosaemia may be suspected clinically from the characteristic symptomatology and by the appearance of the offending monosaccharide in the urine. This can easily be identified as a non-glucose reducing substance with a simple test such as Clinitest tablets or Benedict's solution which are positive, but the specific glucose oxidase test is negative. It must be emphasized that these tests will only be abnormal if the offending monosaccharide has been ingested shortly before the time of testing. It is important to appreciate that patients with galactosaemia often have an overwhelming septicaemic-like illness in the first days of life, and unless specifically looked for the diagnosis of galactosaemia may never be considered in life. A further problem is that some patients with galactosaemia may not have galactosuria even in the first months of life. Similarly, fructosaemic patients may not have fructosuria, even when challenged with a fructose load. These diagnoses must be vigorously pursued since the effect of not treating the patient is devastating, while with appropriate treatment the prognosis is good.

Tyrosinaemia, too, presents diagnostic difficulties, particularly since patients with acute hepatocellular necrosis may have many of the biochemical features of tyrosinaemia in the first month of life. Often a diagnosis of tyrosinaemia must be made initially but revised when the biochemical features resolve as the liver disease improves. Unfortunately, the institution of a low tyrosine, low phenylalanine diet is not associated with improvement in the condition in all patients.

The clinical features and diagnostic investigation in rarer metabolic disorders in which a hepatitis syndrome may occur in infancy are given in *Table 4.4*.

The exact mechanism of hepatocellular injury in these various conditions is far from clear. In some it appears to be part of a complex metabolic derangement which causes hepatocellular necrosis and increased mesenchymal activity. In many, the hepatocellular changes are less damaging than changes in other organs. An exception is the liver disease associated with genetic deficiency of the serum protein alpha-1 antitrypsin (*see* below). Liver disease complicating cystic fibrosis is considered elsewhere (page 269).

LIVER DISEASE ASSOCIATED WITH THE GENETIC DEFICIENCY OF THE SERUM PROTEIN ALPHA-1 ANTITRYPSIN

Alpha-1 antitrypsin is a glycoprotein synthesized in the liver accounting for approximately 90 per cent of the alpha-1 globulin in serum. Its molecular weight is between 50,000 and 60,000. Its genetic control is thought to be by a single autosomal gene responsible for at least 24 different alleles which may be distinguished by acid-starch gel electrophoresis and antigen-antibody crossed immunoelectrophoresis. The variants so recognized are labelled alphabetically in the protease inhibitor (Pi) phenotyping system. PiM is the predominant type occurring in 70–100 per cent of individuals in studies of normal populations; such individuals having a serum alpha-1 antitrypsin concentration of between 200 and 400 mg/dl in health, increasing with infection, pregnancy, oral contraceptives, perinatal diseases and in many acute liver disorders.

Individuals with genetic deficiency have serum concentrations of between 20 and 160 mg/dl which increase little with these stresses and are of phenotypes PiZ or Pi nul in which little or no alpha-1 antitrypsin is found in the serum. Between 50 and 60 per cent of such individuals develop emphysema, with its onset in early adult life; 10–20 per cent develop serious liver disease commonly starting in infancy.

The physiological role of alpha-1 antitrypsin has yet to be determined. In addition to inhibiting the enzyme trypsin, it inhibits elastase, collagenase and leucocyte and bacterial proteases. It may thus have a role in controlling tissue responses in infection and inflammation and particularly in modifying the response to enzymes released from dying bacteria or damaged cells. In addition it may influence both coagulation and fibrinolysis being an effective inhibitor of plasminogen.

TABLE 4.4

Metabolic Disorders Associated with the Neonatal Hepatitis Syndrome

Disorder	Screening investigation	Definitive investigation	Associated clinical features
Galactosaemia	Non-glucose reducing substance may be found in the urine when galactose is ingested (not invariably)	Decreased concentration of R.B.C. Galactose-1-phosphate uridyl transferase	Onset at birth with vomiting, failure to thrive, haemorrhagic diathesis, septicaemia, and later cirrhosis, mental retardation and cataracts
Fructosaemia	Fructosuria may be present when fructose is ingested	Decreased or absent hepatic fructose-1-phosphatase	Onset after introduction of sucrose-supplemented milk. Hypoglycaemia. Haemorrhagic diathesis, hepatomegaly, failure to thrive, anorexia, glycosuria, hyperaminoaciduria
Tyrosinaemia	Positive ferric-chloride test, positive Phenistix	High concentration of serum tyrosine-phenylalanine. Low concentration of parahydroxy phenylpyruvate oxidase in liver	Onset at 1 —4 weeks of age with failure to thrive, hepatocellular failure, bleeding diathesis, renal tubular dysfunction, and vitamin D resistant rickets
Cystic fibrosis	Albumin in meconium	Sweat sodium chloride greater than 70 mmol/litre	Meconium ileus, failure to thrive, malabsorption, anaemia, oedema, respiratory tract infection
Nieman—Pick disease		Sphingomyelinase deficient in leucocytes, lymph nodes or liver biopsy	Hepatosplenomegaly, progressive dementia, blindness

Neuro-visceral storage disease, with ophthalmoplegia	Sphingomyelin accumulation. Sea-blue histocytes in marrow and liver		Hepatosplenomegaly, progressive dementia presenting with supranuclear ophthalmoplegia
Gaucher's disease	Deficient glucosyl ceramide beta-glucosidase in leucocytes, bone marrow or liver biopsy	Cells in marrow	Splenomegaly, hepatomegaly, lymph node enlargement, pulmonary infiltration and central nervous system involvement
Wolman's disease	Deficiency of acid esterase in leucocytes or liver biopsy		Vomiting, diarrhoea, failure to thrive, abdominal distension, hepatosplenomegaly, steatorrhoea, adrenal calcification, developmental delay
Zellweger's syndrome	Mitochondrial abnormalities on liver biopsy	High serum iron with saturation iron-binding capacity	Low birth weight, prominent forehead, with open metopic suture, sagittal suture synostosis, congenital cataracts, hypertelorism, high-arch palate, cirrhosis, cysts of kidney, stippled cartilage in diaphysis and patella
Dubin–Johnson syndrome	Pigment in the liver on biopsy (may not be evident until the age of 4 years)	Bromsulfophthalein Sodium clearance reduced with rebound increase in concentration at 120 minutes	Positive family history
Trihydroxycoprostatic acidaemia (THCA)	Defect of specific THCA hydroxylating enzyme	Very low serum cholic acid	Persistent cholestasis. Biliary hypoplasia progressing to cirrhosis and death by the age of 3 years

TABLE 4.4 *Continued*

Familial neonatal hepatic steatosis	Liver biopsy shows hepatocytes crammed with fat	Usually leads to death: hepatocellular failure by the age of 4 weeks
Hypopituitarism	Hypoglycaemia, decreased serum cortisol and urinary 17 ketosteroids	Metyrapone test. Growth hormone deficiency, low T4 and TSH	Clinical, biochemical and pathological features of idopathic hepatitis in infancy
Hypothyroidism		T4 low, TSH high	*NB.* Characteristically causes an unconjugated hyperbilirubinaemia but may cause jaundice in what would otherwise be an anicteric hepatitis
Alpha-1 antitrypsin deficiency (*see* text)		

Pathological features

Liver biopsy in the acute stages shows features indistinguishable from idiopathic neonatal hepatitis except that giant cell transformation is rarely prominent and the histological features may be very similar to those of extrahepatic biliary atresia. Fibrous tissue in the portal tract is prominent and often gradually increases to cause intralobular fibrosis. When cirrhosis develops, it may be macronodular, micronodular or take a so-called biliary form. Recent research suggests that where there is marked bile duct proliferation and portal tract fibrosis in early infancy, cirrhosis is likely to supervene in the first decade. In contrast, where there is little portal tract fibrosis in initial biopsy cirrhosis may well be delayed.

A distinctive pathological feature is the presence of diastase-resistant, PAS positive, magenta-coloured globules 2–20 nm in diameter seen most prominently in the periportal hepatocytes, but only after the age of 12 weeks. These globules appear to correspond to the amorphous material which on electronmicroscopy is seen to distend the endoplasmic reticulum of some hepatocytes. Other intracellular organelles are normal. The material reacts with the specific fluorescin-tagged antibody to alpha-1 antitrypsin, giving a bright fluorescence not seen in the hepatocytes of non-PiZ subjects. The accumulation of this material, which is antigenically similar to normal (PiM) serum alpha-1 antitrypsin, occurs in PiZ subjects whether liver disease is present or not.

The pathogenesis of liver disease associated with alpha-1 antitrypsin deficiency is at present uncertain. Since the incidence and severity of liver disease is greater in some families than in others, it has been suggested that a second associated genetic factor may be necessary for liver disease to occur. It might have a part in controlling protease/antiprotease balance in tissues, since the most favoured pathogenesis of progressive liver disease is deficiency of tissue antiprotease with an uninhibited action of bacterial, viral or cellular proteases released by tissue damage however initiated. It has been suggested that a factor in causing emphysema could be depressed levels of chemotactic factor inhibitor resulting in an inordinate attraction of neutrophils to the site of tissue injury. It has been suggested also that the alpha-1 antitrypsin deficient individuals who avoid disease have diminished leucocyte proteases. Preliminary research findings suggest that a further aetiological factor could be persistently disturbed cellular immunity, as evidenced by lymphocyte cytotoxicity for isolated rabbit hepatocytes seen in children with alpha-1 antitrypsin deficiency and liver disease (Smith *et al.*, 1977).

If an exogenous factor initiates the liver damage, it must operate *in utero* or in the perinatal period. A large proportion of children with alpha-1 antitrypsin deficiency and liver disease have low birth weights. Very few patients develop significant liver disease without a history of obstructive jaundice in the first months of life.

Diagnosis

Diagnosis may be suspected by visual scanning of the serum protein electrophoresis which shows a deficient or absent alpha-1 globulin. More specifically, the diagnosis may be made by an immuno-precipitation method measuring the actual serum concentration of alpha-1 antitrypsin. Since the various phenotypes of alpha-1 anti-trypsins give a wide range of serum concentrations, in health and disease, most research workers in the field prefer to determine the alpha-1 antitrypsin phenotype using the acid starch-gel electropho-resis and crossed immuno-precipitation technique mentioned previously. With this, liver disease seems to have been associated only with PiZZ state and Pi nul. The observation of liver disease in one family with SZ phenotype may be a chance association.

Clinical features

Liver disease usually presents as an acute hepatitis in the first four months of life with conjugated hyperbilirubinaemia often following directly from neonatal physiological jaundice but sometimes starting as late as four months. Clinical severity of the hepatitis may be very variable. Some infants appear well apart from jaundice and slow weight-gain, while others show irritability or lethargy, marked failure to thrive with vomiting, hypotension, purpura with low platelet counts and prolonged prothrombin time and septicaemia. Serum bilirubin concentrations may rise as high as 340 μmol/litre (20 mg/dl). Aspartate aminotransferase levels vary in the acute stage from 80 to 600 iu/litre with alkaline phosphatase from 150 to 1,300 iu/litre. The jaundice may persist for periods of as little as one week to over a year. Although the serum bilirubin returns to normal aspartate aminotransferase is likely to remain intermittently elevated, while persistent elevations of the alkaline phosphatase and cholesterol are usual. In a few instances the liver disease will have been so severe in infancy that cirrhosis and its complications develop.

The majority of those who survive the acute hepatitis have a period of relative well-being before cirrhosis and its complications appear later in childhood or early in adult life. Although, in general, the degree of irreversible liver damage reflects the clinical severity of the initial hepatitis, cirrhosis in infancy may follow a mild hepatitis. Cases which have a predominantly parenchymal injury with relative sparing of the portal tract seem to have a better short-term prognosis (Mowat *et al.*, 1977). In some instances, cirrhosis may not be present even in the third decade, suggesting that it is not an inevitable outcome in those with cholestasis in infancy, as had been initially suggested.

As well as patients who have symptomatic disease, approximately 40 per cent of infants with alpha-1 antitrypsin deficiency without overt liver disease have persistently elevated serum enzyme levels. The prognosis for such infants is unknown. Very rarely cirrhosis will appear in childhood without any antecedent hepatitis in the newborn period.

Management

Unfortunately, there is as yet no specific treatment for alpha-1 antitrypsin deficiency. Phenobarbitone given as a possible enzyme reducer had no effect on serum alpha-1 antitrypsin concentration, its functional activity or on liver function tests. Corticosteroids and immunosuppressants do not appear to control the hepatitis. Administration of exogenous alpha-1 antitrypsin is impractical since its half-life is only six days. Non-specific measures to mitigate the complications of cholestasis and to control the complications of cirrhosis do, however, add considerably to the patient's comfort. Liver transplantation has been attempted but the patient did not survive.

INFECTIONS ASSOCIATED WITH HEPATITIS IN INFANCY

Although a wide range of agents causing generalized infection of the neonate produce hepatitis as a major or minor component of the illness no infectious cause can be identified in the vast majority of patients. Bacterial infections such as *Escherichia coli* septicaemia and infection with Listeria, cytomegalovirus, rubella virus and hepatitis B virus, have all been associated with extrahepatic biliary atresia as well as hepatitis. In addition, septicaemia may complicate liver disease primarily due to a metabolic abnormality such as galactosaemia. The cytomegalovirus may frequently be found in the urine of infants who are well.

Considerable care, therefore, is necessary before the neonatal hepatitis syndrome can, in an individual patient, be attributed to any of these alleged pathogens, unless the hepatitis is associated with the severe extrahepatic clinical manifestations listed in *Table 4.5*. In clinical management it is essential to exclude bacterial infection, listeriosis,

TABLE 4.5

Infectious Causes of the Hepatitis Syndrome of Infancy

Infecting agents	Screening investigations	Definitive investigations	Principal extrahepatic clinical manifestations
Cytomegalovirus	CF antibody in serum	Isolation from urine and liver with demonstration of virus in liver by IF	Small for dates; microcephaly; meningoencephalitis; intracranial calcification; neonatal thrombocytopenic purpura; splenomegaly; retinitis, deafness
Rubella virus	CF and HAI antibodies in serum	Specific IgM antibody, virus isolation from nasopharynx and liver	Small for dates; cataracts, retinitis; congenital heart defects; microphthalmia, buphthalmos and corneal oedema; myocarditis; neonatal thrombocytopenic purpura; splenomegaly; osteopathy; lymphadenopathy
Hepatitis B virus	Antigen and antibody in mother	Hepatitis B antigen in infant Demonstration of hepatitis B antigen in liver by IF and EM	None described
Herpes simplex virus	Perinatal herpes in mother	Isolation and demonstration of virus from superficial lesions and liver	Splenomegaly; heart failure, pneumonitis; skin vesicles; meningoencephalitis
Coxsackie B virus	Isolation from respiratory tract and faeces	Isolation from liver	Myocarditis; meningoencephalitis; pneumonitis

Varicella zoster virus	Demonstration of virus from superficial lesions	Demonstration of virus in the liver	Disseminated infection as in herpes simplex; skin lesions more obvious
Bacterial infection		Blood culture, urine culture, CSF	Anaemia; any other system may be involved
Listeria		Isolation of organisms from blood culture, CSF or liver	Septicaemia; meningitis; pneumonitis; purpura
Treponema pallidum	VDRL or TPI, particularly in mother	Demonstration of Treponema by dark ground illumination	Rhinitis; skin rash; bone lesions; anaemia; lymphadenopathy; meningoencephalitis
Toxoplasma gondii	CF antibody in serum	Rising antibody titre in infant; specific IgM antibody; isolation of organisms from liver and CSF; visualization of organism from liver and CSF	Microcephaly; macrocephaly; meningoencephalitis; intracranial calcification; choreoretinitis; thrombocytopenia; purpura

CF = Complement fixing; HAI = Haem. agglutination inhibition; IF = Immunofluorescence microscopy; EM = Electron microscopy;
CSF = Cerebrospinal fluid
(Reproduced from *Essentials of Paediatric Gastroenterology* by courtesy of Churchill Livingstone)

toxoplasmosis and infection with *Treponema pallidum* since specific antibiotic therapy for these is available. For viral infections no effective treatment has yet been devised.

Hepatitis viruses The virus causing acute infectious hepatitis A has not yet been implicated in hepatitis in this age group. Hepatitis B surface antigen has been found in a small number of infants with hepatitis, in some cases leading to cirrhosis. More commonly the hepatitis is anicteric and causes no symptoms. Infection is derived either from an asymptomatic carrier mother, a mother who has had hepatitis in the last trimester of pregnancy, or early in the puerperium, and also from hepatitis B antigen positive blood or serum. Where infection is derived from the mother, the exact mode of infection is not clear. It may be transplacental, intrapartum or postpartum. The finding of the antigen in the cord blood increases the likelihood that hepatitis B surface antigen will persist in the infant but it is not inevitable. If the mother has had symptomatic hepatitis in the last trimester of pregnancy or early in the puerperium, there appears to be a 40 per cent chance of hepatitis B antigenaemia in the infant. Preliminary studies suggest that the occurrence of 'e' antigen in the mother is associated with an 80–90 per cent incidence of antigenaemia in the infant. In most instances the disease is mild but there is moderate persistent elevation of the aspartate transaminase and the infant may become a chronic carrier. There is some evidence that such asymptomatic carriers are more prone to significant liver disease, for example, cirrhosis or cancer, later in life.

In infants and mothers who are asymptomatic carriers there is a much lower incidence of infection, approximately only 5–10 per cent having antigenaemia and associated liver disease. In most instances the disease is mild, but fulminant hepatitis has been observed 59–150 days after birth in infants of asymptomatic carriers.

Because of these observations, attempts have been made to modify the possibility or severity of infection in the infant by giving immuno-globulin with a high concentration of antibody to hepatitis B surface antigen. Only a small number of infants has so far been treated. A prospective controlled trial of this form of treatment will be necessary to show whether it is efficacious.

CHROMOSOMAL ABNORMALITIES

In Trisomy 13 and 18, between 20 and 30 per cent of patients have hepatitis. The presence of such trisomies may be suspected clinically from the marked physical abnormalities and can be confirmed by analysis of the chromosomal karyotype. The hepatitis may contribute to failure to thrive. Hepatitis may be slightly more common in infants with Down's syndrome and there is often the suggestion that it occurs more frequently in female phenotypes with Turner's syndrome, but it is difficult to be certain whether there is indeed an increased incidence in these two conditions.

FAMILIAL SYNDROMES

A number of distinct syndromes with familial occurrence of obstructive liver disease in infancy has been described. Obstructive jaundice in infancy, followed by recurrent episodes of jaundice throughout childhood and in later life and *lymphoedema*, has been reported in a group of patients with common ancestry in south west Norway. Liver biopsy in infancy shows changes of the neonatal hepatitis syndrome whereas in adults the main abnormalities are intracanalicular cholestasis (Aagenaes, 1974). Towards puberty these patients develop oedema of the leg with hypoplasia of the lymph vessels in the limbs. It has been suggested that deficiency of intrahepatic lymphatics may contribute to the cholestasis. Families with similar disease have been described from North America and Australia.

Alagille *et al.* (1975) have described a syndrome causing chronic cholestasis associated with characteristic abnormalities outwith the liver. The disease usually presents as a persistent cholestasis in the first three months of life with marked pruritus and a relatively moderate elevation of serum bilirubin. There is hepatosplenomegaly and xanthomata may be found. By the second year of life the serum bilirubin has usually returned to normal or is only slightly elevated at between 4 and 8 mg/dl ($68-136 \mu$mol/litre). In contrast, the serum triglycerides are markedly elevated, often exceeding 2 g/dl ($12.9-25.9$ mmol/litre) while the cholesterol will range from 0.5 to 1 g/dl. Serum lipid electrophoretic pattern shows an absent or flattened alpha lipoprotein peak with a sharply increased beta lipoprotein peak. Liver biopsy in the first months of life shows hepatocellular damage with clarification and ballooning of hepatocytes and prominent bile stasis. There may be some giant cell transformation but little mesenchymal reaction. The characteristic histological abnormality is, however, hypoplasia of intrahepatic biliary ductules. From surgical liver biopsy it is clear that bile ducts are often absent in these portal triads or where present are narrow and may even have no visible lumen.

The facial appearance is characteristic: the forehead is prominent, the eyes are deeply set and somewhat widely separated, there is mild hypertelorism and a straight nose, which in profile is in the same plane as the forehead. The chin is small and pointed. A harsh mid-systolic murmur heard maximally in the third intercostal space at the left sternal border occurred in 13 of the 19 initially described patients. In 9 pulmonary artery stenosis was demonstrated on angiography. Vertebral arch defects were observed in 12 of 19 patients; this was characteristically growth retardation and some of the patients had mild to moderately severe mental retardation. Hypogonadism has been observed in some children. The aetiology is unknown, but the frequency with which similar abnormalities have been noted in siblings of the indexed cases suggests a genetic basis.

The prognosis for such children appears to be rather better in the short term than those with other forms of intrahepatic biliary hypoplasia, most having survived the first decade.

Watson and Miller (1973) have described a somewhat similar syndrome characterized by congenital *hypoplasia and stenosis of the pulmonary arteries*, sometimes with associated cardiovascular malformations, associated with a very heterogeneous pattern of neonatal liver disease, under the term 'arterio-hepatic dysplasia'. From their studies they concluded that the condition may be inherited in an autosomal dominant fashion, with variable penetrance. Ten of these had the neonatal hepatitis syndrome, eight with hypercholesterolaemia, but in only two patients did the levels reach those recorded in Alagille's series. In only two of these patients was intrahepatic biliary hypoplasia documented. These patients were of normal intelligence, but had minor skeletal abnormalities in some instances and were small and thin, only two being above the fifteenth percentile for height and weight. They had a bird-like face with prominent forehead and prominent chin. The ears were malformed in one case and prominent in five others.

In a report emphasizing the cardiovascular abnormalities, Greenwood *et al.* (1975) report 14 cases with intrahepatic biliary dysgenesis (a term which they appear to use synonymously with intrahepatic biliary hypoplasia) and *peripheral pulmonary stenosis*. These patients had a mild neonatal hepatitis syndrome followed by hepatomegaly, hyperlipoproteinaemia, xanthomata, growth retardation and pruritus. There were no abnormalities outwith the cardiovascular and hepatobiliary systems. The aetiology was not clear, but the presence of mild similar features in other family members and the presence of the syndrome in siblings suggested a genetic factor.

Juberg and colleagues (1966) reported four affected siblings in a sibship of eight, with jaundice starting at the age of 3–5 months, hepatomegaly, growth retardation, mild mental retardation, hypercholesterolaemia, and on liver biopsy, hypoplastic bile ducts with increased portal tract fibrosis.

PROGRESSIVE FAMILIAL INTRAHEPATIC CHOLESTASIS WITH HYPERCHOLESTEROLAEMIA

Severe familial intrahepatic cholestasis, proceeding to early death, often in the first decade, together with the absence of hypercholesterolaemia has been described in a number of reports, such as the eight cases in the Amish Byler family, but also in families of smaller sibships. The condition appears to be inherited in an autosomal recessive fashion. In the children in the Byler series, and in those described by Odievre, jaundice occurs intermittently initially, often being provoked by infection, with attacks lasting from a few days to 20 months. Remission is never complete, however; hepatomegaly persists, there is gradually increasing hepatic fibrosis leading to portal hypertension, cirrhosis, and alimentary bleeding. Diarrhoea, steatorrhoea, and failure to thrive are prominent features. Hypoplastic intralobular bile ducts are not a feature of this syndrome. The biochemical abnormality underlying the disorder has not yet been defined. In some instances, it has been shown that there is an accumulation of bile acids in the serum, including the bile acid lithocholic acid, with diminished bile acids in the intestines, but this may be a secondary phenomenon. Cholestyramine has no appreciable effect on the evolution of the disease. Inspissated bile, gallstones, large gallbladders and evidence of pacreatitis, have all been described in such cases. Such abnormalities however, may simply be complications of the liver disease, however initiated. It is clear from the above that it is as yet impossible to authenticate isolated cases as falling within these sub-classifications without a positive family history.

FAMILIAL NEONATAL CHOLESTATIC JAUNDICE WITH HEPATIC STEATOSIS

A number of families have been described in which severe neonatal cholestatic jaundice sometimes causing kernicterus, with a bleeding diathesis, leading to death in the first month of life, has been associated with severe fatty infiltration of the liver. Biochemical abnormality underlying this condition has not be elucidated.

POST-HAEMOLYTIC CHOLESTASIS

Transient conjugated hyperbilirubinaemia occurs during the recovery phase in erythroblastosis in which it appears that the bilirubin is conjugated more rapidly than it can be excreted. Liver function tests are, however, normal. When the unconjugated hyperbilirubinaemia has been protracted and severe, or if there has been marked anaemia at birth, the urine may contain bile and the stools become acholic. Laboratory investigations show typical features of the hepatitis syndrome in infancy. The liver biopsy shows hepatocellular necrosis and giant cell transformation. There may be both hepatocellular and canalicular cholestasis. There is little increased fibrosis, or changes in the portal tracts. Prognosis is good.

ACUTE NEONATAL HEPATIC NECROSIS

Neonatal hepatic necrosis is a rare condition presenting in the first four weeks of life with a haemorrhagic diathesis. Features of liver disease rapidly follow. The aetiology is unknown but in some instances it has been associated with viral hepatitis type B.

The liver shows massive necrosis with collapse of the reticulum. There is marked haemosiderin deposition and scanty giant cell transformation.

The course is one of steady deterioration with marked spontaneous haemorrhage. Vigorous supportive therapy with fresh blood transfusions, clotting factors, vitamin K and steroids is indicated.

CONJUGATED HYPERBILIRUBINAEMIA IN INFANCY ASSOCIATED WITH PARENTERAL NUTRITION

Intravenous alimentation using solutions of aminoacids, dextrose and lipids with added vitamins and electrolytes has become a commonly employed procedure in paediatrics. It has been used for augmenting nutrition in low birth weight, premature infants, infants with gastrointestinal disorders, such as necrotizing enterocolitis, and in infants with protracted diarrhoea.

Conjugated hyperbilirubinaemia with hepatomegaly and other features of hepatitis has been reported sporadically in infants receiving parenteral nutrition, usually for some weeks. It has occurred with regimens which have included lipids and in those with no lipids.

Pathology

Cholestasis, hepatocellular damage and mild to moderate degrees of multinucleated giant cell transformation with hyperplasia of the Kupffer

cells are the main features. Cholestasis is both canalicular and hepatocellular, being more severe towards the central portions of the lobule.
There are no bile plugs in the portal tracts. Hepatocytes are mildly
to moderately swollen with rarification and vesiculation of the cytoplasm. They may show moderate accumulations of glycogen and
haemosiderin. Erythropoietic activity is increased in the hepatic
parenchyma but there is little inflammatory cell infiltrate. The hyper-
plastic Kupffer cells contain PAS positive pigments and bile pigment.

The portal tracts are widened with often chronic inflammatory cell
infiltrate. There is increased portal fibrosis.

Ultrastructural studies show giant mitochondria of varying shapes
and sizes and damaged endoplasmic reticulum. There is increased
collagen fibres in the space of Disse.

Pathogenesis

The exact aetiology is unknown. The majority of cases occur in prematurely born infants. Many have had possibly harmful factors such
as sepsis, hypoxia, intra-abdominal surgery and drugs. The frequency
of the disorder increases with the duration of intravenous feeding.

Both aminoacid solutions and protein hydrolysates cause a
progressive rise in serum alkaline phosphatase concentration in the first
three weeks of administration. Intravenous aminoacid solutions may
cause hyperaminoacidaemia, metabolic acidosis and hyperammoniaemia. Intravenous lipids cause the lipoprotein X concentration to rise
progressively in serum. These and other factors may cause disturbances
of intracellular metabolism. Associated with these changes there is
deposition of unidentified pigment in both Kupffer cells and
hepatocytes. It is unknown whether this deposition is associated with
any toxic or metabolic effects. Lack of essential nutrients, trace
elements or single aminoacids have been postulated as possible contributory factors. In addition, the lack of gastrointestinal stimulation to
bile secretion has been postulated as a possible cause.

Clinical features and laboratory findings

The clinical features are those of hepatitis in infancy. Acholic stools are
unusual.

Serum bilirubin concentration ranges from 34 μmol/litre to 340
μmol/litre (2–20 mg/dl), returning to normal within 7–100 days
of discontinuing intravenous nutrition. The alkaline phosphatase, serum
transaminases, are frequently between two and three times normal.

Blood ammonia may be raised to as much as three times that of normal. The prothrombin time is usually normal.

Treatment and prognosis

When intravenous nutrition is withdrawn jaundice settles and the liver function tests gradually return towards normal. There have been no long-term follow-up studies on these infants. The long-term prognosis is therefore uncertain but the presence of hepatocellular damage and portal tract fibrosis in the short term does cause anxiety about possible long-term effects. It is recommended, therefore, that intravenous feeding should be curtailed as much as possible if jaundice or other features of hepatocellular injury appear. Tests of liver function should be carried out regularly while intravenous feeding progresses.

IDIOPATHIC HEPATITIS IN INFANCY

In most series of cases all aetiological tests are negative in the majority of infants. The percentage in whom no cause can be found in any series is determined by referral patterns, the investigation facilitates available at the time of the study and by the rigidity of criteria for an aetiological diagnosis (*Table 4.6*). Long-term follow-up of such infants may allow more precise diagnosis in a few when new features appear, for example, progressive brain deterioration and sphingomyelin in the bone marrow in patients with Nieman—Pick disease. In others, the birth of a second affected sibling raises the possibility of an unrecognized genetic disorder.

Infants with idiopathic disease of the liver are frequently of low birth weight, born following abnormal pregnancies and come to medical attention because of complications of prematurity or low birth weight, rather than because of the hepatitis. Of 28 such cases studied during a prospective investigation of the hepatitis syndrome in infancy in South East England, five were born before 37 weeks and 11 were light-for-gestational age (below the tenth percentile for age). Eleven came to medical attention for reasons other than jaundice. Jaundice developed in the first two weeks of life in 19 but occurred later in the remainder. It persisted for from 2 to 26 weeks with a mean duration of 10 weeks. Although 15 cases were sufficiently severe to have acholic stools, only two of these died of liver disease in the first six months of life. Short-term follow-up (four to seven years) showed that four have mild disturbances of liver function, or hepatic pathology, and one has cirrhosis. A second sibling in this last family had a very mild apparently non-progressive hepatitis.

INTRAHEPATIC BILIARY HYPOPLASIA

This ill-understood disorder is defined pathologically by the absence or diminution in number and size of intralobular intrahepatic bile ducts. The diagnosis can be made only by wedge liver biopsy at laparotomy. The disorder may arise in association with extrahepatic biliary atresia but also it occurs with intact extrahepatic bile ducts. In the latter circumstances the serum bilirubin, bile salts and cholesterol are elevated, changes taken to indicate diminished bile secretion. It is not known, however, whether the structural abnormalities cause the failure of bile secretion or arise from them.

Aetiology

A genetic or familial cause has been suggested in some instances. Intrahepatic biliary hypoplasia has recently been reported in two siblings who were found to have a deficiency in the 24-hydroxylating enzyme system which converts 3-alpha, 7-alpha trihydroxy-5 beta cholestenoic-26-oic acid (T.H.C.A.) to cholic acid, raising the possibility that the

TABLE 4.6

Causes of Obstructive Jaundice in Infancy: the Influence of Environmental Factors and Diagnostic Facilities on the Apparent Cause in Three Areas

Cause	*King's College Hospital, London, England*	*Royal Childrens Hospital, Melbourne, Australia*[1]	*Verwoerd Hospital, Pretoria, S. Africa*[2]
Extrahepatic biliary atresia	62	55	21
Idiopathic hepatitis	91	88	52
Alpha-1 antitrypsin deficiency	35	8	0
Galactosaemia	2	6	0
Cystic fibrosis	2	2	0
Rubella	2	3	0
Cytomegalovirus	3	13	0
Hepatitis Bs Ag	2	1	0
Syphilis	0	1	28
Toxoplasmosis	1	2	0
Blood group incompatibility	4	6	6
Veno-occlusive disease	0	0	8
Miscellaneous	0	0	13

[1] Danks *et al.* (1977)
[2] Pretorius and Roode (1974)

primary defect may be a genetically determined abnormality in bile acid synthesis (Hanson *et al.*, 1975). The 19 cases with homogeneous clinical features, distinct facies, mental retardation, vertebral abnormalities, cardiac murmurs and hypogonadism, described by Alagille *et al.* (1975) also had a familial tendency, but the biochemical basis of this syndrome has not yet been elucidated. Intrahepatic biliary hypoplasia has also been a feature of intrahepatic cholestasis in siblings (Juberg *et al.*, 1966; Gray and Saunders, 1966; Sharp *et al.*, 1967; Ballow *et al.*, 1973).

Clinical features

This is a heterogeneous group of conditions other than in the children with features similar to those described by Alagille *et al.* (1975), and in cases occurring in siblings in which disease may follow a consistent pattern. The onset of symptoms may occur in the first three months of life or be delayed to beyond three years. In the former, there are usually typical features of the hepatitis syndrome, with hepatosplenomegaly and occasionally pruritus and bile salt retention more marked than would be expected with only moderate elevation of serum bilirubin.

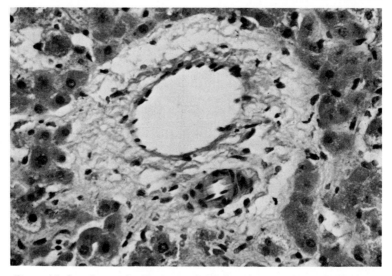

Figure 4.5. Portal tract showing a portal vein branch and, below, a small branch of the hepatic artery. No bile ductules can be seen. The spaces within the portal tract may be lymphatic channels. There is no increased fibrosis or cellular infiltrate. (Percutaneous liver biopsy: haematoxylin and eosin, × 320, reduced to seven-eighths in reproduction)

Liver biopsy at this stage shows typical histological features of hepatitis in this age group with prominent cholestasis. A variety of changes may be noted in the portal tract. There is commonly a morphonuclear neutrophil leucocyte with reduplication of bile ducts and some fibrosis. This is often minimal but in some instances it is already severe and rapidly progresses to a biliary cirrhosis. The extrahepatic bile ducts are patent but of small calibre.

In those cases of late onset, pruritis, hepatomegaly, elevation of serum bile salts, high serum alkaline phosphatase and then elevation of serum bilirubin is the usual progression. Liver biopsy in such cases would usually show in addition to cholestasis, diminished or absent bile ducts in the portal tracts. Varying degrees of fibrosis may be found (*Figure 4.5*).

The subsequent progress is very variable. In patients with marked periportal fibrosis jaundice will in some instances clear, but in others persist. However, portal hypertension and cirrhosis will almost certainly follow, rapidly leading to death by the age of two years.

Where little portal fibrosis occurs jaundice may clear after one to two years, to be followed by a period of well-being in which there are no clinical abnormalities apart from hepatomegaly. In some instances, pruritis and xanthelasma will develop at this stage although the patient is free from jaundice.

For some patients this period of well-being and freedom from jaundice terminates towards the end of the first decade when increasing hepatic fibrosis leads to cirrhosis. Yet other patients remain jaundice-free without evidence of progressive liver disease into the second decade.

Treatment

As well as measures directed towards dealing with the complications of cholestasis mentioned earlier, particularly combating the bleeding diathesis (*see also* page 91), two agents — cholestyramine and phenobarbitone — have a marked influence on the symptoms of this condition.

Pruritus can be controlled with cholestyramine which will also cause a diminution in the accumulation of cholesterol in the tissues and will clear xanthelasma. For reasons that are not understood, cholestyramine also may cause an improvement in liver function tests and in the well-being of the patient. The only well recognized side-effect is folic acid deficiency which can easily be prevented by administering folic acid. Phenobarbitone also has an effect in this condition causing the serum bilirubin to fall, perhaps due to increased bile flow. In some instances, the combination of these two drugs has a beneficial effect.

JAUNDICE IN LATE INFANCY AND CHILDHOOD

Conjugated hyperbilirubinaemia in late infancy and childhood complicates most illnesses affecting the hepatocyte or the biliary system. The
most frequent cause is viral hepatitis type A, but the possibility that
some treatable condition such as chronic active hepatitis, or Wilson's
disease may be responsible, must always be considered. Similarly,
surgically correctable lesions of the biliary system, such as choledochal
cyst, or gallstones, must always come to mind. Very rarely, familial
or genetically determined abnormalities of bilirubin excretion will be
responsible.

BIBLIOGRAPHY AND REFERENCES

Inherited disorders

Arias, I.M. (1961). Studies of chronic familial non-haemolytic jaundice with
    conjugated bilirubin in the serum with and without unidentified pigment
    in the liver cells. *Am.J.Med.* **31**, 510
Shani, M., Seligsohn, U. and Adam, A. (1973). The inheritance of Dubin–Johnson
    syndrome. *Israel J. Med. Sci.,* **9**, 1427

Hepatitis in infancy

Alagille, D. (1972). Clinical aspects of neonatal hepatitis. *Am.J.Dis.Child.* **123**,
    287
Danks, D.M., Campbell, P.E., Jack, I., Rogers, J. and Smith, A.L. (1977). Studies
    of the aetiology of neonatal hepatitis and biliary atresia. *Archs Dis. Childh.* **52**,
    360
Danks, D.M., Campbell, P.E., Smith, A.L. and Rogers, J. (1977). Prognosis of
    babies with neonatal hepatitis. *Archs Dis.Childh.* **52**, 368
Emery, J.L. (1974). Pathology with reference to the bile-retention syndrome.
    Post-grad. med.J. **50**, 344
Landing, P.H. (1974). Consideration of the pathogenesis of neonatal hepatitis,
    biliary atresia and choledochal cyst – the concept of infantile obstructive
    cholangiopathy. *Prog.Pediat.Surg.* **6**, 113
Mowat, A.P., Pscharopoulos, H.T. and Williams, R. (1976). Extrahepatic biliary
    atresia versus neonatal hepatitis. A review of 137 prospectively investigated
    infants. *Archs Dis. Childh.* **51**, 763
Portmann, B., Mowat, A.P. and Williams, R. (1976). Liver histopathology in
    neonates with conjugated hyperbilirubinaemia. *Acta Pediat.Belg.* **29**, 139
Pretorius. P.J. and Roode, H. (1974). Obstructive jaundice in early infancy.
    Aetiological, clinical and prognostic aspects. *S.Afr. med. J.* **48**, 811
Pscharopoulos, H.T. and Mowat, A.P. (1978). An epidemiologic study of hepatitis
    in infancy – aetiological factors and prognosis. In *Proceedings of a National
    Workshop on Neonatal Hepatitis and Biliary Atresia.* Washington, D.C. 1977
    (in press)
Sass-Kortsak, A. (1974). Management of young infants presenting with direct-
    reacting hyperbilirubinaemia. *Pediat. Clins. N. Am.* **21**, 777

Alpha-1 antitrypsin deficiency

Aagenaes, Ø. and Sveger, T. (1976). Clinical aspects of liver disease in children with alpha-1 antitrypsin deficiency. In *Liver Diseases in Infancy and Childhood*, p. 64. Ed. by Berenberg, S.R. The Hague: Martinhus, Nijhoff Medical Division

Fagerhol, M.K. (1976). The genetics of alpha-1 antitrypsin and its implications. In *Aspects of Genetics in Paediatrics*, p. 73. Ed. by Baltrop, D. London: Fellowship of Postgraduate Medicine

Freier, E., Sharp, H.L. and Bridges, R.A. (1968). Alpha-1 antitrypsin deficiency associated with familial infantile liver disease. *Clin.Chem.* **14**, 782

Moroz, S.P., Cutz, E., Balfe, J.W. and Sass-Kortsak, A. (1976). Membrano-proliferative glomerulonephritis in childhood cirrhosis associated with alpha-1 antitrypsin deficiency. *Pediatrics* **57**, 232

Mowat, A.P. (1976). Liver disease in infants and children. In *Recent Advances in Gastroenterology*, p. 261. Ed. by Bouchier, I.A.D. London: Churchill Livingstone

Mowat, A.P., Pscharopoulos, H.T., Williams, R., Portmann, B. and Tait, R.A.J. (1977). Prognosis in childhood of liver disease associated with alpha-1 antitrypsin deficiency, type PiZ. *Gut* **18a**, 978

Odievre, M., Martin, J.P., Hadchouel, M. and Alagille, D. (1976). Alpha-1 antitrypsin deficiency in liver disease in children. Phenotypes, manifestations and prognosis. *Pediatrics* **57**, 226

Sharp, H.L. (1976). Relationship between alpha-1 antitrypsin deficiency and liver disease. In *Liver Diseases in Infancy and Childhood*. p. 52. Ed. by Berenberg, S.R. The Hague: Martinhus, Nijhoff Medical Division

Smith, A.L., Cochrane, A.M.G., Mowat, A.P., Eddleston, A.W.L.F. and Williams, R. (1977). Cytotoxicity to isolated rabbit hepatocytes by lymphocytes from children with liver disease. *J.Pediat.* **91**, 584

Sveger, T. (1976). Liver disease and alpha-1 antitrypsin deficiency detected by screening of 200,000 infants. *N. Engl. J. Med.*, **294**, 1316

Galactosaemia

Hsia, D. Y.-Y. (1969). *Galactosemia*. Springfield, Ill.: Thomas

Isselblacher, K.J. (1966). *Galactosaemia in the Metabolic Basis of Inherited Disease*, p. 178. 2nd ed. Ed. by Stanbury, J.B., Wyngaarden, J.B. and Fredrickson, E.S. New York: McGraw-Hill

Monk, A.M., Mitchell, A.J.H., Milligan, D.W.A. and Holton, J.B. (1977). The diagnosis of classical galactosaemia. *Archs Dis. Childh.* **52**, 943

Oberklaid, F., Danks, D.M. and Davies, H.E. (1976). Problems encountered in the diagnosis of galactosaemia. *Aust.paed.J.* **12**, 14

Fructosaemia

Levin, B., Oberholzer, B.G., Snodgrass, G., J.A.I., Stimmler, L. and Wilmers, M.J. (1963). Galactosaemia an inborn error of fructose metabolism. *Archs Dis. Childh.* **38**, 220

Odievre, M., Gontil, C., Gautier, M. and Alagille, D. (1978). Hereditary fructose intolerance in childhood; Diagnosis, management and course in 52 patients. *Am. J. Dis. Child.* **132**, 605

Fructose-1, 6-diphosphatase deficiency

Bakker, H.D., DeBree, P.K., Ketting, D., Van Sprang, F.J. and Wadman, S.K. (1974). Fructose 1,6-diphosphatase deficiency: another enzyme defect which can present itself with the clinical features of tyrosinosis. *Clinica.chim.Acta* **55**, 41

Tyrosinosis

LaDu, B.N. and Gjessing, L.R. (1972). Tyrosinosis and tyrosinemia In *The Metabolic Basis of Inherited Disease,* p. 296, 3rd ed. Ed. by Stanbury, J.B., Wyngaarden, J.B. and Fredrickson, D.S. New York: McGraw-Hill
La Rochelle, J., Prive, L., Belanger, M., Belanger, L., Trembley, M., Claveau, J.C., Aubin, G. and Paradis, D. (1973). Hereditary tyrosinaemia. Clinical and biological study in 62 cases. *Pédiatrie* **28**, 5
Yu, J.S., Walker-Smith, J.A. and Burnard, E.D. (1971). Neonatal hepatitis in premature infants simulating hereditary tyrosinosis. *Archs Dis. Childh.* **46**, 306

Cystic fibrosis

Oppenheimer, E.H. and Esterly, J.R. (1975). Hepatic changes in young infants with cystic fibrosis. *J.Pediat.* **86**, 683
Taylor, W.F. and Qaqundah, B.Y., (1972). Neonatal jaundice in cystic fibrosis. *Am.J.Dis.Child.* **123**, 161

Neimann—Pick disease

Crocker, A.C. and Farber, S. (1958). Neimann—Pick disease: a review of 18 patients. *Medicine, Baltimore* **37**, 1
Neville, B.G.R., Lake, B.D., Stephens, R. and Sanders, M.D. (1973). Neurovisceral storage disorders with vertical supra-nuclear ophthalmoplegia and its relationship to Neimann—Pick disease. *Brain* **96**, 97

Wolman's disease

Kamalian, N., Dudley, W. and Beroukhim, F. (1973). Wolman's disease with jaundice and subarachnoid haemorrhage. *Am.J.Dis.Child.* **126**, 671

Zellweger's syndrome

Gilchrist, K.W., Gilbert, E.F., Goldfarb, S., Goll, U., Spranger, J.W. and Opitz, J.M. (1976). Studies of malformation syndromes of man, 11b; the cerebro-hepato-renal syndrome of Zellweger; comparative pathology. *Eur. J. Pediat.* **121**, 99

Trihydroxy coprostatic acidaemia

Hanson, R.F., Isenberg, J.N., Williams, G.C., Hachey, D., Szczepanik, P., Klein, P.D. and Sharp, H.L. (1975). The metabolism of 3,7,12-trihydroxy-5 beta cholestan-26-oic acid, in two siblings with cholestasis due to intrahepatic bile duct anomalies. *J.clin.Invest.* **56**, 577

Dubin–Johnson syndrome

Kondo, T., Yagi, R. and Kuchiba, K. (1975). Dubin–Johnson syndrome in a neonate. *New.Engl.J.Med.* **292**, 1029

Hepatitis B surface antigen

Beasley, R.P., Stevens, C.E., Shiao, I.S. and Meng, H.C. (1965). Evidence against breast feeding as a mechanism for vertical transmission of hepatitis B. *Lancet* **2**, 470

Dupuy, J.M., Frommel, D. and Alagille, D., (1975). Severe viral hepatitis Type B in infancy. *Lancet* **1**, 191

Geraty, R.J. and Schweitzer, I.L. (1977). Viral hepatitis Type B during pregnancy, the neonatal period and infancy. *J.Pediat.* **90**, 368

Kohler, P.F., Dubois, R.S., Merrill, D.A. and Bowes, W.A. (1974). Prevention of chronic neonatal hepatitis B virus infection with antibodies to hepatitis B surface antigen. *New.Engl.J.Med.* **291**, 1378

Okada, K., Kamiyama, I., Inomata, M., Imai, M., Miyakawa, Y. and Mayumi, M. (1976). e-Antigen and anti-e in the serum of asymptomatic carrier mothers as indicators of positive and negative transmission of hepatitis B virus to their infants. *New.Engl.J.Med.* **294**, 746

Other viral causes of hepatitis in infancy

Chiba, S., Hori, S., Kawamura, N. and Nakao, T. (1975). Primary cytomegalovirus infection and liver involvement in early infancy. *Tohoku J. exp. Med.* **117**, 143

Madelin, J.-C. (1973). Hepatite virale du Nourrisson. *Revta Pract.* **23**, 55

Rotthauwe, H.W. (1974). Viral hepatitis in infancy and childhood. *Clin. Gastroenterol.* **3**, 437

Sass-Kortsa, A. (1974). Management of young infants presenting with direct-reacting hyperbilirubinaemia. *Pediat. Clins N. Am.* **21**, 777

Non-viral infections

Dommergues, J.P. (1973). Hepatites infectieuses non virales du norrisson. *Revta Pract.* **23**, 4941

Escobado, M.B., Barton, L.L., Marshall, R.E. and Zarkowsky, H. (1974). The frequency of jaundice in neonatal bacterial infections. *Clin.Pediat.* **13**, 656

Familial conjugated hyperbilirubinaemua/biliary hypoplasia

Aagenaes, Ø. (1974). Hereditary recurrent cholestasis with lymphoedema. *Acta paediat. Scand.* **63**, 465

Alagille, D., Odievre, M., Gautier, M. and Dommergues, J.P. (1975). Hepatic ductular hypoplasia associated with characteristic facies, vertebral malformations, retarded physical, mental and sexual development and cardiac murmur. *J.Pediat.* **86**, 63

Ballow, M., Margolis, C.Z., Schachtel, B. and Hsia, Y.E. (1973). Progressive familial intrahepatic cholestasis. *Pediatrics* **51**, 998

Clayton, R.J., Iber, F.L. Ruebner, B.H. and McKusick, V.A. (1969). Byler's disease. Fatal familial intrahepatic cholestasis in an Amish kindred. *Am. J.Dis.Child.* **117**, 112

Exss, R. and Rotthauwe, H.W. (1976). Hypertension and bilateral stenosis of the renal artery associated with congenital hypoplasia of the intrahepatic bile ducts. Eur.J.Pediat. **121**, 125

Gharardi, G.J. and MacMahon, H.D. (1970). Hypoplasia of terminal bile ducts. *Am.J.Dis.Child.* **120**, 151

Gray, O.P. and Saunders, R.A. (1966). Familial intrahepatic cholestatic jaundice in infancy. *Archs Dis. Childh.* **41**, 320

Greenwood, R.D., Rosenthal, A., Crocker, A.C. and Nadas, A.S. (1976). Syndrome of intrahepatic biliary dysgenesis and cardiovascular malformation. *Pediatrics* **58**, 243

Juberg, R.C., Holland-Moritz, R.M. and Henley, K.S. (1966). Familial intrahepatic cholestasis with mental and growth retardation. *Pediatrics* **38**, 819

Linarelli, L.G., Williams, C.N. and Phillips, M.J. (1972). Byler's disease. Fatal intrahepatic cholestasis. *J.Pediat.* **81**, 484

Luders, D. (1974). Hypoplasia of intrahepatic bile ducts and other forms of intrahepatic cholestasis in infancy. *Mschr.Kinderheilk.* **122**, 207

Odievre, M., Gautier, M., Hadchouel, M. and Alagille, D. (1973) Severe familial intrahepatic cholestasis. *Archs.Dis.Childh.* **48**, 806

Watson, G.H. and Miller, V. (1973). Arterio-hepatic dysplasia. *Archs Dis. Childh.* **48**, 459

Williams, C.N., Kaye, R., Bigger, L., Hurwitz, R. and Senior, J.R. (1972). Progressive familial cholestatic cirrhosis and abnormal bile acid metabolism. *J.Pediat.* **81**, 493

Neonatal hepatic necrosis

Dupay, J.M., Frommel, D. and Alagille, S. (1975). Severe viral hepatitis Type B in infancy. *Lancet* **1**, 191

Phillip, A. and Larson, E. (1973). Overwhelming neonatal infection with Echo 19 virus. *J.Pediat.* **82**, 391

Reupner, B.H., Bhagadan, B.S., Greenfield, A.J., Campbell, P. and Danks, D.M. (1969). Neonatal hepatic necrosis. *Pediatrics* **43**, 963

Conjugated hyperbilirubinaemia in infancy associated with parenteral nutrition

Bernstein, J., Chang, C-H., Brough, A.J. and Heidelberger, K.P. (1977). Conjugated hyperbilirubinaemia in infancy associated with parenteral alimentation. *J.Pediat.* **90**, 361

Touloukian, R.J. and Seashore, J.H. (1975). Hepatic secretory obstruction with total parenteral nutrition in the infant. *J.pediat.Surg.* **10**, 353

Rare causes of cholestasis

Herman, S.T., Baggenstoss, A.H. and Cloutier, M.D. (1975). Liver dysfunction and histologic abnormalities in neonatal hypopituitarism. *J.Pediat.* **87**, 892

Pellarin, D., Alagille, D. and Bertin, P. (1971). Conjugated hyperbilirubinaemia and haemangioma of the liver in a newborn. *Archs fr. Pediat* 28, 1093

Rasanen, O., Korhonen, M., Simila, S., Autere, T. and Hakosalo, J. (1971). Familial fatal steatosis of the liver and kidney in two siblings. *Z. Kinderheilk.* 110, 267

Rothauwe, H.W. and Rothauwe, I. (1971). Familial recurrent intrahepatic cholestasis with the onset in infancy. *Z. Kinderheilk.* 110, 292

Taylor, A. (1968). Autosomal trisomy and hepatitis syndromes. *J.med.Genet.* 5, 227

Wadlington, R.W.B. and Riley, H.D. (1973). Familial disease characterised by neonatal jaundice, hepatic steatosis and kernicterus. *Pediatrics* 51, 192

Walker, W. (1971). Haemolytic disease in the newborn. In *Recent Advances in Paediatrics*, 4th ed. p. 131. Ed. by Gairdner, G. and Hull, D. London: Churchill Livingstone

CHAPTER 5

Extrahepatic Biliary Atresia

Introduction

Extrahepatic biliary atresia, the most common of these progressive hepatic disorders, is itself a rare disease affecting approximately 1: 14,000 live-born infants. It is, nevertheless, the most important hepatic cause of morbidity in infancy and early childhood. Until the recent introduction of the biliary drainage procedure – hepatic portoenterostomy – the vast majority of affected children progressed inexorably to a miserable death, usually between 18 months and two years; pruritus adding to the problems caused by cirrhosis and fat malabsorption. Although as paediatricians we have learned to cope with some of the complications of this disorder, we are little nearer to understanding its cause or pathogenesis than was Dr John Thompson who, in 1891, at the end of a masterly treatise on the subject, suggested that the condition might arise from 'a congenital narrowness or irregularity of *the lumen of the ducts* of such a nature as to render *them* unnaturally liable to disease from *its* interference with the proper performance of *their* function'. Hepatic portoenterostomy, with its many problems, is far from the complete solution of the problems of biliary atresia, but at least this operation has given hope and stimulated research in an area of paediatrics in which little progress has been made this century. Further evaluation of this operation will be needed to assess its full value. Liver transplantation, an operation of even greater potential but still a formidable research undertaking with immense difficulties, may also come to have a role in helping such patients.

Definitions

The terminology applied to biliary disorders in childhood is not standardized. The terms used in this text are defined below.

Extrahepatic biliary atresia is characterized by complete inability to excrete bile and by obstruction, destruction, or absence of the bile ducts anywhere between the duodenum and first or second order of branches of the right and left hepatic ducts. The extent and site of the obstruction or absence of the bile ducts is extremely variable. The most common finding is complete obstruction of all the extrahepatic bile ducts with obliteration of the lumina and their replacement by fibrous cords, extending to the portahepatis. Prior to the introduction of hepatic portoenterostomy, such cases were considered surgically non-correctable. The term *'surgically correctable'* is applied where there is distal atresia but the common hepatic duct is patent up to the level of the porta-hepatitis, contains bile and is in continuity with the main intrahepatic bile ducts. If the obstruction is below the junction of the cystic duct the gallbladder is dilated and contains bile.

Intrahepatic biliary hypoplasia is characterized by an absence or reduction in the number of bile ducts seen in portal tracts within the liver substance. Diagnosis requires that in two or three portal tracts normal portal vein and hepatic artery branches can be identified with absent or disproportionately small bile ducts. There is usually increased fibrous tissue in the portal tracts. A wedge biopsy of the liver is usually necessary to establish the diagnosis.

The term (*see* page 69) appears to be used by some authors synonymously with biliary dysgenesis.

The term *extrahepatic biliary hypoplasia* is used to refer to the operative cholangiographic demonstration of a patent but narrow biliary tree with contrast medium extending up into the liver and flowing into the duodenum.

Aetiology and pathogenesis

The aetiology of extrahepatic biliary atresia is unknown. It is unlikely that it arises as a primary failure of development of bile ducts, if only because of the very variable extent of the biliary obstruction in this disorder. It seems certain that the hepatic parenchymal cells develop as outgrowths from the primitive bile duct system. Since hepatocytes are present in abundance in biliary atresia, normal early development of bile ducts presumably occurs. In some infants there is firm post-natal evidence, including cholangiography, that the bile ducts were intact but have subsequently been destroyed. Pathological study of tissues removed from the area of the porta-hepatis and the proximal extrahepatic bile ducts suggests that the condition of the vast majority of infants results from a sclerosing inflammatory lesion initiated in the ductular tissues.

It may start in fetal life, around the time of birth or early in post-natal life. Since in the majority of infants the unconjugated physiologic jaundice of the newborn continues as the conjugated hyperbilirubinaemia of biliary atresia, the exact time of onset is usually uncertain, but in a few infants jaundice is not noticed until they reach the age of between two and six weeks.

The degree of duct involvement is very variable, affecting all or part of the extrahepatic bile duct and frequently the intrahepatic bile ducts. Distension of the intrahepatic bile ducts which occurs in other forms of bile duct obstruction does not occur in the typical case. The progressive degeneration of bile duct epithelium, lumenal obliteration with inflammatory cell infiltrate leading to periductular fibrosis (progressive obstructive cholangiopathy) affecting the extrahepatic bile duct, is followed by marked changes within the liver.

There is widening of the portal tracts with increased activity of fibroblasts leading to the deposition of fibrous tissue, the appearance of numerous bile ducts and the development of angulated, distorted bile ductules showing apparently aimless proliferation near the edges of the portal tract. The bile ducts may contain within their lumen bile plugs, there is prominent cholestasis within the hepatocytes and some giant cell transformation. Without surgical drainage there is increasing fibrosis with a gradual decrease in the number of intrahepatic bile ducts. In cases that survive beyond the age of 12 months the histological appearance may change to that of bile duct hypoplasia. Biliary cirrhosis with portal hypertension is the inevitable outcome. There is considerable case-to-case variation in the rapidity with which portal hypertension and cirrhosis develops. Whether such intrahepatic extension of the lesion occurs primarily or is secondary to the extrahepatic bile duct obstruction is unresolved at present.

In cases in which bile drainage results from surgery, liver biopsy specimens frequently show a similar succession of changes, apparently affecting parts of the biliary system which are not draining effectively. In such instances the prognosis is dependent on whether there are sufficient unaffected segments to maintain liver function and also on whether the haemodynamic changes in the damaged section of the liver lead to portal hypertension.

Aetiological considerations

Relationship with neonatal hepatitis

In view of the many similarities in the clinical and biochemical features of extrahepatic biliary atresia and idiopathic neonatal hepatitis, it has been suggested that both may be caused by the same basic disease process, in some instances the major damage occurring in the bile ducts, but in others in the hepatic parenchyma. To support this hypothesis its protagonists quote the very occasional recovery of alleged causative organisms as rubella, cytomegalovirus, Listeria and hepatitis B surface antigen in both conditions. None of these organisms has in any way fulfilled Koch's postulate; cytomegalovirus in particular, is suspect since, as well as often being an opportunistic infection in the ill-patient it may cause infection without any abnormal clinical features. Further, in most case reports in which this association has been made, there is extensive hepatocellular damage unlike that seen in typical extrahepatic biliary atresia. With such extensive liver injury, bile flow is considerably reduced and the extrahepatic bile ducts may be so narrow that they are considered atretic.

Short gestation and low birth weight are rare in infants who develop biliary atresia, although frequent in infants who develop hepatocellular jaundice in early infancy. Of 103 with 'hepatitis' 23 were born prematurely and 36 were of low birth weight as opposed to only one of 32 infants with atresia (Mowat, Pscharopoulos and Williams, 1976).

Twenty-five per cent of infants with biliary atresia have minor or major congenital malformations elsewhere, but no single abnormality is associated with biliary atresia. Three of 29 children who were considered for liver transplantation were found to have a composite vascular abnormality including absence of the inferior vena cava, a pre-duodenal portal vein and anomalous hepatic arterial vasculature. Biliary atresia has occurred with the polysplenia syndrome. It has affected one of identical twins.

Clinical features in the first two months of life

The onset, clinical features and biochemical findings are similar to those observed in the vast majority of patients with a neonatal hepatitis syndrome. The first indication of cause for concern is prolongation of neonatal jaundice with the appearance of bile-stained urine. In most instances, the date of onset of the jaundice is difficult to define since it is continuous with physiologic jaundice, but in approximately 20 per cent of cases jaundice starts after the second week of life. It is often said that normal meconium is passed by these infants. Unfortunately, by the time the diagnosis is suspected, it is often impossible to determine what meconium was passed since mothers often do not nurse their infants in the first 24 hours of life and there is no record that meconium passed was normal. The stools become acholic in the vast majority of cases within the first six to eight weeks of life but there is, from time to time, some pigment in the stool. In nearly 20 per cent of cases the urine contains bilirubin but no urobilinogen. Rarely, spontaneous haemorrhage, particularly from the umbilicus, may be the first sign of biliary atresia.

Infants with extrahepatic biliary atresia are usually born at term, of good birth weight, and are well nourished in the first two months of life. Hepatomegaly is usual with the liver edge palpable in all instances, in more than 50 per cent of cases being more than 5 cm below the costal margin at the right mid-clavicular line. The left lobe of liver is often enlarged also. It is important to palpate the liver edge throughout its length to assist in the differential diagnosis from choledochal cyst. The liver surface is smooth and its consistency moderately increased. In 70 per cent of cases the spleen is palpable. The mechanism of splenomegaly is unknown but portal hypertension is certainly a factor, being present with levels of greater than 22 cm of water in 30 per cent of cases by the age of two months. There is rarely, however, signs of portosystemic venous shunting and ascites is distinctly unusual. Although slight oedema of the pretibial tissue is commonly seen, other cutaneous features of chronic liver disease, such as palmer erythema or spider naevi, are rare.

Biochemical features in the first two months of life

The serum bilirubin on presentation at the age of two to eight weeks is commonly in the region of 136–204 μmol/litre (8–12 mg/100 ml) with between 50 and 70 per cent of the bilirubin conjugated. Rarely, the total bilirubin may be as low as 110 μmol/litre (6.5 mg/dl) with only 51 μmol/litre conjugated (3 mg/dl), but in over 90 per cent of cases, more than 68 μmol/litre (4 mg/100 ml) of the serum bilirubin will be conjugated in the first ten weeks of life. During the first ten weeks the serum bilirubin level may remain constant with a day-to-day variation of less than 51 μmol/litre but in other instances it may rise progressively. In yet a third pattern there are day-to-day fluctuations with rises and falls of greater than 51 μmol/litre. Levels as high as 340 μmol/litre (20 mg/dl) are occasionally attained during this period.

The serum aspartate aminotransferase and other tests of hepatocellular integrity are always abnormal, the vast majority of cases having serum levels at between two and ten times normal, but rarely high values are obtained. The serum alkaline phosphatase level is also usually elevated but in only 50 per cent of cases does the value exceed 230 iu/litre. The serum albumin is normal, and the cholesterol may be at the upper limit of normal. Anaemia is unusual, but between 5 and 10 per cent of cases would have prolonged prothrombin times which corrects within 6 hours of giving intramuscular vitamin K.

Late clinical features

The child who survives beyond 4–6 months of life with biliary atresia suffers progressively from the effects of cirrhosis and fat malabsorption. The rate of development of these features is variable. All structures, tissue fluids and secretions, including tears, become jaundiced, the child eventually developing a greenish hue. Intestinal secretions pigment the previously acholic stools. The abdomen becomes markedly distended because of hepatomegaly, splenomegaly and ascites. In contrast, the remainder of the body becomes emaciated with lack of subcutaneous fat, muscle bulk and bone structure. Growth is retarded and motor development slowed. Unless vitamin D supplements are given, rickets develops. Pruritus adds to the child's misery. Hypersplenism and alimentary blood loss due to portal hypertension cause anaemia with all its consequences. There is increasing fluid retention which with diaphragmatic elevation and pulmonary oedema causes respiratory distress. Death, due to alimentary bleeding, chronic hepatic failure, systemic

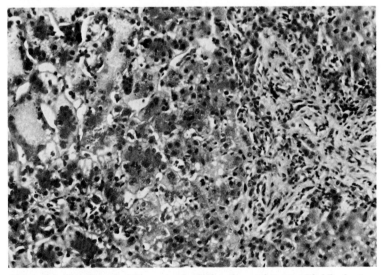

Figure 5.1. Extrahepatic biliary atresia. Widened portal tract with bile duct reduplication, increased fibrosis and cellular infiltrate in an infant aged 7 weeks with extrahepatic biliary atresia. Note that there is extensive giant cell transformation in the hepatic parenchyma (× 320, reduced to seven-eighths in reproduction)

bacterial infection or bronchopneumonia, usually occurs by the age of two years but some infants die within eight months, while a few survive to the age of three years. Exceptional cases may survive to the age of 13 or 14 years.

Differential diagnosis

Biliary atresia must first be distinguished from the known infectious, metabolic and genetic causes of conjugated hyperbilirubinaemia in early infancy. It must then be distinguished from idiopathic neonatal hepatitis, in which laparotomy is not indicated (*see* Chapter 4, page 51). Pre-operative distinction from the rare surgically correctable disorders, such as choledochal cyst (page 332) or spontaneous perforation of the bile duct (page 339), is also important. Ultrasonic echography of the biliary tree, barium meal to show duodenal displacement, and the use of radioactive tagged Rose Bengal to obtain a scan of the biliary tree or to demonstrate its increased concentration in ascites, also assist in identifying these two conditions (*see* page 386).

Diagnostic investigations

Systematic investigation to identify and treat known causes of neonatal hepatitis syndrome must be undertaken, bearing in mind that bile duct lesions have occurred in a number of systemic viral infections. This seems to be distinctly rare. It should be recalled that significant bacterial infection may occur around the time of onset of the jaundice in biliary atresia and, if jaundice does not clear with specific treatment of bacterial infection, biliary atresia should be suspected.

In any child with conjugated hyperbilirubinaemia persisting for more than two weeks, biliary atresia must be considered. However, only one in seven such patients will have biliary atresia. Laparotomy is ultimately required to confirm the diagnosis and to allow its surgical correction. Since laparotomy in patients with hepatitis will almost certainly cause some temporary deterioration in liver function (due to drug effects, changes in blood flow through the liver caused by intermittent positive pressure respiration, loss of fluid and blood) and may even cause an increased incidence of cirrhosis in the long term, it must be avoided as a primary investigation. The introduction of operations which, if undertaken early may cure some patients with complete biliary atresia, which was previously considered non-correctable, makes the early identification of biliary atresia mandatory.

Two investigations are of proven value in this regard.

Percutaneous liver biopsy

There are no unique histological features which distinguish extra-hepatic biliary atresia from infantile hepatitis. Nevertheless, the histo-pathologist with experience of liver biopsies in this age group can provide invaluable assistance in determining whether the cholestasis is due to a bile duct lesion in which there is uniform portal tract involvement, or a disorder of hepatocytes. Bile accumulation within hepatocytes, giant cell transformation, haemosiderin deposition, dis-organization of tubercular pattern in the hepatic lobule, and increased haemopoietic activity occur in both disorders. The main histological abnormalities of diagnostic importance are given in *Table 5.1*. It is

TABLE 5.1
Histological Features of Diagnostic Value
on Percutaneous Liver Biopsy

Bile tract disorders	*Hepatocellular disease*
Enlarged portal tract	Collection of mononuclear cells in the hepatic lobules
Numerous bile ducts	Fatty changes in the hepatocytes
Distorted elongated and angulated bile ductules	Uneven staining of hepatocytes
Increased fibrosis in portal tracts	
Lymphangiectasia of portal tracts	
Infiltration of portal tract with inflammatory cells	

important that the biopsy should contain four or five portal tracts for a diagnosis to be attempted, since in hepatitis individual portal tracts may show features similar to those of atresia but portal tract involvement is not uniform. It should be stressed, too, that hepatitis associated with alpha-1 antitrypsin deficiency will give a histological appearance similar to that of biliary atresia.

In a recently completed analysis of histological data in a series of patients with obstructive jaundice in early infancy, only six per-cutaneous liver biopsies from 82 infants with hepatocellular jaundice were considered to have pathological features consistent with atresia. However, typical pathological features of atresia were found in only 15 of 20 biopsies in patients with atresia (Mowat, Pscharopoulos and Williams, 1976).

Rose Bengal faecal excretion test

A faecal excretion in 72 hours of less than 10 per cent of the injected

TABLE 5.2

Rose Bengal Excretion (R.B.E.) and Liver Biopsy in the
Investigation of Severe Idiopathic Obstructive Jaundice

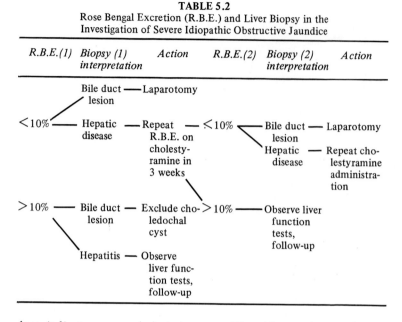

R.B.E.(1)	Biopsy (1) interpretation	Action	R.B.E.(2)	Biopsy (2) interpretation	Action

dose indicates severe cholestasis compatible with extrahepatic biliary
atresia or severe cholestasis. The results of percutaneous liver biopsy
and the Rose Bengal faecal excretion test must be considered together
with the objective of advising early laparotomy in patients with bile
duct lesions and avoiding it in hepatocellular disorders. It may be
necessary to repeat the test after 14—21 days on cholestyramine and
further biopsies may be required to assess the situation. *Table 5.2* gives
a flow diagram of the action required depending on the findings of
these investigations.

Non-invasive tests for biliary atresia

To obviate the need for such invasive and time-consuming investigations
as those referred to above in distinguishing biliary atresia from hepatitis,
a number of investigations on peripheral blood have been claimed to
be of value. A 5′nucleotidase level of less than 30 iu/litre was found
in 35 patients with idiopathic cholestasis, while 24 of 25 with E.H.B.A.
had levels above this value (Sass-Kortsak, 1974). An elevated lipoprotein X concentration which is not lowered by cholestyramine
suggests biliary atresia (Poley *et al.*, 1972). It may be unwise to rely

on such laboratory investigations, if the techniques used are not exactly the same as those described by these authors and the same range of values has been found in normal individuals. The red cell haemolysis test in the presence of perioxidase, serum alpha-fetoprotein concentrations and the ratio of dihydroxy to trihydroxy bile salts, which have been recommended as of value, often give misleading results in the first three months of life and cannot be recommended (Johnston *et al.*, 1976; Manthorpe and Mowat, 1976).

Indications for laparotomy in suspected biliary atresia

Laparotomy is indicated in any infant with persistent conjugated hyperbilirubinaemia and acholic stools in whom: (a) genetic, metabolic and infectious causes have been excluded; (b) the liver biopsy findings are compatible with extrahepatic biliary atresia, and (c) I^{131} Rose Bengal faecal excretion is less than 10 per cent in 72 hours.

With modern surgical techniques *the best results are obtained when surgery is carried out by the age of 60 days.* Suspected cases should therefore be referred as soon as possible to centres with the necessary expertise to make an early presumptive diagnosis. Early laparotomy is also indicated in choledochal cysts and in spontaneous perforation of the bile ducts.

Laparotomy should only be carried out by a surgeon with experience in assessing the condition of the bile ducts of infants at laparotomy. Infants with intrahepatic cholestasis and reduced bile flow have very narrow ducts which may be considered atretic at laparotomy by inexperienced surgeons (and even at autopsy). Cases are on record in which such ducts have been inadvertently removed at laparotomy. Laparotomy is contra-indicated in hepatocellular disorders causing conjugated hyperbilirubinaemia in this age group. It may rarely be indicated in intrahepatic biliary hypoplasia when the therapeutic benefits of the precise diagnosis justifies the risk of laparotomy.

SURGERY

The abdomen is opened using a tranverse laparotomy approach, sectioning both recti muscles, well above the level of the umbilicus at the same horizontal level as the portahepatis. The liver is usually found to be uniformly enlarged but occasionally one lobe may be more enlarged than the other. Even in early cases it feels firm on palpation, but in late cases cirrhosis will have developed. Ascities is rare. In late cases there may be features of portal hypertension.

Most commonly the gallbladder is small and firm and may be partially hidden by hypertrophy of surrounding parenchyma. In these circumstances, it is usually impossible to inject radio-opaque material through the gallbladder. In approximately 25 per cent of cases, the gall-bladder, although small, will contain approximately 1 ml of colourless material, and in these circumstances it may be possible to show a lumen in the gallbladder and common duct but the common hepatic duct is unlikely to be visualized. Further dissection is undertaken towards the portohepatis, examining particularly tissues in front of the right branch of the hepatic artery. Atretic or absent bile ducts will usually be found. In rare instances, the *surgically correctable* abnormality as demonstrated in *Figure 5.2* is found.

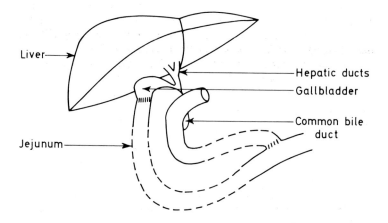

Figure 5.2. Diagrammatic representation of surgically correctable extrahepatic biliary atresia. The distal common bile duct is atretic but the common hepatic duct and main hepatic ducts are patent and are in continuity with the gallbladder via the cystic duct. A cholecystjejunostomy with a Roux-en-Y loop should give satisfactory bile drainage without cholangitis. Unfortunately, long-term cure is exceptional

In individual series of cases between 4 and 35 per cent of cases have a patent segment of extrahepatic bile duct extending into the porta-hepatitis. In these it is possible to fashion an anastomosis between the bile duct and a Roux-en-Y loop from jejunum but only a minority drain bile satisfactorily. Successful surgery is rare after the age of four months. Ascending cholangitis or lymphangitis is a frequent compli-cation. Cirrhosis gradually develops in most cases and prolonged cure is exceptional, although one patient has been reported well at the age of 12 years and another moderately well at the age of 25 years (Berenson, Garde and Moody, 1974).

Surgery of 'non-correctable' lesions

Where no extrahepatic bile duct is available for anastomosis, a wide variety of surgical techniques have been tried with little success. These have included: insertion of various prosthesis linking the liver to the bowel; drainage of lymph from the lymphatic duct to an external fistula or into the oesophagus; direct drainage of hepatic lymph to bowel by anastomosing the portahepatis to the de-peritonized serosal surface of a loop of jejunum; and diligent needling of the liver to find a loculus of bile which can be drained directly to bowel by removing the intervening part of liver.

Hepatic portoenterostomy ('Japanese' operation or Kasai procedure)

In this operation an anastomosis is fashioned between the area of the portahepatis and the bowel. Bile duct remnants or fibrous tissue in front of the right branch of the hepatic artery is carefully dissected free giving a cone of tissue with its base at the portahepatis. This cone of tissue is then cut through at the level of the porta, exposing an area

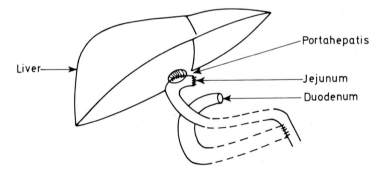

Figure 5.3. Hepatic portoenterostomy for an extrahepatic biliary atresia involving the main right and left hepatic ducts and the common hepatic duct. These have been removed and the area of the portahepatis bared. A side opening in the Roux-en-Y loop of jejunum is anastomosed to the edge of the bared area. Bile is thought to flow from the intrahepatic bile ducts into the bowel but in some patients it is suspected that lymphatic drainage into the bowel may be important

through which bile may drain. A Roux-en-Y loop, at least 20 cm in length is brought up from the jejunum. Its end is closed and a side opening near its end is carefully anastomosed around the bare area of the portahepatis, making no attempt to link bile ductules to bowel mucosa (*Figure 5.3*).

To prevent ascending cholangitis caused by contamination of the area of the portahepatis by bowel organisms, some surgeons have exteriorized the loop of jejunum draining the liver. This fistula allows easy observation of bile flow. The bile has to be reinserted into a distal loop to facilitate digestion. There is as yet no evidence that the incidence or severity of cholangitis is reduced by such fistulae. The exponents of this technique advise that it be closed some months after bile drainage is established, but other surgeons prefer to leave it for as long as two years.

Results

The most impressive results are those reported by Kasai, Watanabe and Ohi (1975). The most recent data from his unit indicates that if surgery is carried out by the age of 60 days, 80 per cent of patients will develop bile drainage, but the percentage falls to 20 per cent if surgery is delayed beyond 90 days. In most other series the percentage developing bile drainage varies from between 30 and 70 per cent.

Kasai has reported that 22 of his patients are alive and well, with normal physique five years after surgery, five being over the age of ten years, and the eldest 22 years.

Complications

The Kasai procedure is obviously one of some complexity, often taking as long as 4 hours. Assessment of the state of the bile ducts at laparotomy is obviously crucial.

In the immediate post-operative period, ileus, bowel perforation, haemorrhage, biliary leakage and wound infections are the main problems. Ascites, persisting for 2–8 weeks, may occur.

In the year following effective surgery, cholangitis occurs in up to 70 per cent of cases with bile drainage. Episodes of cholangitis are characterized by fever and a recurrence of jaundice, with a deterioration in liver function tests. The infecting organisms, Proteus, Klebsiella, *E. coli, S. faecalis* and *Candida albicans* can occasionally be identified by blood culture, but liver biopsy is often required to confirm the presence of the pathogen. Diagnosis is a problem, since during intercurrent viral infections without any direct involvement of the liver, there may be jaundice with a deterioration of liver function.

Cholangitis requires treatment with intravenous antibiotics. Gentomycin, ampicillin, and trimethoprim have been most useful in our experience but the exact antibiotic used should be determined by the culture results, and *in vitro* antibiotic sensitivity.

In spite of good bile drainage, increasing fibrosis within the liver may occur in the first two years following operation. During this time the alkaline phosphatase levels are often considerably elevated to three or four times normal. Cirrhosis may develop in such circumstances. Hepatocellular carcinoma has also been described.

Portal hypertension occurs frequently in survivors, having been found in 20 of 33 cases in one series, two of whom required oesophageal transection for haematemesis. In five out of ten anicteric patients, varices present at the time of surgery were no longer evident on endoscopic examination one year later.

Only long-term follow-up of patients will give us a better idea of prognosis. At present, however, it must be emphasized to parents of children with biliary atresia, that although the operation hepatic portoenterostomy will often give bile-stained stools, the general outlook for the majority of such children must remain guarded, even after apparently successful surgery.

MEDICAL MANAGEMENT OF BILIARY ATRESIA OR PERSISTENT CHOLESTASIS

For disorders in which specific treatment is not available or ineffective the complications listed in *Table 4.3* must be prevented or minimized.

Fat malabsorption due to diminished or absent bile flow, with poor digestion and absorption of fat because of the absence of intestinal bile salts leads to calorie malnutrition and deficiencies of fat-soluble vitamins. Substituting medium chain triglycerides for normal fat mitigates the calorie malnutrition. Fat-soluble vitamins must be given in doses sufficient to keep the prothrombin time normal and to prevent the appearance of rickets. Oral fat-soluble vitamins are given in a dose of between 2 and 4 times the recommended daily allowances but occasionally parenteral vitamins are required. Where rickets results from impaired hepatic hydroxylation of cholecalciferol, 25-OH cholecalciferol, 50 μg per day, will prevent or heal rickets. The exact dose varies a great deal from patient to patient and there is no substitute for measuring serum calcium phosphorus and prothrombin time regularly. Pruritus is a distressing consequence of bile salt retention in these children. It may be ameliorated by giving cholestyramine in the form of Questran in a dose of 4 g per day four times a day. This measure may cause folic acid deficiency and it seems prudent to give prophylactic folic acid. Where pruritus becomes intractable, norethandrolone in a dose of 1−2 mg per day may be effective in controlling it.

Details of the management of cirrhosis (page 256), portal hypertension (page 308) and fluid retention (page 261) are given elsewhere.

Childhood extrahepatic biliary atresia throws a tremendous strain on the family whether surgery is successful or not. Paediatricians have a major responsibility in doing all they can to prevent unnecessary suffering in these children by close attention to details in management. It seems important to give these families full information on the child's hepatic state and on the general prognosis for a particular child.

LIVER TRANSPLANTATION

In view of the dismal prognosis of extrahepatic biliary atresia, many parents are concerned to learn of the prospects for liver transplantation. Successful transplantation requires the availability of a suitable donor, very skilful major surgery, and a carefully monitored drug regimen to prevent immunological rejection. Only two units in the world have significant published experience of this procedure. The group in the Department of Surgery, University of Cambridge, and the Liver Unit, King's College Hospital Medical School, London, under the direction of Professor Roy Calne and Dr Roger Williams respectively, and Dr T.E. Starzl's group based in Denver, Colorado, USA. Only the last named has an on-going research programme in liver transplantation in childhood. The results are far from satisfactory, with the majority of patients dying within the first six months. Eleven of 40 children with biliary atresia survived for more than one year after transplantation, 7 only achieving normal liver function. However, improvements in surgical technique have given in this Unit, a 50 per cent chance of 1 year survival in the most recent patients.

The major problems still persisting are as follows.

(1) Donor availability: this means not only the difficulty in finding a liver of suitable size because of reluctance on the part of clinicians and parents to donate organs for transplantation, but also in finding a donor and recipient who are immunologically compatible as assessed by the H.L.A. antigen system. In practice, immunological compatibility does not seem to have been a major factor in the success of the procedure.
(2) Defective biliary reconstruction causing impaired bile flow, bile sludging and biliary leaks.
(3) Major technical problems related to the vasculature causing impaired perfusion of the donor liver due to kinking of blood vessels, thrombosis or perivascular haemorrhage.
(4) Infection: systemic, viral infection of the biliary tract and liver, septic hepatic necrosis, peribiliary infection.

(5) Immunological rejection: which in spite of the use of prednisolone, azathioprine and/or cyclophosphamide and anti-lympho-
cytic globulin still causes loss of between 1:5 and 1:10 technically
flawless transplants.

In children, particularly infants, the technical problems are greater
because of small vascular size. Paediatricians should be reminded
that in controlling immunosuppression, excluding biliary obstruction,
diagnosing and treating infection, hepatic recipients may require to
spend many many days in hospital, be subjected to many venepunctures
and repeated invasive procedures such as liver biopsy and percutaneous
cholangiography. This may seem a heavy price to inflict on a young
child or his family.

BIBLIOGRAPHY AND REFERENCES

Berenson, M.M., Garde, A.R. and Moody, F.G. (1974). Twenty-five year survival
after surgery for complete extrahepatic biliary atresia. *Gastroenterol.* 66, 260
Howard, E.R. and Mowat, A.P. (1977). Extrahepatic biliary atresia – recent
developments in management. *Archs Dis. Childh.* 52, 825
Johnston, D.I., Mowat, A.P., Orr, H. and Kohn, J. (1976). Serum alphafetoprotein levels in extrahepatic biliary atresia, idiopathic neonatal hepatitis
and alpha-1 antitrypsin deficiency (PiZ). *Acta. paediat. Scand.* 65, 623
Kasai, M., Watanabe, J. and Ohi, R. (1975). Follow-up studies of long-term
survivors after hepatic portoenterostomy for 'non-correctable' biliary atresia.
J.pediat.Surg. 10, 173
Manthorpe, D. and Mowat, A.P. (1976). Serum bile acids in the neonatal hepatic
syndrome. In *INSERM, Paris* 29, 57
Mowat, A.P., Pscharopoulos, H.T. and Williams, R. (1976). Extrahepatic biliary
atresia versus neonatal hepatitis – a review of 137 prospectively investigated
infants. *Archs Dis. Childh.* 51, 763
Poley, J.R., Smith, A.I., Booth, P.J. and Campbell, D.P. (1972). Lipoprotein X
and the double [131]I Rose Bengal test for the diagnosis of prolonged infantile
jaundice. *J. pediat. Surg.* 7, 660
Starzl, T.E., Porter, K.A., Putman, C.W., Beart, R.W., Halgrimson, C.G. and Gadir,
A.F.A. (1976). Liver replacement in children. In *Liver Diseases in Infancy
and Childhood*, p. 97. Ed. by Berenberg, S.R. The Hague: Martinus Nijhoff
Medical Division
Thomson, J. (1891). On congenital obliteration of the bile ducts. *Edinb.med.J.*
37, 523
Weber, A. and Roy, C.C. (1972). Malabsorption associated with chronic liver
disease in children. *Pediatrics* 50, 73

CHAPTER 6

Infections of the Liver

HEPATITIS

Introduction

The term hepatitis indicates an inflammation of the liver, usually associated with hepatocyte degeneration or necrosis. The cause may be infective, toxic, physical, genetically determined or cryptogenic. The course may be acute or chronic. Although it is usual to characterize the hepatitis by the aetiological factor, the wide range of clinical manifestations seen in any of the above types is determined by the severity of the alterations in hepatocyte function. At one end of the scale is an asymptomatic hepatitis in which hepatocellular necrosis is minimal and revealed only by elevation of serum enzyme such as aspartate aminotransferase, at the other end is fulminant hepatitis associated with massive hepatocellular necrosis, hepatic encephalopathy, and spontaneous haemorrhage. Hepatitis in infancy is considered in Chapter 4.

ACUTE HEPATITIS

Although the contagious nature of acute hepatitis was noted in the eighth century A.D., and a viral cause suggested as early as 1908, it has been only in the last 20 years that much progress has been made towards characterizing the agent or agents responsible. Progress in an understanding of the aetiology, pathogenesis and prevention of the most common forms of hepatitis is still severely handicapped by failure to isolate and culture the virus responsible. There is also lack of an easily available suitable experimental model for the isolation and propagation of the responsible agents.

The demonstration in 1969 that Australia antigen, now called the hepatitis B surface antigen, is associated with serum hepatitis gave a much needed stimulus to workers in this field and has produced an avalanche of reports on the antigen and its pathological and clinical effects. A marker for acute hepatitis type A proved more difficult to find. The epidemic hepatitis associated antigen described in Milan in 1970 has subsequently been considered to be a non-specific response to hepatic injury. After a series of unconfirmed reports of a virus associated with acute hepatitis type A, research workers in a number of laboratories have now shown virus-like particles in the faeces early in the illness and have in the last 4 years developed antigen antibody tests which appear to be specific for hepatitis A infection. Indeed, it is already apparent that acute hepatitis may be caused by agents other than hepatitis A or hepatitis B virus or other identified viral causes.

ACUTE VIRAL HEPATITIS TYPE A

Definition

This is an acute inflammation of the liver with varying degrees of hepatocellular necrosis caused by a viral agent – hepatitis A virus (HAV). The above term should replace the many synonyms including infectious or infective hepatitis, I.H. Botkin's disease, short incubation hepatitis, MS-1 hepatitis, and Australia antigen negative hepatitis.

Aetiology

Until 1973, type A hepatitis could be diagnosed clinically only where epidemiological evidence implicated a contagious condition acquired in circumstances in which faecal/oral transmission was possible, and in which there was no evidence of infection by hepatitis type B or other known viral cause of liver damage. In the mid-1970's a number of laboratories demonstrated by immune electronmicroscopy virus-like particles in the faeces early in the illness. A morphologically and immunologically similar antigen derived from human faeces early in the course of the illness, or from marmoset liver infected with human hepatitis A virus, has been used in the detection of antibodies to hepatitis A virus by radio-immunoassay, immune adherence haemagglutination, complement fixation and the ELIZA technique. Using the antibody, antigen can also be demonstrated by similar techniques in serum and liver. Such techniques are costly; the marmoset source is restricted and as yet is only available in a few research centres. Antigen from stools of infected chimpanzees may prove a more useful source.

Current research indicates that the hepatitis A virus is a RNA virus. The morphological and immunological similarity of various classes of particles referred to as hepatitis A antigen, the world-wide consistency of the epidemiology of the condition, and the passive protection afforded by gammaglobulin, obtained in one geographical location but used in other parts of the world, suggests that hepatitis A is caused

Age distribution of IA antibody to HAV

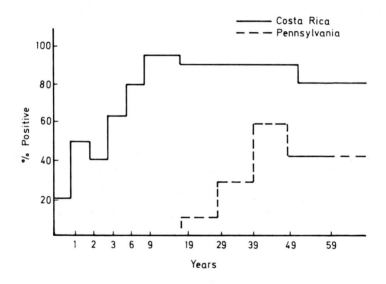

Figure 6.1. Percentage of the population at different ages with hepatitis A immune adherent antibody in the open community in Costa Rica and Pennsylvania (from the data of Villarejos et al. (1976) Proc. Soc. exp. Med. Biol. 152, 524)

by a single viral agent. It may be inactivated by boiling, by radiation with ultraviolet light or by formalin. It has been found in the stools five days before liver damage can be detected by a rise in serum transaminases, but is usually not recoverable by the time the transaminase level is at its peak. Complement fixing antibody titre rises rapidly in the presence of jaundice, but the antibody demonstrated by immune adherence rises more slowly. Both types of antibody may be detected for up to ten years after infection.

Epidemiology

The widespread application of such techniques will give further understanding of the epidemiology of the condition, but preliminary work indicates that in areas where sanitary conditions are poor, and hepatitis is endemic, infection is acquired early in life (*Figure 6.1*). Where standards of hygiene are high, a large pool of susceptible adults exist. The incidence of antibodies in adults in North America is highest in those of lower socio-economic groups. Antibody studies in family epidemics of hepatitis A confirm that approximately 50 per cent of cases are very mild and sub-clinical.

Infection is almost always spread by the faecal/oral route, fingers and feeding utensils contaminated by faeces being the usual mode of spread. The blood and urine are also infective early in the course.

Prior to the development of serological methods of diagnosis, the frequency data related to clinical cases. In less developed countries the maximum incidence appears to be in childhood. Infection seems to spread where there is close family contacts rather than in normal day schools. Epidemics, however, occur in boarding schools and other areas where large numbers are living in close proximity. Sewage-contaminated water and shellfish are responsible for some outbreaks. Chlorination of water is not sufficient to kill the organism.

Pathology

Liver cell damage or necrosis, and inflammatory cell infiltrate in the hepatic parenchyma and portal tracts, with or without bile pigment retention, are the hallmarks of hepatitis. Liver damage occurs throughout the liver in all lobules, but to varying extents and is often most marked in the centralobular areas. Damage may take the form of liver cell swelling with a granular cytoplasm (ballooning degeneration), shrinkage of liver cells (giving a deeply stained cytoplasm), or loss of cells, best appreciated as an irregular collapse of the reticulum network. Such necrosis may be focal, affect groups of liver cells, or confluent. The inflammatory cell infiltrate, both in the parenchyma and portal tracts, is mainly of mononuclear cells but scanty polymorphonuclear neutrophil leucocytes are common. The inflammatory cell infiltrate of the portal tract may extend a little distance into the hepatic parenchyma.

The rate of progression of the pathological changes is very variable. After some weeks or months, features of acute hepatocyte injury regress; but the reticulo-endothelial cellular reaction persists, sometimes with apparent increase in the reaction in the portal tracts. Clumps of cells containing PAS-positive, acid-fast, ceroid pigment and stainable iron are characteristic of this stage. Such changes may persist for many months but healing is eventually complete in most instances.

Variations from this sequence of pathological changes may include the following;

(1) A period of persistent cholestasis.
(2) A period of improvement with a recurrence of cholestasis both proceeding to eventual complete recovery.
(3) A rapid progression to acute fulminant necrosis with hepatic encephalopathy.
(4) Sub-acute hepatic necrosis.
(5) Chronic aggressive hepatitis.

In the last two instances, cirrhosis commonly develops. Following recovery from acute fulminant hepatitis the liver may return to normal.

As well as these intrahepatic changes, a generalized lymph gland enlargement, splenomegaly due to cellular infiltration and inflammatory lesions of the duodenum and kidney are commonly found. Myocarditis, pancreatitis, and aplastic anaemia are rare complications.

Clinical features

The incubation period is from 3 to 40 days. The severity of disease may vary from an asymptomatic sub-clinical infection to rapidly fatal hepatitis; typically the course may be divided into two phases as follows.

The *pre-icteric* phase is characterized by anorexia, nausea, vomiting, lassitude and sometimes intermittent dull abdominal pain felt in the epigastrium or right hypochondrium. There may be fever and headache, particularly in older children. In young infants the stools may be loose, and failure to gain weight is common. Clinical examination may reveal tender hepatomegaly, also splenomegaly and lymph gland enlargement. It is suspected that in many affected children no specific features develop and the disease regresses at this stage.

When jaundice appears at the *icteric phase* there is often a regression of all symptoms and a return of appetite, particularly in young children. In older children, as in adults, there is commonly an exacerbation of the original symptoms with, in some cases, depression and pruritus. The liver is usually enlarged and tender, and the spleen is palpable in 20–30 per cent of cases. The urine is dark because of its bilirubin content, and stools may be pale in up to 30 per cent of cases with significant cholestasis. Jaundice may persist for only a few days but usually fades in the second week. Rarely it may persist for months. Complete recovery is the rule.

Laboratory findings

Serum transaminase levels are elevated from three to four days before the onset of jaundice, returning to normal typically in two—three weeks. The serum bilirubin level rises when the transaminase concentration is already at its peak, which is usually somewhere between 400 and 800 iu/litre, but occasionally will exceed 1,000 iu/litre. Serum alkaline phosphatase levels are rarely more than 50 per cent of the normal value. Further elevation may occur in association with marked cholestasis but should raise the suspicion of extrahepatic bile duct disease. The serum IgM rises at the same time as jaundice develops. A mild leucocytosis may be found in the incubation period often to be followed by leucopaenia and lymphopaenia, often with a few atypical lymphocytes. Haemolysis may occur in patients with glucose-6-phosphate dehydrogenase deficiency but much haemolysis should raise suspicion of co-existing Wilson's disease.

Complications

The following is a list of the complications associated with acute hepatitis.

Fulminant hepatitis
Sub-acute hepatitis
Chronic persistent hepatitis
Chronic active hepatitis
Post-hepatitic cirrhosis

Post-hepatic syndrome
Post-hepatitis hyperbilirubinaemia
Bone marrow aplasia
Pancreatitis
Myocarditis

Cirrhosis (*see* page 246), chronic persistent and active hepatitis (*see* page 215) occur rarely and are considered in detail elsewhere. The most serious is fulminant hepatic failure with massive hepatocellular necrosis (*see* page 126). Atypical features in the course of the hepatitis, which should alert the clinician to the possibility of fulminant hepatitis, are also listed below.

Persistent anorexia
Progressively deepening jaundice
Reappearance of initial features
Reduction of liver size
Ascites
Prolongation of prothrombin time

Low serum albumin concentration
Serum transaminase of greater than
    1,000 iu/litre
Hypoglycaemia
Respiratory alkalosis
Neuro-psychiatric changes

Sub-acute hepatitis

Sub-acute hepatitis is a poorly defined condition. The term is usually used to refer to patients who have presented with a clinically mild hepatitis but in whom recovery is delayed. There is persistent malaise, anorexia, fluctuant jaundice and hepatomegaly which ultimately proceeds to hepatocellular failure with encephalopathy but after a period of more than 8 weeks from the onset. Pathologically there is confluent hepatic necrosis with inflammatory and fibrotic infiltrate joining neighbouring portal tracts and/or hepatic veins. There may be areas of regeneration. The patient may die of hepatocellular failure, alimentary bleeding or bacterial infection. If recovery occurs, cirrhosis is usual.

Prolonged cholestasis

Prolonged cholestasis with conjugated hyperbilirubinaemia when the serum transaminase has fallen towards normal occurs with a frequency which varies from one epidemic to another. Pruritus may be marked. Recovery is complete but differential diagnosis from extrahepatic jaundice causes considerable difficulty. In some instances it may be necessary to proceed to ultrasonic echography of the biliary system or cholangiography (percutaneous or retrograde).

Post-hepatitis syndrome

The post-hepatitis syndrome is characterized by malaise, anorexia with fat intolerance, right upper abdominal discomfort, failure to gain weight, normal liver function tests and a biopsy showing features of the resolving hepatitis. It is rare in the young child but may be seen in the adolescent. After appropriate investigations the patient and the relatives must be reassured about the excellent prognosis.

Post-hepatitic unconjugated hyperbilirubinaemia

This is a rare condition indistinguishable from Gilbert's syndrome (*see* page 29) and may in fact be instances of Gilbert's syndrome brought to light by an acute hepatitis.

Differential diagnosis

In the absence of a readily available test for the laboratory diagnosis of acute type A hepatitis, diagnosis is made on the basis of the clinical features. A history of exposure to a similarly infected individual is most helpful. Recent travel to areas of high incidence of hepatitis raises suspicion of the diagnosis, as does exposure of drinking water of dubious purity or of eating certain shellfish such as mussels or clams. The principal differential diagnosis is from hepatitis type B, but it is important to exclude chronic active hepatitis which should be suspected if the immunoglobulins are raised, the serum albumin is lowered or the prothrombin time prolonged. Drugs, toxins and metabolic disorders, particularly Wilson's disease (*see* page 233) must be considered in any sporadic or isolated case of hepatitis. The possible presence of these treatable disorders must also be considered and excluded in any patient in whom recovery is delayed or the course is atypical.

Management

There is no specific treatment: most patients are adequately cared for at home. It is important, therefore, to outline the probable course of the illness to parents so that they may be alerted to any atypical features heralding the onset of complications. Minimal investigations listed below are necessary to determine the severity of the hepatitis and to exclude other aetiological causes.

Serum bilirubin, total and direct reacting	Full blood count, including reticulocyte count
Serum transaminase	Hepatitis B surface antigen
Serum alkaline phosphatase	Caeruloplasmin
Prothrombin time	Paul Bunnell test
Serum albumin	Cytomegalovirus antibody
Serum immunoglobulins	

It should be stressed that this is a generalized disease. The ill child or teenager will usually elect to go to bed but will gradually increase activity as the disease regresses. There is no evidence that enforced, absolute or partial bed-rest has any bearing on the rate of healing of the liver or that strenuous activity increases the duration of the illness. The patient should be encouraged to choose his own diet, trying to maintain a protein intake of 1 g/kg per day with 4 g of carbohydrate/ kg in the same period. Many patients learn to avoid fats since this intensifies nausea, but when this settles, fat should be taken normally; indeed, one study suggests that healing occurred more quickly when the fat intake was high. Vitamin supplements have not been shown to be beneficial. Anti-emetic drugs such as metoclopramide may be necessary, but it is important to limit the dosage of any drug metabolized by the liver otherwise side-effects, such as dystonic reactions, may appear. Corticosteroids have no place in management. The controlled study which showed that cyanidonal was of value included no children (Blum *et al.*, 1977). To confirm that resolution is complete, liver function tests should be repeated three months after the onset of the jaundice.

Prevention

It has to be appreciated that the virus may be excreted in the stools for at least two weeks before the onset of the jaundice and possibly for as long as one week after its onset. There are likely to be many sub-clinical cases. Measures to block possible faecal/oral spread from recognized cases, however, must be undertaken. These include:

(1) Scrupulous hand-washing before meals and after defaecation.
(2) Sterilization of food utensils.
(3) Steps to prevent faecal contamination of food, milk and water supplies.
(4) Exclusion of potentially affected food handlers from food distribution or kitchens.

Gammaglobulin given intramuscularly is of great value, particularly if given early in the incubation period, but it is helpful at any time before the onset of the disease. Since there are no measures which modify established disease, it is recommended for family contacts and for use in institutions in which hygienic standards are difficult to apply. Its protective action wanes after four months and disappears after six or seven months. In areas of high risk, six-monthly injections are recommended. A dose of 200 mg of human normal immunoglubulin injections (BP) should be given to children of up to the age of ten years, and 500 mg to those aged eleven years or older.

ACUTE VIRAL HEPATITIS TYPE B

Definition

This is an acute inflammation of the liver with hepatocellular necrosis caused by a viral agent, hepatitis B virus. The term replaces serum hepatitis, haemolysis serum jaundice, innoculation hepatitis, post-transfusion hepatitis, long incubation hepatitis, MS2 hepatitis, Australia antigen positive hepatitis.

Aetiology

Hepatitis B virus (HBV) is a DNA virus which is host and organ specific, having been found to date only in infected hepatocytes of man and a few primate species. As yet, no *in vitro* system of propagation of HBV has been discovered. The discovery in 1965 of Australia antigen, now termed the hepatitis B surface antigen (HBsAg), its subsequent association with hepatitis B virus infection in 1969, and the development of sensitive specific measures for its detection has made it possible to gain a great deal of information about hepatitis B virus, its epidemiology and clinico-pathological consequences. The presumed infective form of HBV is a 40–42 nm particle known as the Dane particle, which consists of an inner nucleocapsid core, termed the hepatitis B core antigen (HBcAg), and an outer lipoprotein coat composed of hepatitis B surface antigen. The respective antibodies for the two components for HBV are anti-HBc and anti-HBs. Four major virus-determined subtypes of hepatitis B surface antigen termed adw, ayw, adr, and ayr, which breed true in infected people and experimental animals, have also been identified. Simultaneous infections with these can occur. No clinico-pathological correlates of these viral sub-types have been determined but they are useful epidemiological markers. In serum two additional indicators of HBV infection are HBV specific DNA polymerase and the 'e' antigen, present in sera containing large numbers of Dane particles. Although linked with HBV infection, e antigen is not related to the HBsAg or the HBcAg. It may be an additional antigen on the surface of the Dane particle or an unrelated protein manufactured by the host in response to HBV. Hepatitis B virus components are listed in *Table 6.1*.

The full significance of these two markers will probably have to await the development of more sensitive methods of detection and perhaps the availability of a more easily accessible experimental model. Much of the work in humans related to these two antigens has been done in patients with chronic disease. In such patients the core can be seen in the nucleus of the hepatocytes where DNA replication or multiplication of the viral genome occurs. The protein coat of hepatitis B surface antigen appears to be synthesized in the endoplasmic reticulum of infected hepatocytes. The complete virion is formed when the core leaves the nucleus and becomes surrounded by its protein coat. How it migrates to the plasma membrane and into the tissue fluid and bloodstream as a Dane particle is not known.

In acute hepatitis, the Dane particle, the DNA polymerase and the hepatitis B surface antigen appear in the serum one to two weeks before the illness commences. The e antigen may also be found transiently in serum at this time. Hepatitis B core antigen has not, however, been

TABLE 6.1
Hepatitis B Virus Terminology and Abbreviations

HBV	Hepatitis B virus
Dane particle	A 42nm particle including HBsAg and HBcAg, considered to be the complete DNA virion
HBsAg	Hepatitis B surface antigen found in the Dane particle, as 20nm rods and 42nm spheres in serum, and in infected hepatocytes
HBcAg	Hepatitis B core antigen found in Dane particles and in nuclei of infected hepatocytes
HBV specific DNA polymerase	DNA in the core of Dane particles
Anti-HBs	Antibody to HBsAg
Anti-HBc	Antibody to HBcAg
'e' antigen	Antigen found in some sera which contain hepatitis B surface antigen, (HBsAg) and in the nuclei of infected hepatocytes
Anti-e	Antibody to 'e' antigen
S antigen	Antigen found in nuclei of infected hepatocytes
Anti-S	Antibody to S antigen: found in sera of HBsAg carriers with liver damage

seen in the serum. Fluorescent antibody studies indicate that, in the pre-necrotic stage of disease, the hepatitis B surface antigen is present in all hepatocytes near or on the sinusoidal membrane. There its presence produces cellular and humoral immune responses, the outcome of which determines whether the cell dies, is damaged, retains the virus and its products, or harbours the viral core in its nucleus. At present it is uncertain whether the immune responses are directed against the virus or viral products on the plasma membrane, against altered plasma membrane, or against liver specific cell surface lipoprotein. Where hepatocellular necrosis occurs the antigen-containing cells are eliminated. What determines the outcome of the viral host interaction is at present the subject of much research.

A number of studies in children suggest that if they are infected with the hepatitis B virus other than by injection, they are liable to become chronic carriers with little or no necrosis. While such children produce large amounts of hepatitis B surface antigen, they tend to have few Dane particles in the serum and are thus rarely highly infectious, their blood being infectious in transfusion amounts only. It seems that some children go on to develop chronic hepatitis because they fail to eliminate completely the cells which are programmed to produce hepatitis B surface antigen, often without any evidence of the core antigen in the nuclei.

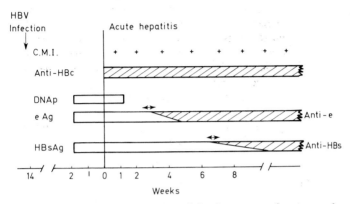

Figure 6.2. Diagrammatic representation of the time course of antigen and antibody changes in peripheral blood following exposure to the hepatitis B virus (HBV). HBsAg, 'e' Ag and HBV specific DNA polymerase (DNAp) are detectable in the blood before there is any biochemical evidence of hepatocellular damage. The concentration of these antigens often falls before there is clinical hepatitis. Anti-HBc appears early in the disease but the timing of the appearance of anti-e and anti-HBs is variable. Both antigen and antibody can be detected at the same time. The duration of detectable antibody following acute infection is uncertain but current evidence suggests that anti-HBc is the most long lasting

A stylized diagram of the time course of the appearance of hepatitis B surface antigen, its antibody and the other antibodies mentioned is presented in *Figure 6.2.*

Carriers of hepatitis B surface antigen

In Western Europe, the United States of America and Australia, approximately 0.6 per cent of the population are asymptomatic carriers of hepatitis B surface antigen; but in the Mediterranean basin tropical Africa, South East Asia, and parts of the Far East, the incidence of carriers varies from 3 to 10 per cent of the total population. The carrier state may last for a few years or for the whole lifetime of the individual. The host-related factors which predispose to persistent hepatitis

B surface antigen carrier state are poorly understood, but they seem to include infection at an early age, mild or anicteric infection, and a depressed immune response because of age, Down's syndrome, underlying disease or immunosuppressive therapy.

It is estimated that between 1 and 4 per cent of adults in North America infected by hepatitis B virus become chronic carriers and the carrier state incidence in infants and children infected is between 30 and 40 per cent. Some carriers have relatively normal livers and low infectivity. The hepatitis B surface antigen carrier who also has the e antigen in the serum is not only more likely to have Dane particles and be very infective, but also to have progressive liver disease. The presence of e antigen in the sera of hepatitis B surface antigen-positive mothers in pregnancy is associated with a very high risk of hepatitis B virus infection in their infants. The chronic carrier does not appear to be able to produce sufficient amounts of antibody to hepatitis B surface antigen and those who are developing progressive liver disease also fail to produce antibody to the e antigen.

Epidemiology

The application of tests for hepatitis B surface antigen and its antibody have given an important and surprising insight to the epidemiology of hepatitis B virus infection. It is now clear that therapeutic transfusion or injection of blood products is a relatively uncommon mode of transmission. The major sources of infection are chronic carriers of hepatitis B surface antigen and patients with acute hepatitis which may be asymptomatic. Person-to-person spread by close contact is now well documented. Hepatitis B surface antigen has been detected in many body fluids including urine, saliva, tears, sweat, breast milk and semen. Blood-sucking arthropods may play a role in the spread of disease.

Hepatitis B virus infection in infancy is most likely to be acquired from a mother who has had hepatitis B surface antigen-positive acute hepatitis in the last three months of pregnancy or in the puerperium, or who is an e antigen-positive carrier of the hepatitis B surface antigen. Infection in the neonate may cause a sub-clinical infection, an acute hepatitis followed by recovery, or go on to cirrhosis or even acute fulminant hepatitis. Hepatitis B in late infancy or childhood, is distinctly rare in North Western Europe and North America when compared with the frequency in adults. When it is seen it occurs usually in a family epidemic where an adult relative has a hepatitis B virus infection. Other sources are patients on renal dialysis or drug addicts. It occurs also in up to 40 per cent of institutionalized children in North

America, particularly those with Down's syndrome. Haemophiliacs who have received infusions of anti-haemophylic globulins (Factor VIII) as cryoprecipitate are at particular risk, perhaps because this concentrates antigen a great deal. With the screening of all donor blood, blood transfusion is now a rare cause.

In some Mediterranean countries infection in early childhood causes a specific papular acrodermatitis and generalized lymph gland enlargement with hepatitis of very varying severity. This has not been reported in adults. Where the incidence of hepatitis B surface antigen carriers in adults is high, acquired hepatitis B antigen infection does occur relatively frequently in childhood. The disease is likely to be clinically evident in only about 50 per cent of cases. Such infection seems to be particularly frequent in India.

Pathology

The pathological responses in type B hepatitis are similar to those in viral hepatitis type A, with the exception that the patient may fail to clear the virus from the hepatocytes and become a chronic carrier. Such carriers may have normal hepatic histology, chronic persistent hepatitis, chronic aggressive hepatitis, cirrhosis or may go on to develop hepatocellular carcinoma in adult life.

Clinical features

The incubation period varies from a few weeks to 5 months but is often around 120 days. Many patients are asymptomatic. Urticaria, arthralgia and abdominal pain may occur in the prodromal phase, to be followed by hepatitis; this is clinically and biochemically indistinguishable from viral hepatitis Type A, except that the illness may last longer and long-term sequelae or complications are more commonly recognized. The diagnosis is confirmed by the finding of hepatitis B surface antigen or antibody in the peripheral blood. The management of hepatitis B viral infection is similar to that of hepatitis A infection except that the clinical and laboratory staff must be alerted promptly to the persistent risk of blood-borne infection. In adults the flavonoid, (+)-cynidanol-3, accelerates the rate of disappearance of HBsAg from the blood, a fall in serum bilirubin and relief of nausea, anorexia and pruritis (Blum et al., 1977).

Prevention

All blood for transfusion in whole or part must be screened by the most sensitive tests available and, if positive, rejected. Blood or blood products should be used only when necessary. The infectivity of human anti-haemophilic globulin (Factor VIII) has been emphasized since the preparation of this product concentrates the hepatitis B antigen. All equipment coming into contact with blood must be destroyed or thoroughly cleansed and sterilized by heat, that is, by boiling for at least 10 min, autoclaving at 15 lb or dry-heat sterilization at 170°C for 30 minutes.

Since oral infection can occur, scrupulous hand-washing is necessary.

Patients at high risk of infection, such as those requiring long-term renal dialysis, should have their serum checked regularly for antigen-aemia and, if positive, separate facilities provided for their care. This mode of management has virtually abolished hepatitis B surface antigen infection in renal dialysis units in the United Kingdom.

Gammaglobulin with high concentration of antibody to hepatitis B surface antigen has been used to try to minimize the risk of infection following accidental innoculation and to protect individuals working in areas of high risk, such as renal dialysis units, and those caring for patients who carry the antigen. The evidence that such protection is effective is still not yet convincing. Standard human gammaglobulin is ineffective.

Preliminary reports of active immunization with heat-treated and formalin-treated preparations of hepatitis B surface antigen, in experimental animals and in man, are encouraging both in the serological response and in the apparent protection afforded to patients at high risk of infection. Further studies are required, however, before these can be made generally available.

VIRAL HEPATITIS NOT IDENTIFIABLE AS A OR B

The documentation of up to four attacks of acute hepatitis in single individuals and the failure to find evidence of infection with hepatitis A or hepatitis B virus in all instances, particularly in hepatitis following blood transfusion, raises the possibility that there may be other hepatitis viruses as yet unidentified. Hepatitis in these circumstances seems to be as variable in severity as in classical type A or B. Management is similar. The incubation period tends to be similar in duration to acute viral hepatitis type B. Viral hepatitis not identifiable as A or B is principally a problem following blood transfusion. There is some epidemiological evidence that such hepatitis in patients receiving massive blood transfusion may be prevented by gammaglobulin administration immediately following transfusion.

HEPATITIS ASSOCIATED WITH SYSTEMIC VIRUS OR VIRUS-LIKE ILLNESSES

In the disorders listed below the predominant clinical manifestations are those of a systemic infection with particular features related to the aetiology. There may be focal or diffuse hepatic involvement.

Yellow fever	Coxsackie virus
Infectious mononucleosis	Arena virus
Cytomegalovirus infection	Reovirus
Human herpes virus 1	Psittacosis
Mumps	Toxoplasmosis
Adenovirus	

Jaundice is rare, although the serum bilirubin is often marginally raised and there is moderate elevation of the serum transaminases. Only the hepatitis complicating cytomegalovirus infection, infectious mononucleosis and yellow fever will be considered in detail.

YELLOW FEVER HEPATITIS

Hepatitis may occur as part of the generalized illness caused by the Group 4 arbovirus (*Flavivirus febricus*). The infection is transmitted in enzootic areas in Africa and South America by the mosquito. Infection is endemic but, rarely, epidemics may occur. The incubation period is four to six days. The disease varies in severity from a subclinical infection to a fatal illness: 5–10 per cent of cases die.

Pathology

The characteristic hepatic lesion is a diffuse severe necrosis of hepatocytes in mid-zone of the hepatic lobule with little inflammatory change. Occasionally, the hepatic necrosis may be diffuse. Some fatty change may occur in the hepatocytes. The connective tissue does not proliferate and no permanent scarring occurs if the patient recovers. Similar changes in the myocardium and renal tubules are equally important clinically.

Clinical aspects

Jaundice appears on the fourth to fifth day of the illness. The liver is tender but not enlarged. Splenomegaly is unusual. In the malignant form, haemorrhagic diathesis occurs.

The diagnosis may be suspected on the basis of prolonged fever with a slowing of the pulse rate due to cardiac involvement, albuminuria, and hepatitic features in the absence of hepatosplenomegaly. Leptospirosis is the main differential diagnosis. Confirmation may be made by antibody tests (complement fixation test and haemagglutination test) or by the intracerebral innoculation of monkeys or mice.

There is no specific treatment. Supportive care, correction of hypotension, and conservative management of renal failure may be required.

From the age of six months the disease may be prevented by vaccination which provides protection for at least ten years. With currently available vaccine reactions are rare, but allergy to egg is a contraindication to their use.

INFECTIOUS MONONUCLEOSIS HEPATITIS

This disorder, typically seen in adolescents and young adults is caused by the human herpes virus IV, (Epstein—Barr virus). The incubation period is 30—40 days. It leads to a generalized disturbance of the reticulo-endothelial system with enlargement of lymph nodes, pharyngeal lymphatic tissue, splenomegaly (75 per cent), palatal enanthema (50 per cent), peri-orbital oedema (30 per cent) and a variable exanthem. Pneumonitis and central nervous involvement with benign aseptic meningitis, encephalitis, or infectious polyneuritis, may also occur. The temperature may rise to 39°C and settle by lysis over a variable period usually averaging six days. In severe cases, however, it is not unusual for the temperature to rise to 40—41°C and to remain at this level for more than two weeks.

Hepatic features

Hepatic involvement with inflammation and necrosis as evidenced by raised serum transaminase levels, occurs in over 90 per cent of cases. Histologically there is dense accumulation of large mononuclear cells in and around the portal tracts and within the hepatic parenchyma. The Kuppfer cells are large and numerous. There are foci of liver cell necrosis but these are less diffuse than in viral hepatitis. Cholestasis is absent or slight. Recovery is associated with conspicuous mitotic activity in the hepatocytes, sometimes taking as long as eight months to resolve.

The clinical course is often mild with minimal hepatic enlargement and tenderness, although occasionally this may be severe. Jaundice occurs in 5—15 per cent of cases. Prolonged severe jaundice and even fatal hepatocellular necrosis has been recorded.

Diagnosis

The diagnosis is made by finding atypical lymphocytes in the peripheral blood, a positive heterophil antibody test (Paul—Bunnell), or by a specific antibody test for EB virus. Where hepatic features are prominent, cytomegalovirus infection and acute hepatitis types A and B are the main differential diagnosis.

Treatment

There is no specific treatment for this self-limiting disease. In severe cases, however, the administration of corticosteroids has a dramatic effect in reducing the size of the hypertrophied lymphoid tissue and should be used in instances of severe hepatitis. In the mild case they are not indicated.

CYTOMEGALOVIRUS (HUMAN HERPES VIRUS, TYPE V)

Infection may cause hepatonecrosis and inflammation. The outstanding pathological change observed in all forms of the disease are the pathognomonic greatly enlarged cells. Such changes occur primarily in epithelial cells, for example, in the cells lining the small bile ductules. There may also be a parenchymal reaction in the liver.

Clinical features

In infants symptomatic infection is most commonly associated with generalized multi-system disorder acquired *in utero*. In older children and adolescents symptoms resembling mild acute viral hepatitis or infectious mononucleosis may occur but often infection is asymptomatic or results in only a mild non-specific febrile illness. Jaundice is unusual, but more frequently elevation of serum transaminases can be recorded.

Symptomatic disease is most commonly associated with the administration of immuno-suppressive or cytotoxic drugs, or following major cardiovascular surgery with cardiopulmonary by-pass techniques.

Diagnosis of cytomegalovirus infection is established by the isolation of the virus from the urine, blood or liver, or by antibody tests showing serum conversion and/or by the presence of IgM antibody to cytomegalovirus. It should be noted, however, that cytomegalovirus may cause a chronic viraemia or viruria and that it may be provoked from latency by immuno-suppressive drugs and debilitating illness. Some caution is necessary, therefore, in assuming an aetiological relationship between clinical features and the recovery of the virus from the urine or blood.

JAUNDICE DURING OTHER SYSTEMIC INFECTIONS

Hepatomegaly, jaundice and impaired hepatic function with abnormal liver function tests may occur during the course of many other infections, but usually the hepatic features are of minor clinical importance. The mechanism of hepatocellular injury is probably complex, it ranges from direct tissue invasion to damage by exotoxins. Haemolysis may add to the jaundice.

Pathological features range from marked hyperplasia of the reticuloendothelial system through hepatocellular damage which may only be manifest on electronmicroscopy, to portal tract infiltration or features of bile duct obstruction. The possible causes include viral agents such as Coxsackie virus, arbovirus, rickettsia; bacteria such as *S.typhi*, *E.coli*, pneumococci, tuberculosis; protozoa, for example malaria, leishmaniasis, toxoplasmosis; and helminths, such as Trichinella, Toxocara, and Ascaris. The last may cause biliary obstruction by lodging in the common bile duct.

Treatment is that of the underlying disease. Rarely, specific supportive measures may be necessary if there is marked hepatocellular damage. Parasites in the biliary tree require surgical removal.

PYOGENIC ABSCESS OF THE LIVER

Abscess formation within the liver is fortunately rare in children. When they occur, they may be single or multiple.

Aetiology

Abscesses may occur as a complication of generalized septicaemia, particularly in children with depressed immunity. These are often children with serious underlying disease, such as leukaemia, who are also receiving immuno-suppressive drugs. In some instances, defective leucocyte function (chronic granulomatous disease) or dysgammaglobulinaemia are predisposing factors. Intra-abdominal sepsis, such as peritonitis following perforated appendicitis, are now rarely complicated by hepatic abscess formation presumably because of improved surgical techniques and the effective use of antibiotics. Abscess formation still occurs following suppurative cholangitis, penetrating injuries of the liver and direct extension of infection from neighbouring organs.

The infecting organisms include Staphylococcus, Streptococcus (aerobic and anaerobic), *E.coli*, Klebsiella, and Enterobacteriaceae species, *Pseudomonas aeruginosa* and Proteus. In some parts of the world *Salmonella typhi* are frequently responsible. Mixed infections also occur. Actinomyces, Nocardia and *Candida albicans* are also occasional causes.

Pathology

Abscesses may be large, single and well encapsulated with fibrous tissue. If multiple, they are usually closely related to the portal tracts. They cause disintegration of the surrounding hepatic structures and are associated with a marked polymorphonuclear leucocyte infiltration. Where infection has occurred via the bile ducts the lesions are concentrated around the bile tracts. The majority of abscesses arising from intra-abdominal causes or from septicaemia are in the right lobe of the liver.

Clinical features

The initial clinical features are often very non-specific such as malaise, nausea, weight-loss, fever, and vague upper abdominal discomfort. A previous history of intra-abdominal sepsis, trauma to the abdomen or surgery to the biliary tree, should raise suspicion of the diagnosis. Unfortunately, many cases are still first diagnosed at autopsy.

Hepatomegaly with tenderness on deep palpation is the most useful clinical sign. Tenderness may be difficult to ascertain in young children. Mild jaundice, pallor, features of recent weight-loss and decreased range of respiratory movements are occasionally noted.

Laboratory investigations

Standard tests of liver function are relatively unhelpful. In some instances, the serum bilirubin is raised, the albumin depressed and the alkaline phosphatase raised. A high vitamin B_{12} is said to be a useful indicator of liver abscess. Unfortunately, it is not an investigation that is frequently carried out unless this disorder is suspected. The white cell count may be raised with an increased proportion of polymorphonuclear neutrophil leucocytes but this is not invariable. The most helpful investigations are liver scanning and angiography. A liver scan using technetium 99 will show a filling defect if the lesion is more than 2 cm in diameter. A gamma scan using gallium may show the abscess as an area of increased uptake of radioisotope. Ultrasonic scan of the liver may be helpful in that it can show a fluid-filled cavity. Hepatic arteriography is the most helpful investigation showing a relatively avascular area around which the blood vessels are stretched. The abnormality may be most obvious in the sinusoidal phase of the study.

Treatment

Once an abscess has been localized to the liver, it must be drained surgically. Many patients, however, in a 'poor' general condition require transfusion of blood, plasma or albumin before surgery can be undertaken. Broad spectrum antibiotic therapy in high doses is given intravenously. Full radiological investigation should proceed surgery. At laparotomy the liver is needled and pus aspirated for culture. The antibiotic therapy may have to be modified following the completion of these studies.

If the lesion is single, drainage via an extraperitoneal route is advised. A drainage tube is left in the abscess cavity to promote free drainage and to allow irrigation. If the lesions are multiple but localized to one part of the liver, partial or complete lobectomy may be required. If there are abscesses throughout the liver, effective surgical drainage is rarely possible.

LEPTOSPIROSIS

Leptospirosis is an acute infectious disease of very varying severity caused by any one of many serological types of Leptospira, for example, *L.icterohaemorhagiae* (Weil's disease), *L.canicola* (canicola fever), *L.autumnalis* (pre-tibial fever).

Epidemiology

Rats, cattle, household pets such as dogs and hamsters, and many wild animals, reptiles and birds are the sources of the disease. Excreta, particularly urine, are infected. Leptospiral spirochaetes can survive for a long period outside their animal vectors, so infection can occur without direct contact. Infection is transmitted to humans in food, drinking and bathing water. Only a minority of cases occurs now in adults in occupations previously considered high risks for leptospirosis. Children, students and housewives are more frequently infected.

Pathology

Leptospirosis is characterized by an extensive vasculitis affecting small blood vessels in the skin, myocardium, kidney, brain and liver. The hepatic changes are those of a mild and diffuse hepatitis with portal infiltration, but little evidence of hepatocellular necrosis. Acalculous cholecystitis and pancreatitis may also occur.

Clinical features

Contrary to earlier reports, the course of the disease is not related to the leptospira serotype. Many infections are asymptomatic. Others cause biphasic illnesses which are self-limited and are not unlike many other viral or bacterial illnesses. Only 10 per cent of recognized cases are icteric. The overt disease is characterized by any or all of the following.

After an incubation period of 3–21 days there is an abrupt onset of fever, muscular pains, headache and vomiting. A maculo-papular petechial or purpuric rash, may develop. Albuminuria with casts, red and white cells and uraemia may occur because of renal involvement. Pneumonitis and myocarditis may be evident. An aseptic meningitis may be found.

In the second week of the illness, these features may settle but in some cases damage to the myocardium, kidneys or liver becomes more marked. Death may occur due to renal failure, or arrhythmia.

Laboratory findings

Laboratory tests reflect the degree of organ involvement. Leptospira can be recovered in the blood or cerebrospinal fluid in the first ten days of the illness and in the urine from the 7th to 30th day. The diagnosis may be by leptospira antibody tests using a complement fixation technique. A rising antibody titre can usually be demonstrated although this can be suppressed by therapy.

Treatment

If given early during the infection, penicillin appears to be effective in limiting the development of the disease. Supportive therapy will be required for congestive heart failure, renal failure or hepatic failure. If the vasculitis causes gangrene, amputation may be required.

HEPATIC AMOEBIASIS

The protozoal parasite *Entamoeba histolytica* causes liver damage when it is carried to the liver in the portal venous system from ulcerative lesions in the colon.

The amoebae multiply and block small intrahepatic portal vein branches causing focal necrosis and lysis of liver tissue. The necrotic areas vary in size from a few millimetres up to 10cm in diameter. The large ones contain thick, red-brown liquid. The lesions are focal, not generalized. Surrounding liver tissue is normal. The lesions heal with some scar formation but cirrhosis does not develop.

Epidemiology

Although the amoebae have a world-wide distribution, the disease appears to occur principally in the tropics and sub-tropics. The reasons for this are at present not clear. Different strains may exist with different powers of invasion. Invasion may only occur in the presence of some other unrecognized factor.

Clinical features

Although *E.histolytica* infection of the liver occurs secondary to infection of the large bowel, patients frequently give no history of significant gastrointestinal symptoms. High fever, rigors and profuse sweating are the main symptoms. Pain in the shoulder, neck and upper abdomen are occasional complaints.

Physical examination shows an ill-looking child, with diminished respiratory movements, hepatomegaly with tenderness on palpation and percussion. Jaundice is rare.

Laboratory investigations

Liver function tests are usually normal. The leucocyte count is raised with a predominence of polymorphonuclear neutrophil leucocytes. There may be mild anaemia. Cysts and vegetative forms of *E.histolytica* may be found in fresh stool specimens. A fluorescent antibody test on the patient's serum is of great value in establishing the diagnosis. Antibodies persist for up to 3 years after acute infection.

Treatment

Chloroquin (20 mg/kg per day up to a total of 500 mg daily) for at least two weeks or metronidazole in a dose of 50 ml/kg per day for ten days are the drugs of choice. Some authors have advised that these drugs be given in sequence.

Secondary infections are said to occur in between 10 and 20 per cent of cases. In these, surgical drainage will be indicated. Surgery is also indicated where the lesion ruptures through the diaphragm into the right chest, or into the pericardium.

HYDATID DISEASE

Hydatid disease is caused by the larval stage of infection by the dog tapeworm *Echinococcus granulosus*. Man is infected by contact with the excreta of dogs. Sheep, pigs and camels, like man, are intermediate hosts.

The ova is ingested, burrows through the intestinal mucosa and is carried in the portal vein to the liver where it develops into the adult cyst. A few ova will by-pass the liver and be trapped in the lungs. A few will get into the general systemic circulation.

Pathology

Within the liver, the Echinococcus slowly develops into a large adult cyst, surrounded by thickened compressed tissue which may eventually calcify. The surrounding layer of fibrous tissue is thin, however, and frequently daughter cysts are formed around the main cyst and eventually multiloculated cysts develop. These are usually found in the right lobe of the liver.

Epidemiology

The disease is common in sheep-grazing countries. It is also frequently found in Southern Europe, particularly in the Mediterranean Basin. The disease appears to be rare in Great Britain, but cases are reported from Wales and the Scottish Islands.

Clinical features

The diagnosis is suspected when hepatomegaly is discovered. There may be a distinct round and smooth swelling affecting part of the liver. The patient is not ill but may have a dull ache in the right upper quadrant. Urticaria or anaphylactic shock may occur if hydatid fluid is released into the peritoneum or into the circulation. The peripheral blood count may show an eosinophilia. Technetium scan of the liver will show a filling defect. Ultrasonic scanning shows this to be a fluid-filled cavity. A plain radiograph of the abdomen may show a calcified lesion.

The diagnosis is confirmed by serological tests. A complement fixation test and a haemagglutination test appear to be more sensitive and more specific than the intradermal (Casoni) test.

Treatment

Uncomplicated hepatic hydatid cysts carry a good prognosis. The risks of complications are always present. If the cyst is large it should be removed surgically, great care being taken to avoid spillage of its contents into the peritoneal cavity.

LIVER FLUKES

The liver and biliary system may be damaged as a result of infestation with *Fasciola hepatica* (sheep) *Clonorchis sinensis* (freshwater fish) and *Opisthorchis felineus* and *Opisthorchis viverrini* (cat). It is thought that man is usually infected by eating plants to which the cercaria are attached. The larvae eventually reach the liver and biliary system interfering with biliary flow. Cholangitis with fever, right upper quadrant pain, hepatomegaly and eosinophilia are the main features. There may be complicating suppurative cholangitis.

Diagnosis

Diagnosis is established by recovery of the ova in the faeces. A tanned red cell agglutination test is highly specific for antibodies to *Clonorchis sinensis*.

Treatment

Treatment is by daily injections of emetine in a dosage of 1 mg/kg of bodyweight for ten days. This may have to be followed by two weeks of chloroquine in a dosage of 300 mg per day for a child aged seven years, and 600 mg for a child aged 12 years. For *fascioliasis*, Bithionol (50 mg/kg on alternate days for 2 weeks) is the treatment of choice.

SCHISTOSOMIASIS (BILHARZIASIS)

This disorder is caused by one of three blood flukes. Two invade the intestine, *Schistosoma japonicum* and *S.mansoni*, and the third the bladder (*S.haematobium*).

Epidemiology

Blood flukes are widely distributed throughout the world. *S. haematobium* occurs mainly in the Near East, Iran, Iraq and Egypt. while *S.japonicum* occurs in China and *S.mansoni* in Africa, the Arabian Gulf and Brazil.

The intermediate host is a freshwater snail. In the snail the parasite produces cercariae which escape into water and gain access to a human host in the next 48 hours by penetrating the unbroken skin or buccal mucosa. The parasites pass via the bloodstream and lungs to the liver where they develop within about two months into adult male and female worms. These produce eggs which traval against the blood flow to take up positions in the venous plexus of the rectum, colon or bladder. Eggs are passed in the stool or in the urine, and if they gain access to the intermediate host the cycle is complete.

Pathology

Eggs become deposited in many tissues. They produce a granuloma with intense infiltration with round cells, eosinophils and some giant cells. Healing takes place with the production of fibrous tissue. This occurs characteristically in the bladder, ureter and the liver. In the liver the lesions are around and in the portal tracts. They cause intense fibrosis with little or no bile duct proliferation. There is little or no nodular regeneration, although there may be some disturbance of the hepatic architecture. There is portal venous obstruction as a result of the fibrosis. Splenic enlargement and portosystemic collateral channels are numerous.

Clinical features

Schistosomiasis can occur in any age group. It is rare in the first 18 months of life, but in endemic areas most children become infected during childhood. The course is extremely variable.

The first stage is characterized by itching around the area of the entry of the organism into the skin. This stage is commonly missed. In the second stage, fever, urticaria and eosinophilia are the most prominent features as well as vague symptoms such as malaise, lack of interest in school work, weight-loss and poor appetite. The third stage may see a continuation of these symptoms but with, in addition, features due to involvement of the urinary tract, the bowel or the liver.

The hepatic features are those of cirrhosis, but hepatocellular function is usually well maintained.

The diagnosis is made by the recovery of ova in the stool, liver biopsy or rectal biopsy. Serological and intradermal tests are available but they are not entirely specific.

Treatment

The response to treatment with various anti-bilharzia remedies depends a great deal on the degree of infestation of the individual, the duration of the illness and the severity of complications. Complications such as anaemia, genito-urinary surgery or portal hypertension may require specific management. Encephalopathy often develops following porto-caval anastomosis.

Drug treatment

If therapy is started in the acute or early chronic stages, the prognosis is good. In the presence of liver disease, chemotherapy is difficult. Oral therapy with lucanthone and niridazole is contra-indicated. Parenterally administered antimonials remain the drugs of choice, although they do have serious cardiac toxicity. Intramuscular Stibophen in a dosage of 0.05 ml of a 6.3 per cent solution/kg per day for three days, followed by 0.1 ml/kg on alternate days for ten injections will often produce parasitological cure. Unfortunately, reinfection may occur.

HEPATIC INVOLVEMENT IN ULCERATIVE COLITIS AND CROHN'S DISEASE

In both ulcerative colitis and Crohn's disease there is an increased incidence of hepatic and biliary disease. Although there is no good evidence that this is due to infection of the liver, bacteraemia or bacterial toxins may play a part in its aetiology. It is therefore considered in this section.

Liver disease may occur more frequently in ulcerative colitis and Crohn's disease when these have their onset in infancy or childhood. Hepatic symptoms may not appear until adult life (Toghill, Benton and Smith, 1974). Paradoxically, some children may have features of hepatic disease years before gut symptoms occur.

Aetiology

Little proof exists concerning the causes of ulcerative colitis. Crohn's disease or the hepatic dysfunctions associated with these. Hepatic involvement which occurs with these disorders may simply be a part of the multi-system involvement which in the case of ulcerative colitis, particularly, has an auto-immune basis.

The findings of portal pyaemia in patients undergoing colectomy suggests that the liver disease may be due to bacteria from the diseased colon. Against this hypothesis is the observation that liver biopsies are usually sterile in this condition and broad-spectrum antibiotics have not been shown to influence the course of liver disease.

Similarly, there is no good evidence relating the liver disease to an adverse reaction to drugs used in treatment of the bowel disease or to toxins, such as bile salts, which may be absorbed through the diseased colon.

Pathology

The most frequent abnormality is a *pericholangitis* in which there is periductular inflammation of the interlobular bile ducts. Portal tracts have a dense and often focal infiltrative lymphocytes with occasionally polymorphs and eosinophilic cells. There may be ductular proliferation and periportal cholestasis. Piecemeal necrosis of periportal hepatocytes also occurs. Eventually, periportal fibrosis and biliary cirrhosis may develop. A similar process may affect the extrahepatic ducts giving a *sclerosing cholangitis*. The gallbladder may be involved in this process.

The hepatic parenchyma frequently shows fatty change and a non-specific reactive hepatitis. Rarely, the appearances are those of chronic active hepatitis or a non-biliary cirrhosis.

Clinical features

Hepatic involvement is frequently asymptomatic. It is suspected by the finding of hepatomegaly and abnormal liver function tests, particularly a raised alkaline phosphatase and gammaglutamyltranspeptidase. Rarely, episodes of cholestasis occur with fever, and jaundice. This may last for weeks or months. Such patients require careful follow-up since they do have more frequently rapid progression of their liver disease than asymptomatic patients. In some instances, liver disease first is suspected when cirrhosis and its complications present. Liver disease is most frequently reported years after the first onset of bowel symptoms but in some instances liver disease may precede bowel symptoms by two to three years.

Sclerosing cholangitis is suggested by prolonged cholestasis. Diagnosis can only be made by demonstrating the narrow extrahepatic bile ducts by percutaneous cholangiography or by endoscopic retrograde cholangiopancreatography. In some cases, operative cholangiography through the gallbladder is required to show full details of the biliary anatomy.

Features of chronic active hepatitis and cirrhosis are similar to those described elsewhere (pages 221 and 249).

Because of the very wide spectrum of hepatic involvement both liver biopsy and cholangiography are frequently essential to make a complete diagnosis of the extent of hepatic involvement in inflammatory disease of the large bowel.

Treatment

There is no specific treatment for pericholangitis. Control of the under-lying bowel disorder or its resection may cause an improvement in symptoms. In one series of adult patients resection of the diseased bowel and ulcerative colitis was followed by a marked reduction in pericholangitis (Eade, Cooke and Broke, 1970). I know of no such data in children but it would seem reasonable at this time to regard evidence of progressive liver involvement as an indication for surgical resection of the diseased bowel.

In sclerosing cholangitis surgical relief of areas of focal obstruction is helpful, if this is possible. If the whole of the extrahepatic biliary system is narrowed, a period of T-tube drainage of the common bile duct may be helpful. Corticosteroids and antibiotics are both ineffective. Long-term prognosis must be very guarded but periods of freedom from cholestasis for as long as 5 years are reported.

Chronic active hepatitis should be treated as described in Chapter 12. The response to treatment is less predictable than in chronic active hepatitis without clinical evidence of multi-system involvement.

In adult patients, bile duct carcinoma, hepatocellular carcinoma and intrahepatic granulomata have been reported.

BIBLIOGRAPHY AND REFERENCES

Viral hepatitis

Blum, A.L., *et al.* (1977). Treatment of acute viral hepatitis with (+)-cyanidonal-3. *Lancet* 2, 1153

Dienstag, J.L., Schulman, A.N., Garaty, R.J., Hofnagle, J.H., Lorenz, D.E., Borcell, R.H and Barker, L.F. (1976). Hepatitis A antigen isolated from liver and stool; immunologic comparison of antisera prepared in guinea-pigs. *J.Immunol.* 117, 876-881

Dupuy, J.M., Kostewicz, E. and Alagille, D. (1978). Hepatitis B in children: analysis of 80 cases of acute and chronic hepatitis B *J.Pediat.* 92, 17

Fienstone, S.M., Kapikian, A.Z., Porcell, R.H., Alter, H.J. and Holland, P.V. (1975). Transfusion-associated hepatitis not due to viral hepatitis type A or B. *New Engl.J.Med.* 292, 767

Geraty, R.J., Hoofnegle, J.H., Markenson, J.A. and Barker, L.F. (1974). Exposure to hepatitis B virus and development of chronic HBsAg carrier state in children. *J.Pediat.* 84, 661

Krugman, S. (1973). Viral hepatitis. In *Infectious Diseases of Children and Adults*, p. 76. Ed. by Krugman, S. and Ward, R. St. Louis: Mosby

Le Bouvier, G.L. (1973). Subtypes of hepatitis B antigen: clinical relevance. *Ann.intern.Med.* 79, 894

Maupas, P., Coursget, P., Goudeau, A., Durcker, J. and Bagros, (1976). Immunization against hepatitis B in man. *Lancet* 1, 1367

Maynard, J.E., (1976). Hepatitis A. *Yale J.Biol.Med.* 49, 227

Mowat, A.P. (1975). Dystonic reactions to drugs. *Dev.Med.Child Neurol.* 15, 654

Schaffner, F. (1976). Hepatitis B virus infection in children. In *Liver Diseases in Infancy and Childhood*, p. 163. Ed. by Berenberg, S.R. The Hague: Martinhus Nijhoff, Medical Division

Seminar on Viral Hepatitis (1972). *Am.J.Dis.Child.* **123**, 275

Villarejos, V.M., Provest, P.J., Ittinshon, O.L., McLean, A.A. and Hilleman, M.R. (1976). Sero-epidemiologic investigations of human hepatitis caused by A, B and a possible third virus (39432). *Proc. Soc. exp. Biol. Med.* **152**, 524–528

Yellow fever

Francis, T.I., Moore, E.L., Eddington, G.M. and Smith, J.A. (1972). Clinico-pathological study of human yellow fever. *Bull.Wld Hlth Org.* **46**, 659

Kilpatrick, Z.M. (1966). Structural and functional abnormalities of the liver in infectious mononucleosis. *Archs intern.Med.* **117**, 47

Madigan, N.P., Newcomer, A.D., Campbell, D.C. and Taswell, H.F. (1973). Intense jaundice in infectious mononucleosis. *Mayo Clin. Proc.* **48**, 857

Cytomegalovirus

Henshaw, J.B., Betts, R.F., Simon, G. and Boyton, R.C. (1965). Acquired cyto-megalovirus infections. *New Engl.J.Med.* **272**, 602

Pyogenic abscess of the liver

Johnston, R.D. and Baehner, R.L. (1971). Chronic granulomatous disease: correlation between pathogenesis and clinical findings. *Pediatrics* **48**, 730

Nebesar, R.A., Tefft, M. and Colodny, A.H. (1970). Angiography of liver abscess in granulomatous disease in childhood. *Am. J. Roentg.* **108**, 628

Rubin, R.H., Swartz, N.M. and Malt, R. (1974). Hepatic abscess: changes in clinical, bacteriological and therapeutic aspects. *Am.J.Med.* **57**, 601

Wong, M.L., Kaplan, S., Dunkie, L.M., Stechenberg, B.W. and Feigan, R.D. (1977). Leptospirosis: a childhood disease. *J.Pediat.* **90**, 532

Hepatic amoebiasis

Brandt, H. and Tamayo, R.P. (1970). Pathology of human amoebiasis *Hum.Path.* **1**, 351

Cohen, H.G. and Reynolds, T.P. (1975). Comparison of metronidazole and chloroquin for the treatment of amoebic liver abscess. A controlled trial. *Gastroenterology* **69**, 35

Jesse, W.F. and Hendley, C.W. (1975). Amoebic liver abscess in childhood. *Clin.Pediat.* **14**, 134

Hydatid disease

Joske, R.A. (1974). The changing pattern of hydatid disease with special reference to hydatid disease of the liver. *Med.J.Austr.* **1**, 129

Gelfand, M. (1970). Schistosomiasis. In *Diseases of Children in the Tropics and Sub-Tropics*, p. 847. 2nd ed. Ed. by Jelliffe, J.B. London: Edward Arnold

Hepatic disease accompanying chronic inflammatory disease of the bowel

Coperman, A.M. and Judd, E.S. (1972). The role of colectomy in hepatic disease accompanying ulcerative and granulomatous colitis. *Mayo.Clin.Proc.* 47, 36

Eade, M.N., Cooke, W.G. and Broke, E.N. (1970). Liver disease in ulcerative colitis. (2). The long-term effect of colectomy. *Ann. intern. Med.* 72, 489

Shmerling, B.H. (1978). Ulcerative colitis. In *Progress in Pediatric Surgery,* p. 1, Vol, 11. Ed. by Rickham, P.B., Hecker, W.H. and Provot, J. Baltimore and Munich: Urban and Schwazenberg

Toghill, P.J. Benton, P. and Smith, P.G. (1974). Chronic liver disease associated with childhood ulcerative colitis. *Postgrad.med.J.* 50, 9

CHAPTER 7

Fulminant Hepatic Failure

Definition

Fulminant hepatic failure is a complex syndrome in which severe impairment of hepatic function is associated with progressive mental changes. These may start with confusion or delirium and pass rapidly into stupor or coma. Only patients who develop signs of encephalopathy within eight weeks of the onset of liver disease, and in whom there is no evidence of previous liver disease, are included in this definition. The mortality in children under the age of 14 years is almost 30 per cent in reported series. Those who survive may develop cirrhosis, but a substantial number regain normal hepatic structure and function and have no neurological impairment.

Pathogenesis

The initial liver injury is in most instances, presumed to be viral hepatitis type A. Hepatitis type B, infectious mononucleosis, mushroom poisoning, hepatotoxic drugs, or apparently hypersensitivity reactions to drugs such as monoamineoxidase inhibitors or halothane, may be responsible in other cases. The factors which determine the severity of the hepatic injury are not known. Nor is it clear what limits the liver's ability to recover or regenerate. If part of the liver is resected either in the experimental animal or in man, because of trauma or tumour, rapid regeneration occurs. In fulminant hepatic failure in many cases no signs of regeneration are found.

Pathology

Liver biopsy during life, or immediately following death, shows widespread hepatocellular necrosis or total absence of hepatocytes, except for a few surviving in some periportal zones. Little or no regeneration may be evident. The hepatocyte 'volume' normally accounting for approximately 85 per cent of the area on the slide is frequently reduced to between 15 and 35 per cent of the area in the section.

Very numerous bile ducts are seen because of the collapse of the reticulin framework allowing marked crowding of portal tracts. Bile ducts may also be prominent because of regeneration. There is a marked acute cellular infiltrate, both in the portal tracts and in the hepatic parenchyma.

There are no characteristic morphological abnormalities in the brain except oedema which may be present in up to 40 per cent of fatal cases and cause herniation of the temporal lobe or cerebellum. Secondary changes due to hypoxia and vascular insufficiency also occur.

The mechanisms of hepatic encephalopathy

The absence of structural changes within the brain (other than oedema) the rapid onset of coma and its reversibility suggest a metabolic origin. In spite of intensive study of the complex biochemical features of this syndrome, as yet there is no adequate explanation for such features, nor have the biochemical data provided a rational basis for the comprehensive management of this disorder and its complications.

Hepatic encephalopathy is usually attributed to the abnormal retention of nitrogenous metabolites or toxins secondary to impaired hepatic function. There is considerable evidence that substances involved in causing the syndrome arise from the gut. In addition, intrahepatic shunting of portal blood directly into the systemic circulation, without contact with hepatocytes, may be important. Intestinal bacteria, ingested protein and the presence of blood in the alimentary tract, play a major part in the production of encephalopathy by increasing ammonia absorption. Serum ammonia levels determined in venous blood are elevated to a degree which reflects the cerebral state but is not directly correlated with it. However, some patients who are in deep coma have normal serum ammonia. Current experimental evidence indicates that although ammonia is possibly a major factor in the pathogenesis of coma it is not responsible for all the neuro-psychiatric symptoms and signs.

In addition to alimentary factors causing the coma the continuing hepatic necrosis, with incomplete hepatic metabolism and the effects of the initiating illness on other organs, makes the metabolic consequences of this syndrome very different from those of sub-total hepatectomy.

Other metabolic factors which have been implicated in the pathogenesis include short-chain fatty acids, such as butyrate, valerate and octinoate, which are increased in the blood and cerebrospinal fluid in hepatic encephalopathy, possibly because of ineffective hepatic metabolism. The levels attained are not in themselves sufficient to cause coma, but they may do so by acting synergistically with ammonia.

Considerable interest has recently been directed to abnormalities in serum aminoacid concentrations in fulminant hepatic failure and to the possible role of changes in the concentration within the brain of neuro-transmitters. The straight chain aminoacids phenylalanine, tyrosine, methionine and tryptophan are increased, while the branched chain aminoacids valine, leucine and isoleucine are decreased.

Neuro-transmitters are chemicals which mediate the post-synaptic action of neurones. The 'false' neuro-transmitters are chemicals structurally related to neuro-transmitters but interfering with synaptic function. Neuro-transmitters are metabolized from aminoacids (*Table 7.1*). Thus, the abnormalities in aminoacids may lead to secondary

TABLE 7.1
Amino acid – Catecholamine Metabolic Pathways
within the Brain

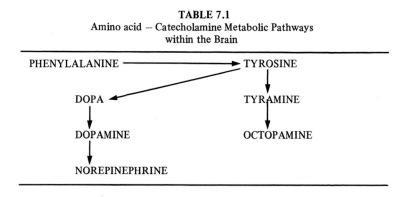

changes in neuro-transmitters. Data relating to the concentration of these true or false neuro-transmitters in blood or cerebrospinal fluid must be interpreted with caution. There may be wide variation in the concentration of these substances in various parts of the brain. The site of critical concentration of these metabolites is not known, but it is considered that an important site of action may be the reticular formation.

A very important metabolic abnormality which may complicate the encephalopathy is profound hypoglycaemia. In addition, changes in the serum concentration of hydrogen ion, sodium, potassium, phosphate, magnesium and calcium may contribute. In the initial stages, there is commonly a respiratory alkalosis, due to hyperventilation, leading to a decrease in cerebral perfusion and oxygen consumption. A metabolic alkalosis may arise secondary to hypokalaemia which is often present early in the course. Alkalosis increases the cerebral uptake of ammonia.

Tissue necrosis both within the liver and in sites of secondary infection and tissue hypoxia may give rise to a metabolic acidosis. Hyponatraemia, may develop spontaneously or be aggravated by salt-losing diuretics (*Table 7.2*). Osmotic diuretics such as hypertonic glucose, given for nutritional reasons or to reduce intracranial pressure, may cause hypernatraemia, particularly if the urinary sodium excretion is low.

Cerebral blood flow may be decreased in part due to hypercapnia. In part, encephalopathy has been attributed to reduced cerebral blood flow and reduced glucose utilization, but the data relating to this do not indicate whether these changes are primary or secondary.

Clinical features

Development of fulminant hepatic failure during the course of infective or toxic hepatitis may be heralded by the features given in *Table 7.2* (*see also* Chapter 6). Features of liver injury may have been present for hours or weeks. The disease course may be one of progressive or increasingly severe jaundice, anorexia and vomiting, followed by clouding of consciousness. In other patients after a typical initial onset

TABLE 7.2
Biochemical Abnormalities in Fulminant Hepatic Failure

Serum bilirubin elevated both total and direct reacting
Aspartate transaminase often increased to values of between 20 and 80 times normal, but may fall to normal range in the late stages
Alkaline phosphatase increased to values of between 1 and 8 times normal
Prothrombin time is always prolonged
Albumin may be normal initially, but falls with the duration of the illness
Hypoglycaemia
Serum urea is often low initially but both it and the creatinine rises if renal failure develops
Serum concentrations of sodium, potassium and hydrogen ion are variable and require repeated monitoring
Serum concentrations of phosphate, magnesium and calcium often fall

---

of hepatitis, there is a period of improvement followed by the occurrence of fever, anorexia, abdominal pain and vomiting. In such patients rapid decrease in liver size in the absence of clinical improvement is a very serious sign. Rarely encephalopathy may develop before jaundice is apparent.

Spontaneous haemorrhage into the skin or gastrointestinal tract may occur. Ascites may develop. The respiratory rate usually increases

Table 7.3
Grades of Hepatic Coma

(1)	Minor disturbances of consciousness or motor function
(2)	Drowsy but responsive to commands
(3)	Stuporose but responsive to pain
(4)	Unresponsive to painful stimuli

early in the encephalopathy, with typical deep and forceful respiration which may lead to a respiratory alkalosis.

The initial neurological features may be lethargy, verbal confusion or combative, irrational hyperactivity. Restlessness, disorientation, repeated yawning and sucking movements progress to apathy, stupor and coma (*Table 7.3*). Eventually, the respiratory and vasomotor centres fail.

The neuromuscular state varies with the degree of encephalopathy. In minor degrees, incoordination and tremor may be evident. Asterixis or flapping tremor, that is, rapid flexion and extension movements of

TABLE 7.4
Complications of Hepatic Coma

Cerebral oedema	Electrolyte imbalance
Renal failure	Respiratory difficulties
Acid-base disturbances	Cardiac lesions
Bleeding diathesis	Pancreatitis
Hypoglycaemia	Bone marrow depression
Increased susceptibility to infection	Ascites (late)

the wrist and metacarpal phalangeal joints on sustained posture with the forearm fixed, is typically seen, although not pathognomonic. Tendon reflexes may be increased and as the coma deepens the Babinski response becomes positive. Clonus can be demonstrated. Eventually, decerebrate rigidity or decorticate posture may occur. With progressive brain stem involvement 'doll's-eye' movements are lost, the pupils become fixed and unresponsive. Hypotonia and areflexia occur terminally.

Complications (*Table 7.4*)

Cerebral oedema Cerebral oedema is a frequent complication occurring in between 30 and 40 per cent of fatal cases.

Renal failure Renal failure with severe oliguria, inappropriately low sodium excretion, or anuria, tends to develop, particularly in the later stages. Both acute tubular necrosis and functional renal failure may occur. The mechanism leading to functional renal failure is not known.

Acid-base disturbances Acid-base disturbances occur in nearly all cases. Hyperventilation is a constant feature during the early stages of coma, causing a respiratory alkalosis. Metabolic alkalosis also occurs due to potassium deficiency, administration of alkalis or continuous gastric aspiration.

Hypoxia Hypoxia occurs frequently. It may be due to pulmonary infection or oedema, secondary to abnormal capillary permeability, resulting in interstitial and alveolar oedema. Intrapulmonary shunts may contribute to the hypoxia. A respiratory acidosis may occur.

Bleeding diathesis A bleeding diathesis is almost always present. Its severity varies from patient to patient. The incidence of clinical haemorrhage varies in reported series from between 40 and 70 per cent and is a contributory factor to death in between 10 and 60 per cent. The most common coagulation defect is a decrease in Factors II, V, VII, IX and X; all except V are measured by the prothrombin time. An increase in Factor VIII is occasionally seen and is unexplained. Severe hypofibrinogenaemia is rare and the mechanism of the decrease is uncertain. Although evidence of disseminated intravascular coagulation has been found, heparin therapy is not helpful. Development of severe gastrointestinal haemorrhage is frequently a major contributory factor to death. It may occur when the generalized bleeding diathesis is improving. Severe thrombocytopenia may contribute to this. Many patients bleed from localized erosions in the oesophagus, stomach or duodenum.

Metabolic abnormalities Hypoglycaemia, low serum sodium, phosphate, magnesium and potassium may occur.

Susceptibility to infection A major problem is increased susceptibility to infection. This may take the form of a Gram-negative septicaemia, peritonitis or localized infection. In the unconscious state, inadequate ventilation favours respiratory tract infection. Infection greatly increases the metabolic demands by causing tissue breakdown. It may lead to increased accumulation of aminoacids and short-chain fatty acids, thereby aggravating the encephalopathy.

Circulatory problems Circulatory disturbances are common. The cardiac output is high due to decreased peripheral resistance. In the late stages, unexplained hypotension is very common. It may arise from central vasomotor depression. Sinus tachycardia occurs in 75 per cent of cases. Bradycardia, is a late development. Sudden, unexpected cardiac arrest occurs in up to 25 per cent of cases.

Other complications *Pancreatitis* occurs in a small percentage of cases. *Bone marrow depression* may affect all components or only platelets, white blood series or the red blood cell series. It occurs rarely but is usually irreversible. *Ascites* occurs as a late complication, in cases following a prolonged course.

Treatment

Other causes of coma such as subdural haematoma, must be considered and if necessary excluded.

The basis of treatment is to maintain homeostasis as satisfactorily as possible and to support life until spontaneous regeneration of the liver can occur. Complications should be anticipated and prevented if possible. Ammonia absorption from the gut must be minimized. The patient must be protected from sedation (*Table 7.5*).

Patient monitoring

Fulminant hepatic failure is a syndrome of considerable variability. Different therapeutic measures are applicable in different patients and different stages in the development of the disorder. The care of the patient with fulminant hepatic failure requires intensive nursing support

TABLE 7.5
Aggravating Factors in Hepatic Encephalopathy

Gastrointestinal haemorrhage	Uraemia
Hypovolaemia	Infection
Potassium depletion	High protein intake
Hypoglycaemia	Constipation
Sedatives and anaesthetics	

and observation by medical staff familiar with the range of metabolic abnormalities and complications which have to be anticipated or prevented. As part of supportive therapy, intensive monitoring of the cardiovascular, respiratory, central nervous systems, and of fluid and electrolyte balance is essential. As well as clinical assessment, this requires initial and serial determination of pulse, blood pressure, central venous pressure, bodyweight, serum and urinary concentration of electrolytes, urea, creatinin and osmolarity. The blood pH and concentrations of glucose, phosphate, calcium and magnesium must be measured regularly. Standard tests of liver function, peripheral blood count and prothrombin time should be performed daily, with serum amylase.

An ECG should be performed to assess the intracellular potassium status with continuous recording to detect arrhythmia. EEG monitoring adds to information available on the state of the central nervous system. Because of the frequency of cerebral oedema, without papilloedema, intracranial pressure monitoring has been introduced but its value in modifying therapy is uncertain.

Food, fluids and electrolytes

All protein must be stopped and the bowel emptied by an enema. Neomycin and lactulose should be given by naso-gastric tube.

Intravenous fluids in the form of 5 or 10 per cent dextrose at a rate of 1.5 litres/m^2 per day are given. There is likely to be serious potassium depletion which must be replaced by oral or intravenous potassium in a dose of 3 mmol/kg per day. If acidosis is present, it should be corrected by sodium bicarbonate. Sodium, however, has to be given with care, because even if the concentration in the serum is low, this may be due to inappropriate water retention rather than a low total body sodium. In some patients the blood glucose will be low on this regimen and higher concentrations of glucose will be required. If these are used, the urinary glucose must be carefully monitored. To try to minimize endogenous protein catabolism, high concentrations of intravenous glucose have been used to provide calories. If there is no risk of vomiting, calories may be given also in the form of Caloreen by naso-gastric tube.

Respiration

Hypoxia must be corrected by increasing the environmental oxygen concentration but often endotracheal intubation is required. Regular chest physiotherapy is essential.

Circulation

Patients are extremely sensitive to volume depletion. A central venous line is essential in monitoring and the blood pressure must be maintained to achieve maximum hepatic perfusion. This may require the careful infusion of salt-poor albumin, fresh frozen plasma or whole blood, depending on the serum albumin concentration or the haemoglobin concentration.

Bleeding diathesis

One of the most difficult problems lies in preventing major bleeding. Intravenous vitamin K may be given but is likely to be ineffective in the presence of fulminant hepatic failure. When there is no bleeding, fresh frozen plasma may be given prophylactically if the prothrombin time is prolonged by more than 35 seconds. It may be helpful if assays can be done of Factors II, V, VI, IX, XI, and fibrinogen, since it is known that at least 30 per cent of normal concentrations of these factors is essential for homeostasis. Fresh frozen plasma contains all the essential factors in a concentration of 1 unit (100 per cent of normal)/ml. Thus, up to 30 per cent of plasma volume may have to be given to bring the concentration of these factors up to that required for normal coagulation. This produces great problems with fluid overload and for that reason Factor concentrates have been used. Most commercially available concentrates contain no Factor V. An additional problem is that these concentrates may carry hepatitis B virus or non-A, non-B Hepatitis virus.

If spontaneous haemorrhage has occurred it will require replacement with fresh compatible blood. Alimentary haemorrhage is a major complication since as well as causing hypotension, it does add to the protein in the gut and thereby aggravate the encephalopathy. There is some evidence that the frequency of this complication can be reduced by the use of cemitidine.

Thrombocytopenia complicated by purpura may be corrected by platelet transfusion. Unfortunately, it is difficult to predict *in vivo* viability or functional effectiveness of transfused platelets.

Avoidance of sedation

In the early stages of encephalopathy, chidlren are often extremely difficult to control and the temptation to give sedation is great. It should be resisted as far as possible, since even half the standard therapeutic dose appropriate for a child of that age and weight is likely to have a profound and prolonged effect. Excessive uncontrolled activity tends to be short-lasting and may be rapidly followed by deep coma. If sedation must be given, for example, when a patient is being transferred to another hospital, one-half of the normally appropriate dose of diazepam may be used. Even then the patient will need detailed supervision to correct depressed or arrested respiration.

Secondary infection

Respiratory tract infection, urinary tract infection, septicaemia and peritonitis may all be present with few overt signs. A high index of suspicion and frequent bacteriological investigations is necessary for early diagnosis. Awareness of this danger with asepsis as far as practicable, is probably better than prophylactic broad-spectrum antibiotics in such patients. If, however, the patient deteriorates and no other parameters have changed it is reasonable to use broad-spectrum antibiotics while awaiting the results of bacteriological investigations.

Renal failure

If renal failure develops it is best treated by early peritoneal dialysis. This would be indicated by a plasma creatinine of > 0.4 μmol/litre, potassium > 6 μmol/litre, or by marked fluid retention. In some cases, haemodialysis may be necessary.

Cerebral oedema

A major unsolved problem is the control of cerebral oedema. Neither corticosteroids, including dexamethasone in conventional doses, nor osmotic agents such as mannitol or glycerol, have overcome this problem. In the monitoring of such patients the introduction of devices for directly measuring intracranial pressure has led to the more rational use of these agents and may yet lead to advances in treating this complication. Experimental work with dexamethasone suggests that if given early in the course it may prevent the development of cerebral oedema.

Experimental measures

In addition to supportive care, many other measures have been

TABLE 7.6
Forms of Therapy Which Are Not Well Established

Corticosteroids	Total body washout
Exchange transfusion	Hyperbaric oxygen
Haemodialysis using cuprophane or cellophane membranes	L-Dopa
Haemodialysis using polyacrylonitrime membrane	Infusion of aminoacids
Haemoperfusion of charcoal column	Extracorporeal perfusion of liver from pig, calf, baboon or human cadaver
Haemoperfusion of XAD-2 resin	Cross-circulation with an animal, for example, a pig
Plasmaphaeresis	Cross-circulation with a human volunteer

advocated in the treatment of this serious condition. Some of which are listed in *Table 7.6*.

In none of these measures has any controlled trials providing evidence that therapy is advantageous. Limited trials have shown the mortality to be slightly greater in those patients treated with corticosteroids or with exchange transfusion. In none of the other measures in *Table 7.6* has a controlled trial been reported. When a series of cases is reported, often the data does not contain sufficient information to allow the assessment of prognosis if only supportive therapy had been offered. In assessing therapy and prognosis the following factors must be considered.

(1) The age of the patient.
(2) The cause of the liver disease.
(3) The severity of liver involvement in particular epidemics.
(4) The grade and duration of coma when therapy was commenced.
(5) The morphometric assessment of hepatocyte volume.
(6) Quantitative liver function tests, for example, conjugation of cholic acid or galactose elimination capacity.
(7) Prothrombin time.

BIBLIOGRAPHY

Berk, P.D., Martin, J.F., Scharschmidt, B.F. and Plotz, P.H. (1976). Current status of artificial hepatic support systems. In *Progress in Liver Diseases*, p. 398. Vol. 5. Ed. by Popper, H. and Schaffner, F. New York: Grune and Stratton

Fischer, J.E. and Baldessarini, R.J. (1976). Pathogenesis and therapy of hepatic coma. In *Progress in Liver Diseases*, p. 363. Vol. 5. Ed. by Popper H. and Schaffner, F. New York: Grune and Stratton

Loening, W.E.K., Coovadia, H.M. and Parent, M.A. (1974). Exchange transfusion in fulminant hepatic failure in Children. *S.Afr.med.J.* **48**, 128

MacDonnel, R.C. *et al.* (1973). Cross-circulation between children in hepatic coma and chimpanzees. *J.Pediat.* **82**, 591

Silk, D.BA. *et al.* (1977). Treatment of fulminant hepatic failure by Polyacrylonitril-membrane haemodialysis. *Lancet* **2**, 1

Williams, R. (1976). Hepatic failure and development of artificial liver support systems. In *Progress in Liver Diseases*, p. 418. Vol. 5. Ed. by Popper, H. and Schaffner, F. New York: Grune and Stratton

Zacarias, J., Brinck, P. and Guidobro, J.G. (1971). Treatment of hepatic coma with exchange transfusion *Am.J.Dis.Child.* **122**, 229

CHAPTER 8

Reye's Syndrome

(Encephalopathy and fatty degeneration of the viscera)

Definition

Reye's syndrome is an acute disorder occurring in children of any age and characterized by a severe encephalopathy with marked cerebral oedema (without cellular infiltration or demyelination) and diffuse fatty infiltration of the viscera. Typically it occurs in a very small percentage of children during the recovery phase of what appears to be a mild, unremarkable, respiratory tract infection or an exanthematous illness such as chickenpox. Liver function is very disturbed but there may be no clinical features indicating hepatic involvement. Death from cerebral oedema has occurred in approximately 40 per cent of reported cases. If the patient survives the acute illness, the hepatic and cerebral pathological changes are completely reversed, but there may be long-term neurological handicaps if cerebral hypoxia has occurred.

Incidence

The incidence of Reye's syndrome appears to be increasing. The first reported case was probably in 1929. Reye, Morgan and Baral (1963) in a report from Australia highlighted the disorder. Since then, over 800 cases have been reported. Review of autopsy files for the years prior to 1960 reveal very few cases. Since the aetiology of this condition is unknown the pathological, clinical and biochemical abnormalities will be considered before discussing aetiology.

Pathology

Hepatic changes

The severity and speed of evolution of hepatic changes correlate with the severity of the encephalopathy. In the first 24 hours after the onset of vomiting or neurological features, hepatic changes are often limited to glycogen depletion and cytoplasmic swelling most evident at the periphery of the hepatic lobule. In severe cases the glycogen depletion may be panlobular and is likely to be associated with a high incidence of hypoglycaemia and a high death rate. Lipids are abundantly seen in frozen sections stained with Sudan dyes, the lipid droplets being smaller in the inner part of the lobule than at the periphery. No cytoplasmic vacuolation may be detected in haematoxylin and eosin stained paraffin sections at this time.

As fat accumulates the lipid droplets appear to coalesce; other cytoplasmic constituents are condensed and displaced to the perinuclear region of the cell or are arranged in linear strands running from the nucleus to the periphery of the cell. A characteristic micro-vacuolization of the parenchyma becomes evident. This may take from one to four days to develop. Mitotic activity may be evident in the periphery of the lobule within ten hours of onset, but is more evident three days later. Hepatic necrosis is absent or inconspicuous. In severe cases portal tract inflammation is evident after the first 24 hours.

Lipid may clear in two to five days in mild cases, but persist up to nine days in severe ones. By one month the liver has returned to normal.

Histochemical studies show a reversible severe reduction in the mitochondrial enzymes succinic dehydrogenase and cytochrome oxidase. Electronmicroscopic examination shows progressive alteration in liver ultrastructure – particularly the mitochondria – which parallel the clinical severity of the disease. Electronmicroscopic examination of biopsy material early in the course of the encephalopathy shows the hepatocytes to be swollen and universally affected by a process causing swollen, pleomorphic mitochondria with loss of dense bodies as well as small droplet triglyceride accumulation and loss of glycogen. There is proliferation of the smooth endoplasmic reticulum and a great increase in peroxisomes. Chromatographic studies of the lipids in liver indicate that both triglycerides and free fatty acids are increased.

Fatty changes are also seen in the epithelial cells of the loop of Henle and of the proximal convoluted tubule of the kidney, in the heart, the pancreas and the lymph nodes.

Cerebral lesions

Cerebral oedema, usually evident grossly, is manifested as a heavy brain with swollen, flattened gyri and narrow sulci, There may be herniation of the brain through the foramen magnum and secondary compression of the brain stem. There is no significant inflammatory reaction in the brain or meninges. Microscopic changes are secondary to cerebral oedema and hypoxic neural changes. Ultrastructural studies of brain biopsies show unusual diffuse mitochondrial swelling, similar to those seen in the hepatocytes. In addition, blebs or vesicles are found in myelin sheaths and there may be moderate astrocyte swelling.

Clinical features

The majority of cases are reported in children between the ages of six months and 15 years, but any age between two months and 18 years may be affected. One patient, aged 29 years, appears to have had this disorder. Early reports suggested that there was a concentration of children aged less than two years but this has not been confirmed. The sex distribution is equal.

The patient is commonly recovering from a mild unremarkable, 'prodromal' illness such as a respiratory tract infection, or exanthemata, for example, chickenpox. Vomiting develops and becomes persistent and profuse, which may coincide with, or be rapidly followed by, a change in the mental state leading to a progressive deterioration in consciousness. Initially the child may simply be unusually quiet and withdrawn. A period of irrational behaviour, sometimes with visual hallucinations develops, proceeding in some children to agitated delirium. The patient becomes progressively lethargic. Gross motor actions such as walking become increasingly clumsy. Neurological examination may show the presence of intermittent clonus or a positive Babinski response. The respiratory rate is typically rapid at this stage. Coma with decerebrate posturing, opisthotonos, dilated, slowly responsive pupils, and retinal features of increased intracranial pressure supervene. Respiration is both rapid and deep. Convulsions occur in about 30 per cent of cases. They are usually generalized. Eventually brain death will occur.

The rate of progression through these various stages is variable, ranging from three to four hours to between 48 and 60 hours. The more rapid the progression, the worse the prognosis. Cases may stabilize, improve and recover completely, spontaneously or with therapy, at any stage short of brain death. There are no focal neurological signs or features indicating meningeal irritation.

There is commonly no clinical evidence of visceral disease. The liver may be palpable but is rarely noted to be strikingly enlarged.

Diagnostic laboratory findings

Serum aminotransferases are elevated from levels of between twice normal to up to one-hundred times normal. Prothrombin time is prolonged. Hyperammoniaemia is common early in the course. Hypoglycaemia is a feature in severe cases, particularly in those aged less than two years, but it is not a constant finding. The cerebrospinal fluid is normal apart from a low sugar in some cases. These clinical features and laboratory findings are sufficiently distinctive to allow a presumptive diagnosis of Reye's syndrome until liver biopsy can be performed (*Table 8.1*). There are, however, other encephalopathies of unknown cause which mimic this disorder without having the distinctive hepatic pathology.

Biochemical abnormalities

As well as the biochemical abnormalities detailed above, a welter of metabolic abnormalities have been documented in children with clinical Reye's syndrome (*Table 8.2*). They may partly be explained by transient reversible deficiency of mitochondrial enzymes, ornithine transcarbamylase and carbamyl phosphate synthetase. These enzymes facilitate the conversion of ammonia to urea. Enzyme activities are maximally

TABLE 8.1
Diagnosis of Reye's Syndrome

Mild antecedent illness	Biochemical evidence of hepatic dysfunction
Profuse vomiting	Absence of other possible causes
Objective central nervous system dysfunction	Characteristic liver biopsy findings (*see* text)

reduced on the first days of the illness, recovering to normal by the seventh day. Massive tissue breakdown occurs in Reye's syndrome, which results in enormous losses of protein nitrogen in the urine but very little of this is in the form of urea. Serum citrulline is low, but the substrates of these enzymes accumulate – amongst these is carbamyl phosphate. It diffuses from the mitochondria into the cytoplasm where it is changed to orotic acid, a substance which decreases lipoprotein synthesis and may thereby contribute to the fatty acid accumulation within the liver. Fatty acids themselves have many potentially toxic effects including impaired glycolysis and pyruvate degradation. In addition they may have a direct disruptive effect on mitochondrial membranes (*Figure 8.1*).

TABLE 8.2
Biochemical Abnormalities in Reye's Syndrome

The degree of change in these substances varies with the severity of the condition and with the stage of illness

Substances increased

Ammonia	Glucose (rarely)
Aminoacids (except L-citrulline)	Insulin
Free fatty acids	Glucagon
Glycerol	Growth hormone
Aceto-acetate	Cortisol
Pyruvate	Potassium
Lactate	Hydrogen ion concentration

Concentrations decreased

Glucose	L-citruline
Alpha and pre-beta lipoproteins	Hydrogen ion concentration (rarely)

A further group of metabolic disorders are related to the increased lipolysis in adipose tissue stores. This is perhaps caused by the very high concentrations of glucocorticoids, growth hormones and glucagon sometimes found in this syndrome. Lipolysis causes high serum free fatty acids and a raised serum glycerol level. The presentation of these to viscera incapable of metabolizing them could result in accumulation of triglyceride in the parenchymal cells and the development of ketosis.

These metabolic disturbances are not limited to brain and liver but affect skeletal and cardiac muscle and kidneys. The precise role in pathogenesis of abnormalities in fatty acid metabolism, ammonia retention and the many other metabolic aberrations found in this syndrome has not as yet been unravelled. The confusion may, in part, be due to observers failing to relate their findings to the stage of the disease. There may be very different metabolic effects depending on the relative degree of hepatic involvement and tissue destruction.

Epidemiological and pathogenic considerations

The exact aetiology remains unknown. As already mentioned, the incidence of Reye's syndrome is increasing. In part, this is due to increasing awareness of the disorder rather than a true increase. There is an equal sex incidence, and it is predominantly a disease of childhood. It is of worldwide distribution. It occurs in minor epidemics, particularly in urban areas. In North America, three of these have been epidemiologically and geographically related to influenze B epidemics.

It is estimated that one case of Reye's syndrome occurs for every 1,700 cases of influenza B infection. Endemic cases have been associated with a variety of viral infections, for example, varicella-zoster, influenza A and para-influenza. Virus is not recovered in the brain, liver or muscle of affected individuals.

Toxins considered in the aetiology include salicylates, pteridines, isopropyl alcohol, hypoglycins, and 4-pentenoic acid, but the current evidence associating any of these with Reye's syndrome is weak.

More important perhaps are aflatoxins. These are mycotoxins produced by many species of fungi which generally require an environmental temperature of $25-30°C$ to grow well, on foodstuffs. In Thailand

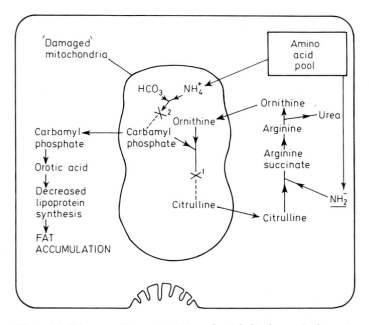

Figure 8.1. Diagrammatic representation of metabolic changes in the acute stage of Reye's syndrome. Within the hepatocyte the major abnormality is a defect in the intramitochondrial part of the urea cycle which converts ammonia to urea. The enzymatic activity of ornithine transcarbamylase and carbamylphosphate synthetase is decreased, leading to impairment of the metabolic changes in the cycle at the points $X1$ and $X2$ respectively. Both defects cause accumulation of ammonia and decreased L-citrulline production; Carbamylphosphate accumulates within the mitochondria and diffuses into the cytoplasm where its metabolism leads to decreased lipoprotein synthesis and hence fat accumulation. These effects are exaggerated by the increased tissue breakdown and release of nitrogen and increased lipolysis occurring in other tissues. The combined effect of these two lesions is to produce the serum changes shown in Table 8.2

it has been shown that a degree of aflatoxin contamination of food follows the seasonal and geographic incidence of encephalopathy and fatty degeneration of the viscera. Chemical assay of the tissue of patients with Reye's syndrome shows a higher concentration of aflatoxin than in those who die of other disorders or accident. Yet family or even village outbreaks are rare, although contaminated food is presumably shared. In part, this may be attributable to the amount of aflatoxin ingestion or to the increased sensitivity of the young. The administration of aflatoxin to young monkeys has produced features somewhat similar to Reye's syndrome. Possibly aflatoxin alone will not produce the syndrome but will only do so in the presence of other recognized factors.

The apparent concentration of cases of Reye's syndrome in an area of Canada which has recently been heavily sprayed with insecticide was followed by an interesting experimental study in young mice. An encephalopathy with fatty infiltration of the viscera, very similar to that seen in Reye's syndrome, was produced in mice which had DDT or Fenitrothion applied to the skin for 11 days prior to exposure to sub-lethal concentrations of an encephalo-myocarditis virus. Neither insecticide alone or in combination nor the virus caused similar pathological features.

Several well characterized genetic metabolic abnormalities with features similar to those seen in the acute stages of Reye's syndrome have now been described, for example, ornithine transcarbamylase deficiency, hypervalinaemia. In a few cases relapses of Reye's syndrome have occurred after a prolonged period. A mild, protein-tolerant deficiency of ornithine transcarbamylase has been found in two such cases, one of which had recurrent attacks of Reye's syndrome. Such abnormalities have not been found in sporadic cases of Reye's syndrome. The electronmicroscopic, biochemical and enzymatic studies indicate an acute reversible, structural and functional mitochondrial abnormality. The effect of the mitochondrial abnormality is exaggerated by tissue destruction and lipolysis.

The cause of the encephalopathy is undetermined. There is no evidence of primary central nervous system infection. The neural mitochondrial lesions may occur through some direct toxic effect or may be secondary to some metabolic abnormality. Hypoglycaemia may be important in the initial stages. Hyperammonaemia and increased fatty acids, singly or in combination, may also be important.

These epidemiological, clinical, biochemical, electronmicroscopic and experimental data suggest that: (a) Reye's syndrome may arise from an unusual combination of effects – toxic, infective, age-related – on children who have no detected metabolic abnormality; or (b) that in some instances environmental factors will only precipitate the disorder in the presence of a latent genetic abnormality in the metabolism of aminoacids, urea or fatty acids.

Treatment

Therapy in Reye's syndrome is aimed at preventing, minimizing and correcting the recognized metabolic abnormalities and at controlling cerebral oedema. It is essential that treatment be instituted before irreversible brain damage occurs. The overall mortality in recognized cases is around 40 per cent. Although advances in management have occurred, failure to delineate the exact cause has hampered progress. Assessment of the relative efficacy and importance of different aspects of treatment is a major problem. Clinically, the disorder follows a continuum of severity from relatively mild cases which never progress beyond Grade 1 or 2 and ultimately recover, to cases which progress to decerebrate behaviour within a few hours of onset and die of cerebral oedema. Factors observed early in the course which indicate a poor prognosis are given in *Table 8.3*. Unless such parameters are carefully

TABLE 8.3
Factors Indicating Poor Prognosis

Rapid progression of symptoms to Stage IV	SGOT/SGPT ratio of less than 1
Ammonia greater than 300 μmol/dl	EEG: marked slowing
Creatinin phosphokinase greater than 500 iu/litre	Non-esterified fatty acids greater than 0.85 mEq/litre

assessed in evaluating different forms of treatment, misleading interpretations of their efficacy may be made. Adequately documented controlled trials investigating the role of more hazardous forms of therapy are urgently required. Nevertheless, units with particular expertise in the management of this disorder do so with negligible mortality. The outline of management described below is based on the recommendations of such units. Some principles of therapy can be advocated at this time.

(1) Early diagnosis and treatment with intravenous glucose may prevent deterioration in the cerebral state.
(2) Mortality is least in children admitted to units which can provide intensive nursing and medical support.
(3) Tissue hypoxia must be prevented by intubation with or without mechanical ventilation and by maintenance of the systemic blood pressure.

TABLE 8.4
Clinical Assessment of Severity of Encephalopathy in Reye's Syndrome

	Mild (1)	Moderate (2)	Severe (3)	Very severe (4)	Brain death (5)
Mental state	Quiet, normal response to verbal commands	Lethargic, slow mental processes such as difficulty in counting	Agitated delerium, out of contact with environment, but responds to pain	Coma, decerebrate rigidity, pain produces exacerbation of decerebrate posture	Coma, spinal reflexes preserved
Muscular activity	Wishes to lie down but no other abnormality	Clumsy	Poorly controlled gross movements, intermittent clonus	Opisthotonos, extensor spasms of arms and legs	Flaccid paralysis
Respiration	Normal	Normal or increased rate	Normal or increased rate	Increased rate and depth	None
Pupillary responses	Normal	Normal	Dilated, but rapidly responsive	Dilated, but slowly responsive	Dilated and unresponsive
Fundi	Normal	Normal	Venous engorgement	Marked venous engorgement, discs blurred, papilloedema	Variable

(4) Metabolic complications should be rapidly corrected.

(5) Increased intracranial pressure – the cause of death – must be controlled.

When the diagnosis of Reye's syndrome is suspected, an intravenous glucose infusion should be started immediately and continued when the diagnosis is confirmed. As well as attempting to correct hypoglycaemia, it minimizes protein breakdown and lipolysis and thereby the accumulation of ammonia and fatty acids. The exact concentration of glucose and the rate of infusion is still a matter of debate. A 10 or 15 per cent glucose solution at a rate of 1.2 litres/m^2 per day has been advocated while other groups have had satisfactory results using 20–30 per cent glucose with 40mEq sodium chloride and 30mEq potassium phosphate/litre given at a rate of 1.6 litres/m^2 per day. The latter group aim to keep the blood sugar at levels of between 200 and 400 mg/100 ml. Such concentrations, as well as having a possible direct effect in diminishing cerebral oedema may, in theoretical grounds, be helpful in causing decreased proteolysis and also promoting the uptake of aminoacids by muscle.

The severity of the disease should be assessed, recorded and graded (*Table 8.4*).

If it is technically feasible blood should be taken for determinations mentioned in *Table 8.5*. The patient should be transferred to a unit able to offer intensive care, after discussion of immediate care with the staff of that unit.

If the patient has evidence of neurological impairment intravenous mannitol in a dose of 1–2 g/kg of bodyweight over a 30-minute period should be given.

From the studies using intraventricular or epidural intracranial pressure monitoring, it is clear that the cranial pressure may be markedly increased even in the absence of papilloedema. It is certainly present when there are signs of upper brain stem compression, for example, pupillary asymmetry, decreased pupillary reflexes or the development of extra-ocular palsies. Maintaining the serum osmolality at greater than 320 mmol/litre may help to prevent cerebral oedema.

Hypoxia is frequently present in Reye's syndrome, even when there is no cyanosis or hypoventilation. Elective endotracheal intubation, in all except Grade 1 cases, is advised to ensure effective toilet of the upper airway, and correction of hypoxia by adminstration of oxygen of ventilation if it becomes necessary. The PaO_2 should be maintained at between 100–200 mmHg.

A central venous line should be inserted and the central venous pressure maintained at between +2 and +4 cm. This line can be used for the infusion of hypertonic solutions and also to facilitate the

TABLE 8.5
Investigations Required at the Time of Initial Assessment

Blood group determination and cross-matching of blood	SGOT (AST)
Serum sodium, potassium, chloride, bicarbonate, magnesium, calcium and phosphate determinations	SGPT (ALT)
Blood sugar	Creatinine phosphokinase
Serum osmolarity	Ammonia
Blood gas and hydrogen ion concentrations	Non-esterified fatty acid concentration
Haemoglobin, total white blood count, platelet count	Viral antibody titre
Prothrombin time	Serum, urine and faeces to be stored for virological and toxicological studies

collection of blood specimens. Pain and struggling on the part of the child may increase the intracranial pressure. An indwelling intra-arterial catheter greatly facilitates the collection of samples for blood gas determinations.

If facilities exist, continuous intracranial pressure monitoring, using an epidural pressure transducer, should be established. Changes in blood gas values, ventilatory pressures, the patient's response to nursing procedures and physiotherapy, as well as metabolic derangements can all contribute to marked increases in intracranial pressure, which cannot be assessed in any other way. Such increases can be rapidly reversed by modifying or treating the precipitating factor. It is desirable to keep the serum osmolality high at between 310 and 330 mmol/litre as compared with the normal of 285 mmol/litre. Uncorrected rises of pressure must be treated by intravenous mannitol in a dosage of 1–2 g/kg of bodyweight given over a 45-minute period. This has to be repeated as required. Occasionally, this does not control increase in intracranial pressure. Satisfactory recovery has occurred following bitemporal cranial decompression. Hypophosphataemia, hypokalaemia, and hypocalcaemia are particular metabolic abnormalities which frequently require correction. The serum concentration of these ions should be checked regularly. Vitamin K, 5 mg intramuscularly or 1 mg intravenously, may prevent a bleeding diathesis. Fresh frozen plasma or fresh whole blood will be required on occasions. No food is given by mouth. The bowel is cleansed by an enema and by the administration of oral neomycin as used in hepatic encephalopathy.

Four additional forms of therapy unproven by controlled trial, but perhaps slightly more hazardous, have to be considered. Peritoneal dialysis which is an effective way of correcting metabolic abnormalities, was proposed as a means of removing alleged toxins. Studies, however, have failed to show that the use of peritoneal dialysis produces results substantially better than with less invasive techniques.

The addition of insulin to glucose infusion, had what seemed a sound theoretical basis until it was shown that hyperinsulinaemia was usually present in this syndrome. It is not known how active the

TABLE 8.6
Clinical Observations to Assess Progress

Pulse rate	Neurological grading:
ECG monitoring	(a) state of consciousness;
Blood pressure	(b) pupillary size and reactivity:
Central venous pressure	(c) fundi;
Respiratory rate and pattern	(d) neuromuscular
Fluid output monitoring	Intracranial pressure

endogenous insulin is. Impaired liver function may limit its conversion to an active form. Insulin and glucose therapy, however, has yet to be shown to be of value.

Exchange transfusion was introduced into the management of this syndrome as a means of removing potential toxins. It has other possible benefits. If fresh whole blood is used, it provides glucose citrate, liver-dependent clotting factors and very low density lipoproteins as well as other factors. These may play a role in correcting the ultrastructure

TABLE 8.7
Investigations Required to Monitor Progress

Serum sodium, potassium, chloride, bicarbonate magnesium, calcium and phosphate determinations	Prothrombin time
Blood sugar	SGOT (AST)
Serum osmolality	SGPT (ALT)
Blood gas and hydrogen ion concentration	Creatinin phosphokinase
Haemoglobin, total white blood count, platelet count	Ammonia

abnormalities in Reye's syndrome and in causing an improvement in the patient's clinical condition with exchange transfusion. Early diagnosis, careful medical support on the lines detailed above and exchange transfusion using a volume of blood equivalent to twice the total blood volume, is used as an integral part of therapy in one experienced unit with 100 per cent survival rate in 27 patients with Grade IV severity and with 15 who had Grade III severity.

Because of the intramitochondrial block in the urea cycle the production of L-citrulline is limited. The administration of this amino-acid has therefore been advocated to try to promote the extramito-chondrial conversion of ammonia to urea. It has yet to be shown that this agent has any effect on the disease.

Repeated and frequent clinical and biochemical assessment (*Tables 8.6 and 8.7*) is necessary to monitor the course of the disease, the response to treatment and to detect and correct biochemical abnormalities.

BIBLIOGRAPHY AND REFERENCES

Bobo, R.C., Schubert, W.K., Partin, J.C. and Partin, J.S. (1975). Reye's syndrome: treatment by exchange transfusion with special reference to the 1974 epidemic in Cincinnati, Ohio. *J. Pediat.* **87**, 881

Bove, K.E., McAdams, J., Partin, J.C., Partin, J.S., Hug, G. and Schubert, W.K. (1975). The hepatic lesion in Reye's syndrome. *Gastroenterology* **69**, 685

Brain, W.R., Hunter, D. and Turnbull, W.M. (1929). Acute meningoencephalitis in childhood. *Lancet* **1**, 221

Reye, R.D.K., Morgan, G. and Baral, J. (1963). Encephalopathy and fatty degeneration of the viscera: a disease entity in childhood. *Lancet* **2**, 749

Reye's syndrome (1975). Proceedings of a Symposium: Diagnosis, Pathology, Aetiology and Management, p. 1–470. Ed. by Pollack, D.J. (Over 450 references.) New York: Grune and Stratton

Shaywitz, B.A., Leventhal, J.M., Kramer, M.S. and Vanes, J.L. (1977). Long continuous monitoring of intracranial pressure in severe Reye's syndrome. *Pediatrics* **59**, 595

Thaler, M.M. (1976). Reye's syndrome: cause and affect relationships. In *Liver Disease in Infancy and Childhood*, p. 72. Ed. by Berenberg, S.R. The Hague: Martinus Neijhoff Medical Division

CHAPTER 9

Liver Disorders Caused by Drugs or Toxins

Definition

Liver damage may be attributed to a drug or toxin, as follows.

(1) When the agent produces liver disorder at a constant time after exposure to the drug has started and in a predictable dose-related fashion.

(2) In the case of drugs which cause liver disease in only a proportion of individuals taking the drug, the liver disorder regresses when the agent is withdrawn and recurs when it is reintroduced (other causes of liver disease having been excluded).

The second part of this definition is rarely completely applicable. The hepatic reaction is frequently indistinguishable from viral hepatitis (HBs Ag negative) of which there is no readily available test. There is no specific test for drug-induced hepatic injury. In practice, the clinician must be aware that certain drugs have been incriminated in causing a wide range of hepatic disorders and that sporadic unexplained liver disease could be due to drugs. Having identified a possible drug cause, the only safe course is to stop the drug and not use it again.

A vast majority of drugs and toxins are capable of causing liver injury (*Tables 9.1 and 9.2*): 8 per cent of drug reactions reported to the Committee on Safety of Medicines in Britain were of jaundice; 5 per cent of drug exposures are complicated by adverse reactions; in 1 per cent of these reactions hepatic failure occurs.

The great susceptibility of the liver to injury has a number of possible causes; its strategic position astride the portal blood exposing

TABLE 9.1
Drugs Causing Liver Damage

Antibiotics	*Analgesic and anti-inflammatory agents*
Tetracycline	Phenylbutazone
Erythromycin estolate	Indomethacin
Nitrofurantoin	Paracetamol
Ampicillin	Aspirin
Sulphonamides	Dextropropoxyphene
Lincomycin	Ibuprofen
Anti-tuberculous drugs	*Anti-thyroid drugs*
PAS	Methimazole
Isoniazid	Carbimazole
Rifampicin	Thiouracil
Pyrazinamide	
Ethionamide	
Ethambutol	
Anti-metabolites	*Beta-adrenergic blockers*
Methotrexate	
6-mercaptopurine	Propranolol
Azathioprine	Oxprenolol
Anaesthetics	
Halothane	
Chloroform	
	Oral hypoglycaemic agents
	Chlorpropamide
	Tolbutamide
Anti-convulsants and anti-depressants	
Phenobarbitone	*Other agents*
Diphenylhydantion	Methyltestosterone
Trimethadione	Anabolic steroids
Chloridiazepoxide	Methyldopa
Tricyclic anti-depressants,	Oxyphenisatin
(e.g. amitriptyline)	Intravenous nutrients
Monamine oxidase inhibitors,	
(e.g. Iproniazid)	
Phenothiazine	

it to absorbed materials; its ability to concentrate drugs; its importance in their metabolism and excretion. The end-product of metabolism is usually a water-soluble product which can be excreted in bile and urine. The metabolic changes within the liver may convert a drug from a toxic to a non-toxic state or vice versa. This ability can be modified by drugs such as phenobarbitone, alcohol, rifampicin, which non-specifically alter the concentration of drug metabolizing enzymes in the liver.

Lower incidence in children

The slightly lower activity of these drug metabolizing enzymes in children may account for the less frequent recognition of drug-related liver disease in childhood. Less preoccupation with health, absence of self-prescription of drugs, and of drug dependence as well as less alcohol intake, may be more important causes of the lower incidence than any

TABLE 9.2
Poisons Affecting the Liver

Biological	Chemical	Physical
Aflatoxin	Carbon tetrachloride	Hyperthermia
Senecio alkaloids	Tetrachlorethane	Burns
Hypoglycins (Ackee fruit)	Chlorophenithone (DDT)	Irradiation
Amanita mushrooms	Benzine derivatives	
Crotolaria	Trinitrotoluene	
Lupinous	Tannic acid	
Heletropium	Phosphorus	
	Iron	
	Beryllium	
	? Arsenic	

TABLE 9.3
Hepatic Reactions to Drugs or Poisons

Clinico-pathological features	Example of drug or poison
Cholestasis without cellular change	Anabolic steroids
Hepatocellular necrosis:	
Direct	Tetracycline
Metabolite related	Paracetamol
Metabolite + immunological mechanism	Isoniazid
Cholestatic hepatitis	Phenothiazines
Venous thrombosis	Senecio, irradiation
Increased fibrosis	Methetrexate
Chronic active hepatitis	Methyldopa
Fibrosis and angiosarcoma	Vinyl chloride
Adenoma and carcinoma	Anabolic steroids
Gallstones	Oral contraceptives

intrinsic biological reason. Enzyme induction can increase or decrease the toxicity of drugs. Enzyme induction can occur from the effect of such environmental factors as DDT and other insecticides. Thus, drugs and environmental factors must be considered in all types of unexplained liver disease.

The degree of injury (*Table 9.3*) varies from alteration of only one metabolic function without structural change; from asymptomatic elevation of transaminases to fulminant hepatic necrosis; from increased fibrosis to malignant change. Because liver injury may progress to chronic liver disease, fulminant hepatic failure, cirrhosis or malignancy, it is vital to take a complete history of all possible toxins and drugs in isolated sporadic liver disease of unknown cause.

Patterns of liver injury (pathology of suspected mechanisms)

Cholestasis without cellular change

17-Alpha-alkyl-substituted steroids such as methyltestosterone, anabolic steroids such as norethandrone, and oestrogens cause cholestasis without any hepatocellular necrosis or cellular change in the portal tract. The disorder appears to be rare and may only occur in those with a genetic predisposition. The mode of action is not known but it is thought to be because these agents cause a decrease in bile-salt-dependent bile flow. There is complete recovery when the drug is withdrawn.

Hepatocellular damage due to direct cytotoxic injury

A wide range of hepatic cellular injury has been associated with drugs. The exact pathogenesis is frequently unknown. While certain patterns of injury can be recognized, pathologically and clinically, there is often considerable overlap.

Hepatocellular necrosis may occur as the result of a drug or its metabolites interfering directly with a vital function within the cell or by damaging intracellular membrane. Necrosis occurs without much inflammatory cell infiltration as, for example, in paracetamol over-dosage and with carbon tetrachloride. The earliest change seen is an inhibition of protein synthesis associated with a fragmentation of the endoplasmic reticulum and mitochondrial injury leading to a loss of energy.

Fat accumulates and as the effects of injury become more widespread within the cell, lysosomal membranes disintegrate releasing hydrolytic enzymes. General cell lysis follows. With some drugs such injury is proportional with dose and duration of administration occurring within days of starting the drug and can be reproduced in man and experimental animals. With drugs or poisons causing direct injury it may be possible to demonstrate the drug in tissue or body fluids.

In other instances, the pathological process is more complex, with *immunological mechanisms* playing a part in cell damage. The drug or one of its metabolites may change cell membranes so that they become immuno-reactive. It is postulated, for example, that isoniazid and methyldopa, both of which cause temporary elevation of transaminases with mild hepatocellular necrosis in up to 10 per cent of individuals, cause liver injury only in those subjects who mount an inappropriate immunological response. With such drugs, significant liver disease rarely starts until the drug has been taken for three weeks and may not occur for as late as 12 months. The pathological changes within the liver can range from classical centrilobular necrosis, as occurs with paracetamol, to a subacute or chronic aggressive hepatitis, or even a periportal necrosis, for example, caused by methyldopa. The concomitant administration of drugs which induce microsomal enzymes involved in drug metabolism may increase the frequency and severity of such liver injury, for example, when rifampicin is given with izoniazid.

Some drugs appear to produce a predominantly *cholestatic* picture with an inflammatory infiltrate in widened portal tracts. There may be a high proportion of eosinophils in the infiltrate. There is only slight oedema and slight bile duct proliferation. Cholestasis is mainly centralobular and is usually not accompanied by much liver cell necrosis or inflammatory cell infiltrate. The liver cells, however, may be swollen and show variation in nuclear size.

Portal tract reaction tends to fade after a few weeks but in some instances appearances are those of chronic aggressive hepatitis. In other patients granulomata may appear in the portal tracts.

Hepatocellular damage may also occur with features of *generalized hypersensitivity*. Fever, arthralgia, rash and eosinophilia with sometimes generalized lymph gland enlargement precede the onset of liver disease. The hepatic reaction may be predominantly of hepatocellular necrosis with cellular infiltrate. Occasionally granulomata will occur. The mechanism of this liver injury is imperfectly understood.

In adults, further pathological changes have been reported. Androgens and oral contraceptives have been implicated in causing adenomas and hepatocellular *carcinoma*. Increased hepatic *fibrosis* and cirrhosis has followed the use of methotrexate for psoriasis and leukaemia. Hepatic fibrosis and angiosarcoma have occurred following ingestion of arsenic, inhalation of vinyl chloride and Thorotrast injection.

Clinical features

The essential clinical feature is a history of exposure to a toxin or drug. This may have occurred on only one occasion as, for example, with paracetamol overdosage; continuously for from 3 to 52 weeks, for example, with isoniazid; or at intervals of months or years, as with halothane. The liver disorder may mimic almost any form of hepatic disease in childhood. Frequently there is a period of vague malaise or anorexia or even abdominal pain. Rash, fever, eosinophilia and other blood dyscrasia may occur when hypersensitivity is a mechanism of liver damage. There may be other toxic effects on other organs such as kidney, gastrointestinal tract, bone marrow or brain, which overshadow the hepatic features. The hepatic features are thus those of the whole range of liver damage considered in the section on pathology above. A list of drugs which have been associated with liver disease in children is given in *Table 9.1*. Toxins which may be responsible are given in *Table 9.2*.

Treatment

The drug under suspicion must be withdrawn, and other causes of hepatic injury must be considered. There are no specific measures which can be taken; supportive care and symptomatic treatment may be required depending on the severity of the liver damage and/or damage to other organs. If pruritus is severe, cholestyramine may be helpful. There are no specific agents which mitigate the toxic effects of the drugs listed in *Table 9.2*. Cysteamine may be of value in preventing liver damage to paracetamol overdosage, but if it does it must be given within ten hours of ingestion before liver damage is apparent.

Particular clinical features of liver diseases caused by hepatotoxic drugs commonly used in children are considered below. The examples chosen also exemplify the difficulties in relating liver disease to drugs and some of the important clinical implications.

HALOTHANE-RELATED HEPATITIS (unexplained hepatitis following halothane)

The title of this section typifies the controversy surrounding the association between the use of halothane as an anaesthetic agent and subsequent liver disease. All concede that in a few individuals hepatocellular damage with a characteristic constellation of features, such as fever and eosinophilia before the onset of liver damage, has been provoked by deliberate exposure to halothane, sometimes in minute quantities. Anaesthetists concede that halothane causes some cases of hepatitis following exposure to this anaesthetic but argue that many cases have other possible explanations and that this drug is one of the safest anaesthetic agents available. Hepatologists, on the other hand, see patients with liver disease who give a history of repeated exposure to halothane, particularly within a period of less than 28 days.

Clinical features

Typically, 8–13 days after the anaesthetic the patient develops fever anorexia and malaise. Jaundice may subsequently develop 2–15 days later. In other instances, the history is obtained of post-operative fever, for which no explanation has been forthcoming, but has been followed by another exposure to halothane where fever occurs nearer the time of administration of the anaesthetic and is rapidly followed by jaundice. Hepatocellular necrosis is much more frequent after multiple anaesthetics.

The total white count is usually normal but there may be an absolute eosinophilia in the peripheral blood and there is often an excess of eosinophils in the liver biopsy. It is stated that if the jaundice occurs the mortality for this condition is 20 per cent.

HEPATITIS DUE TO ANTI-TUBERCULOUS DRUGS

Tuberculosis is probably the commonest condition in which paediatric patients develop signs of liver damage which can be confidently attributed to drugs. Streptomycin is the only commonly used antituberculous drug which has not been associated with hepatic injury. The range of injury extends from slight asymptomatic rises in the serum transaminases to fulminant hepatic necrosis. In most instances, the patient has been receiving more than one drug in order to minimize the risks of possible bacterial resistance to the antibiotics.

Isoniazid becomes hepatotoxic when it is acetylated. Hepatotoxicity is more likely to occur when the rate of acetylation is increased as may occur for genetic reasons, or be caused by drugs which induce the acetylating enzymes. Amongst these are rifampicin and phenobarbitone. Approximately 10 per cent of individuals receiving isoniazid develop asymptomatic elevation of these serum transaminases and mild hepatitis. These abnormalities settle in the vast majority over the course of two–three weeks, but in a few patients the liver function tests remain abnormal. If this occurs, or the transaminase elevation is greater than six times normal, or if jaundice develops, the drug must be stopped.

A boy aged 12 years was admitted to hospital with a four-week history of fever, lassitude, anorexia and cough. A chest radiograph showed extensive consolidation of the right middle lobe and a right-sided pleural effusion. The total white blood count was 3,500 with 80 per cent polymorphonuclear neutrophil leucocytes. No acid-fast bacilli could be found in the sputum (culture was subsequently positive for *Mycobacterium tuberculosis*), but later acid-fast bacilli were recovered from the sputum of one of five siblings who had had a productive cough for eight weeks. Anti-tuberculous therapy was therefore commenced with rifampicin 20 mg/kg of bodyweight per day, isoniazid 20 mg/kg per day, ethambutol 25 mg/ kg per day and pyradoxine 50 mg per day. The patient's clinical condition improved over the next 48 hours and the fever settled completely in seven days. Thereafter he made a progressive gain in weight and remained asymptomatic but the hepatic problems developed summarized in *Table 9.4*. The patient and his parents were reluctant to use streptomycin by intramuscular injection. It was for that reason that a test dose of rifampicin was given. This did produce a slight rise in the transaminase to 49 iu/litre but the significance of this was not certain. It was therefore recommended daily for a week with checks of liver function tests on every second day. The transaminase rose significantly. The parents therefore accepted the necessity for intramuscular therapy. No liver biopsy was performed, the child had a normal cerebrospinal fluid and had no choroidal tubercles, but he may well have had tuberculosis in his liver.

Para-aminosalicylic acid causes fever, rash and lymphadenopathy in approximately 5 per cent of individuals; 2 per cent of these are likely to have a raised transaminase. If the drug is not withdrawn a fulminant hepatitis may appear with a mortality of 20 per cent.

Rifampicin causes asymptomatic rise in transaminases in 20 per cent of individuals, of whom 8 per cent become jaundiced. The hepatitis is usually mild and resolves when the drug is withdrawn. When two drugs are given together the incidence of asymptomatic elevation of transaminases and hepatitis increases. For example, in patients treated with izoniazid and rifampicin, 35 per cent develop raised transaminases. Some of these will be self-limited but a small percentage do go on to significant hepatitis. Ethambutol and izoniazid together cause elevated aspartate transaminases in some 12 per cent of individuals. Pyrazinamide and ethionamide cause hepatitis in between 5 and

TABLE 9.4

Anti-tuberculous drugs	Days since onset of therapy	Bilirubin μmol/litre (N<20)	A.S.T. iu/litre (N<40)	Prolongation of prothrombin time (N<3 seconds)
Ethambutol				
Rifampicin	1	NT	NT	NT
Isoniazid				
	3	30	62	NT
	16	190	160	16
	19	210	154	19
Rifampicin and isoniazid stopped	23	195	118	19
	24	195	56	0
	43	26	29	0
Test dose of rifampicin	50			
	54	18	49	0
Rifampicin daily for 1 week	56			
	63	20	152	4
Rifampicin stopped and streptomycin added	90	<10	40	0

NT = Not tested

10 per cent of recipients. It should be noted that isoniazid, pyrazinamide and ethionamide are chemically related and if one causes hepatic toxicity, the others should not be used.

Management

Should liver damage occur in a patient with tuberculosis on anti-tuberculous treatment, the tuberculosis may be considered so severe that therapy must be continued. Streptomycin and either ethambutol, cycloserine, or capromycin which have little propensity for liver damage, should be given.

If the tuberculosis seems well controlled, all drugs may be stopped and the patient watched until the transaminase returns to normal. A single test dose of one of the agents should then be given and liver function tests repeated every second day for one week. If no abnormalities are observed a full dose is given for a further week while monitoring of liver function tests is continued. This procedure is then repeated with each of the drugs under suspicion. When the offending agent has been identified it is best excluded from therapy but if it has to be used, disensitization with very small doses which are gradually increased if tolerated, may be successful.

IRRADIATION HEPATITIS

The liver is relatively resistant to damage by irradiation. There is circumstantial evidence in man that irradiation given following cytotoxic drugs may be more injurious with damage likely to follow doses in excess of 2,000 rad.

Pathology

The essential area of damage appears to be in the venous walls. There is a loosely arranged fibroblastic reaction which spreads to the endothelium causing venous obstruction. Liver biopsy therefore shows extreme hepatic congestion with dilated sinusoids and haemorrhage into the walls of hepatic veins. There may be loss of hepatocytes and reticulum collapse, particularly around the central area. The liver is frequently reduced in size. When healing occurs there is marked fibrosis occasionally with cirrhosis and portal hypertension.

Clinical features

Clinical features of liver injury may appear at between seven days and five months following irradiation. In acute cases there may be fever, anorexia, vomiting followed by the rapid onset of jaundice and ascites. Biochemical investigations show raised transaminases with low serum albumin and elevated prothrombin time. Liver scan shows decreased liver size and reduced hepatic uptake. In some instances the onset is insidious with hepatomegaly being a striking feature. Biochemical features may be less severe, but follow a similar pattern. The disease may proceed to total hepatocellular necrosis but more commonly over the course of three to four weeks, liver function improves and returns to normal over three to four months. There may, however, be persistent reduction in the size of the right lobe and compensatory hypertrophy of the left. Portal hypertension may develop.

BIBLIOGRAPHY

Berthelot, P. (1973). Mechanisms and prediction of drug-induced liver disease. *Gut* 14, 332

Harris, F., Cullity, G. and Lister, J. (1974). Hepatitis following actinomycin D and radiation. *Proc.R.Soc.Med.* 67, 26

Maxwell, J.D. and Williams, R. (1973). Drug induced jaundice. *Br.J.Hosp.Med.* 9, 193

McIntosh, S., Davidson, D.L., O'Brien, R.T. and Pearson, H.A. (1977). Methotrexate hepatotoxicity in children with leukaemia. *J. Pediat.* 90, 1019

Mitchell, J.R. and Jollow, D.J. (1975). Metabolic activation of drugs and toxic substances. *Gaestroentrology* 69, 392

Pessarye, D. *et al.* (1977). Isobiazid-rifampicin fulminant hepatitis: a possible consequence of enhancement of isoniazid hepatotoxicity by enzyme induction. *Gastroenterology* 72, 284

Ruymann, F.B., Mosijczuk, A.D. and Sayers, R.J. (1977). Hepatoma in a child with methotrexate-induced hepatic fibrosis. *J.Am.med.Ass.* 238, 2631

Tolman, K.G. (1977). Drugs and the liver. *Med. J. Austr.* 2, 655

Walton, B., Simpson, B.R., Strunin, L., Doniach, D., Perrin, J. and Appleyard, J. (1976). Unexplained hepatitis following halothane. *Br. med. J.* 1, 1171

CHAPTER 10

Inborn Errors of Metabolism Causing Hepatomegaly or Disordered Liver Function

This chapter is restricted to inborn errors of metabolism in which hepatomegaly and/or disturbance of liver function are part of the clinical syndrome but rarely cause major clinical problems. The emphasis will be on diagnosis with only sufficient biochemical details to assist in this and to provide a rational basis for therapy.

GLYCOGEN STORAGE DISEASES

Definition

Glycogen storage diseases (GSD) are inherited metabolic disorders in which the concentration and/or molecular structure of glycogen is abnormal in any tissue of the body. Liver, heart, skeletal muscle, kidney, bones and brain may be involved. In most of these disorders there is excess glycogen but deficient storage can occur. Data at present available indicate that these disorders are inherited in an autosomal recessive fashion, one varient being possibly X linked.

Biochemistry

Glycogen is formed from glucose postprandially and is broken down during periods of fasting to maintain the blood glucose level within a strict range. The core of the glycogen molecule is glucose units linked in an α 1—4 configuration, with branching side chains linked in an α 1—6 fashion after every 4, α 1—4 linkages. A large molecule, with molecular weight between 6 and 60 millions, with multiple branches is formed. Glycogen is stored in the cytoplasm primarily in hepatic and muscle cells. It is metabolized also in lysosomes. Liver glycogen is broken down to glucose. Muscle glycogen is metabolized to lactic acid or carbon dioxide and water. Many enzymes are involved in glycogen synthesis and breakdown. Some of those steps are indicated in *Figure 10.1*. It is likely that other steps have yet to be identified.

Since the biochemical and pathological features, including the long-term prognosis and to some extent treatment, are dependent on which enzymatic activity is defective or deficient, glycogen storage diseases are now classified according to which enzyme, and organ, shows defective activity. Not all disorders can be so classified, however.

In a detailed study of 23 patients with glycogen storage disease, six showed no demonstrable enzymatic defect, three having clinical features of Type I glycogen storage disease, two were Type III GSD, and 1 Type VI GSD (Spencer-Peet *et al.*, 1971). Hug (1976) also

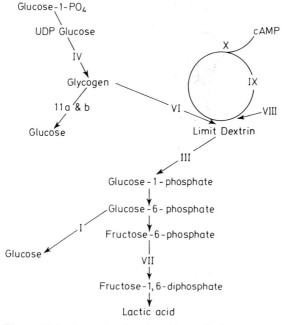

Figure 10.1. Steps in the formation of glycogen and glycolysis. Numbers in roman figures indicate the type of glycogenosis in which this metabolic step is ineffective

TABLE 10.1

Hepatic Involvement in Glycogen Storage Disease

Type	Hepatomegaly	Splenomegaly	Aspartate transaminase	Biopsy	Fibrosis	Cirrhosis
I	+ (Hepatoma)	–	Usually normal	Uniform hepatocellular distension with glycogen, except where interrupted by lipid vacuoles. Mosaic appearance due to cellular enlargement with collapse of sinusoids	0	0
II	+	0	Usually normal	Liver cells are mildly distended with glycogen in membrane-bound vacuoles	0	0
III	+	Rare	Always raised (normal in adults)	As in Type I	+	±
IV	+	+	Raised	Pale amphophilic hyaline material in cytoplasm throughout lobule. It may have a fibrillary birefringent appearance. Cryostat sections stain blue with Lugol's iodine due to amylopectin content	+	+

V	0	Raised	Normal	0	0
VI	+	Raised	Irregular sized hepatocytes with maximal distension by glycogen at periphery of hepatic lobule	+	0
VII	0	0	Normal	0	0
VIII	+	Raised	More irregular distension of hepatocytes by glycogen than seen in Type VI	0	0
IX	+ (normal in adults)	Raised	As in Type VI	+	0
X	+	Raised	As in Type VI	+	0

included a category described as pseudo GSD Type I with normal glucose-6-phosphatase activity and a further group with similar clinical features and a Fanconi syndrome, but no enzymatic defect.

Since many glycogen storage diseases are indistinguishable clinically, precise biochemical diagnosis using biopsy specimens is essential if new modes of treatment are to be advised and assessed. Such diagnosis is beyond the scope of all but a few laboratories. If meticulous care and attention to detail is used specimens can be transported, after due consultation, to distant laboratories with diagnostic facilities. Percutaneous liver biopsy will often yield enough tissue for diagnosis particularly if the amount of tissue used for histological diagnosis is limited. This is best done by cutting cryostat sections of frozen unfixed tissue to provide a few thin sections for histology, while the remainder of the tissue can be used for biochemical studies.

A wide spectrum of clinical severity can occur within each category. Different types are frequently clinically indistinguishable. Current classifications, particularly for the rarer disorders, are likely to be modified as these are further characterized biochemically. In some families more than one enzymatic activity has been shown to be decreased. This increasingly complex classification does not immediately commend itself to the clinician, but it is essential if appropriate treatment is to be given and, more importantly, if inappropriate and possibly injurious treatment is to be withheld.

Clinical features

Glycogen storage disorders must be considered in any infant or child who presents with hepatomegaly, or with cardiac, muscular or neurological dysfunction. Symptoms often start at birth or soon afterwards. The presenting feature may be disturbed behaviour due to hypoglycaemia, or hepatomegaly. The large liver, which may extend to the iliac crest, is typically smooth with only minimal increase in firmness. If hypoglycaemia is severe or persistent, convulsions and mental retardation may occur. Acidosis, vomiting and diarrhoea are prominent in some patients. Failure to thrive is usual. Malabsorption may occur. As the patient becomes older, short stature and adiposity with particularly fat cheeks is a striking feature. In some patients xanthoma develop. Gouty tophi occur. The hepatomegaly becomes less prominent throughout childhood especially in Type VI disease. By adolescence the liver may not be palpably enlarged. Metabolic disorders other than hyperuricaemia also becomes less troublesome with increasing age. Hepatic features are summarized in *Table 10.1*.

Biochemical abnormalities

Hypoglycaemia on fasting is a feature of nearly all GSD's. Hyperlipidaemia is marked in Types I and II and to a lesser extent in all other hepatic forms. Lactic and pyruvic acid are frequently elevated in Type I in the fasting state. Uric acid may be raised. Raised serum transaminases are frequently found (*Table 10.1*). Carbohydrate tolerance tests with glucose, galactose, fructose, insulin or epinephrine are potentially dangerous. As they are frequently uninformative or give equivocal results they are best omitted. Glucagon given intravenously in a dose of 0.7 mg/m^2 with determination of blood sugar at 15 minute intervals, to 60 minutes, and then at 90 and 120 minutes, tests the amount of glycogen stored and the ability to release it. It is usual to fast the children for 10–12 hours before the test, but when severe hypoglycaemia occurs after a short fast, the test may have to be made three or four hours after a meal. In normal patients a rise of > 35 mg/100 ml in the first hour is found. The rise in blood sugar is less in GSD Type I and GSD Type III (in the fasting state). In GSD Type VI the response is often decreased but not invariably so.

Diagnosis

The diagnosis of glycogen storage disease is suspected on the basis of the clinical findings. Hypoglycaemia on fasting is important supporting evidence. Diminished response of blood sugar to glycogen also supports the diagnosis. In GSD Types III and VII erythrocyte glycogen is increased. Specific enzyme defects *may* be demonstrated in leucocytes in Types II, III, IV, VI and IX. If these investigations are not diagnostic, and if clinical features are sufficiently severe to merit trials of therapy, muscle and percutaneous liver biopsy as indicated in *Table 10.2* are necessary.

Treatment

GSD Type 1 Hypoglycaemia must be prevented by frequent meals. Carbohydrate in the form of glucose, D-maltose or starch is used. Fructose and galactose are omitted since either may aggravate lacticaemia. The protein content of the diet is normal, the fat content low, but calories are appropriate for height and weight. Bicarbonate may be required for acidosis. Allopurinol in a dose of 10–20 mg/kg of bodyweight per day may be required if the serum uric acid becomes elevated.

In some infants, hypoglycaemia and acidosis are intractable. Diazoxide starting with a dose of 5 mg/kg of bodyweight per day divided into three doses and increased according to the blood sugar response may control the hypoglycaemia. Chlorothiazide in a dose of 10 mg/kg per day may increase the effect of diazoxide.

TABLE 10.2
Enzymatic Classification of Glycogen Storage Diseases

Type	Enzymatic activity decreased or absent	Affected tissue	Diagnostic tissues
I	Glucose 6-phosphatase	Liver, kidney, intestine	Liver
II	Lysosomal $\gamma-1$, 4 & $\gamma1$, 6 glucosidase	All tissues	Leucocyte, liver or muscle
III	Amylo$-1-6$ glucosidase ($\pm$ phosphorylase kinase deficiency)	Liver, muscle, heart in various combinations	Leucocyte, liver or muscle
IV	Amylo$-1-4\rightarrow1-6$ transferase	? Generalized (abnormal glycogen)	Leucocytes, liver
V	Phosphorylase	Muscle only	Muscle
VI	Liver phosphorylase deficiency (as opposed to complete absence)	Liver	Leucocytes, liver
VII	Phosphofructokinase	Muscle and erythrocytes	Erythrocyte and muscle
VIII	?Inactive liver phosphorylase (normal activating system)	Liver, brain	Liver
IX	Liver phosphorylase kinase	Liver	Erythrocyte, leucocyte, liver
X	Cyclic 3, 5 AMP-dependent kinase	Liver, muscle	Liver, muscle

Side-effects such as hypotension and exacerbation of hyperuricaemia can be troublesome but often the degree of control achieved corrects the metabolic tendency to hyperuricaemia. In some instances, continuous naso-gastric feeding or even intravenous feeding may be necessary to control hypoglycaemia. In intractable cases, portocaval shunting has been performed to improve metabolic control. In older children continuous naso-gastric feeding even intravenous feeding, and porto-caval anastomosis have been used to promote growth in stunted children. There are considerable technical difficulties with all of these and results cannot be predicted.

Other GSD's In GSD's Types III, IX and X, the blood sugar can only be maintained with frequent feeding of a diet rich in carbohydrate. In Type IV disease frequent feeding is also necessary but the diet may contain rather more protein since gluconeogenesis is unimpaired. In all of these disorders hypoglycaemia and acidosis are less difficult to control than in GSD Type I. In GSD Types II, IV and VIII there is, at present, no effective treatment.

HEPATIC INVOLVEMENT IN DIABETES MELLITUS

Carbohydrate is stored in the liver in the form of glycogen. Complex carbohydrate storage disorders associated with hepatomegaly are listed in *Table 10.3*. In health, glycogen is broken down into glucose and helps to maintain the blood sugar in narrow range during fasting or excessive utilization. In diabetes mellitus, if control of blood sugar is poor, excessive glycogen is deposited in the liver causing hepato-megaly. The liver is typically soft and enlargement may be missed without careful examination. The amount of glycogen stored may surpass that found in the liver in glycogen storage disease. In part, the excess of glycogen deposition may arise because of a failure to release glucose. Intravenous administration of exogenous glucagon frequently causes a less marked rise in blood sugar than occurs in normal individuals.

Hepatomegaly in diabetes occurs both as an acute phenomenon, for example in diabetic ketosis, and also as a chronic abnormality when diabetic control is persistently poor. In acute hyperglycaemia with diabetic ketosis the liver may enlarge so rapidly as to cause abdominal pain, usually attributed to stretching of the liver capsule.

Poor diabetic control and persistent hepatomegaly may be associated with growth retardation. In severe cases, a protuberant abdomen, moon-shaped face and fat deposition on the shoulders and abdomen complete the full *Mauriac syndrome*. With more satisfactory 24 hour control of diabetes by dietary means and long-acting or twice-daily soluble insulin, this syndrome is now distinctly rare, but is unfortunately not extinct (*see* page 196).

Social and educational factors — affecting the child, the family and what is euphemistically described as Health Care Services — were

TABLE 10.3

Complex Carbohydrate Storage Disorders Causing Hepatomegaly

Disorder	Material stored	Enzyme deficient	Age at onset	Splenomegaly	Other clinical features	Diagnostic investigations
Mucopolysaccharidosis I (Hurler)	Heparin and dermatan sulphates	Alpha-L-iduronidase	6–18 months	Moderate	Cloudy cornea, gibbus, joint deformity, respiratory infections, progressive mental deterioration	Dermatan and heparin sulphate in urine or enzyme deficiency in leucocytes
II (Hunter)	Heparin and dermatan sulphates	Sulpho-iduronate sulphatase	1–3 years	Moderate	As in Type I but no corneal clouding	Dermatan and heparin sulphate in urine
III (San Filippo)	Heparin sulphate	Not known	1–3 years	Minimal	As in Type I but mental retardation is extremely marked	Heparin sulphate in urine
IV (Maroteaux-Lamy)	Dermatan sulphate	Arylsulphatase B	1–3 years	Minimal	Growth retardation, skeletal abnormalities, corneal opacities, normal intelligence	Dermatan sulphate in urine
Oligosaccharide storage disorders						
Mannosidosis	Manno-rich oligosaccharides	Acid alpha-mannosidase	12–18 months	Moderate	Psychomotor retardation, coarse facies, skeletal abnormalities, lens opacities, vacuolated lymphocytes	Deficient enzymatic activity in leucocytes

considered responsible for the high incidence of this syndrome in a recent series in North-East England (Court, 1978). In some patients, the syndrome arises because of the nature of the diabetes in the individual patient, rather than because of any observed environmental factor.

In adult patients cirrhosis has been found more frequently in patients with diabetes, but no specific cause for the cirrhosis has ever been associated with diabetes and the apparent association may be spurious.

LIPID STORAGE DISORDERS

Definition

Lipid storage disorders are a genetically determined group of disorders in which fatty acids, cholesterol or complex lipids are abnormally stored. Those considered in this chapter are believed to be inherited in an autosomal recessive fashion, with the possible exception of some cases of Gaucher's disease which may be inherited in an autosomal dominant fashion with incomplete penetrance.

Biochemistry

Compound lipids may be classified into main types; as follows.

Glycerophosphate   In these a single fatty acid residue in a triglyceride is replaced by phosphate which is linked with choline to form phosphatidyl choline or lethicin or is complexed with ethanoalamine to form phosphatidyl ethanoalamine or (cephalins).

Sphingolipids   Sphingosine rather than glycerol is the basic molecule. When complexed with a fatty acid, this is termed a ceramide.

		Choline + phosphoric acid	→	Sphingomyelin
		Hexose or trisaccharide	→	Cerebroside
Ceramide	+	Galactose + sulphuric acid	→	Sulphatide
		N-acetyl galactosamine + glucose + galactose	→	Gangliosides

Clinical features

Although hepatomegaly and/or splenomegaly are prominent features

TABLE 10.4

Lipid Storage Disorders causing Hepatomegaly

Disorder	Material stored	Enzyme deficient	Age at onset	Splenomegaly	Other clinical features	Diagnostic investigations
Tay-Sachs disease	Ganglioside G_{m2}	Ganglioside G_{m2}, hexosaminidase (hexosaminidase A)	1st year, 5–10 years, 10 years	Absent	Dementia, tetraplegia, cherry-red spot in macula	Enzyme deficient in serum and leucocytes
G_{m1} Gangliosidosis Type 1	Ganglioside G_{m1}	β Galactosidases	Infancy	Absent	Motor and mental retardation	Enzyme deficient in leucocytes
Gaucher's disease	Glucosyl ceramide	Glucosyl ceramide β glucosidase	Acute in Infancy, chronic in later childhood	Marked	Skin pigmentation, bone and lung involvement, hypersplenism	Enzyme deficient in leucocytes, bone marrow or liver biopsy
Neimann–Pick's disease	Sphingomyelin	Sphingomyelinase	Infancy	Moderate	Convulsions, blindness, tetraplegia, pulmonary infiltration	Enzyme deficient in leucocytes
Fucosidosis	Fucose containing glycolipids and polysaccharides	α Fucosidase	Childhood	Moderate	Dementia, spasticity, cardiomyopathy	Enzyme deficient in leucocytes

Disease	Stored material	Enzyme	Age of onset		Clinical features	Laboratory findings
Wolman's disease	Cholesterol esters and triglycerides	Acid esterase	Infancy	Moderate	Vomiting, diarrhoea, developmental delay, calcified adrenals	Enzyme deficient in leucocytes, liver biopsy
Cholesterol ester storage disease	Cholesterol esters and triglycerides	Acid esterase	Late childhood	Moderate	Malabsorption	Enzyme deficient in leucocytes
Familial hyperlipoproteinaemia Type I	Fat	Lipoprotein lipase	1st decade	Absent	Xanthoma, abdominal pain, lipaemia retinalis	Massive chylomicronaemia
Type IV	Fat	Unknown	1st–3rd decade	Absent	Xanthoma and premature atherosclerosis	Very low density lipoproteins increased
Type V	Fat	Unknown	Usually adult life		Xanthoma and severe abdominal pain	Massive chylomicronaemia and very low density lipoproteins increased

in lipid storage disorders, gastrointestinal symptoms and hepatic dys-function are of little clinical significance in the majority of cases compared with nervous system involvement. These disorders do require consideration in the differential diagnosis of hepatomegaly. Clinical, biochemical, enzymatic and diagnostic information in the most important of these disorders is given in *Table 10.4*. A more detailed account is given here of gastrointestinal and hepatic aspects of clinical relevance.

Gaucher's disease

Gaucher's disease takes three main forms, as follows.

Type 1 describes a chronic non-neuropathic disorder, and has its onset at any time between birth and old age. Its rate of progression is very variable but frequently is slow.

Type 2 (acute neuronopathic) starts in the first six months of life and leads to a neurological death by the age of two years.

Type 3 (sub-acute neuronopathic) presents with visceral features but neurological features develop usually in the first five years of life and are gradually progressive thereafter. Death usually occurs in the third decade.

Gastrointestinal aspects

Groups of Gaucher cells – large, multinucleated cells with a reticular pale-staining cytoplasm – surround the central hepatic veins and obstruct liver capillaries. The liver architecture is often deranged and hepatic fibrosis may be severe. This may be complicated by portal hypertension and ascites in all three types of the disease.

Liver function tests are frequently abnormal but there is no specific pattern. Jaundice is not a feature. Hypersplenism eventually occurs in nearly all patients with Type 1 or Type 3 disease. It may be aggravated by an associated haemolytic anaemia or by displacement of erythrocyte precursors from the bone marrow by Gaucher's cells. Splenectomy may occasionally be indicated where features of hypersplenism are severe or where there are symptoms due to massive splenomegaly. Such procedure should only be undertaken after detailed investigation to exclude portal hypertension, hepatic fibrosis and other causes of anaemia. Although it may give relief from the haematological problems, splenectomy may aggravate deposition of ceramide in other vital tissues.

Niemann–Pick disease

In this disorder, sphingomyelin accumulates in the viscera or brain. Five distinct variants have been described on the basis of clinical features. These are summarized in *Table 10.5*. In Type A there is usually no clinical and biochemical evidence of visceral involvement. Two sibs, however, did have persistent jaundice and disruption of

TABLE 10.5
Sphingomyelin Storage Disorders

Type	Sphingomyelinease activity	Organ involved	Age of onset	Clinical features Course
A	Decreased	Brain	<6 months	Rapid deterioration – death at 2 years
B	Decreased	Viscera	Infancy or early childhood	Slowly progressive to death by the age of 10 years
C	Decreased or normal	Brain and viscera	1–6 years	Gradual deterioration to death by the age of 10 years
D	Normal	Viscera and brain	Infancy	Gradually progressive to death by the age of 10 years
E	Normal	Viscera	Infancy	Uncertain
With sea-blue histiocytes	Normal	Viscera and brain	Infancy and childhood	Persistent splenomegaly and progressive neurological deterioration between the ages of 8 and 20 years

liver architecture. In Type B there is hepatomegaly with raised transaminases and alkaline phosphatase but no other evidence of hepatic dysfunction. In Type D disease there is persistent jaundice and disruption of liver architecture.

Included with the Niemann–Pick disorders, but with a sphingomyelin which is different from that stored in Niemann–Pick disease is the disorder which is characterized by the sphingomyelin storage and the presence of sea-blue histiocytes in the bone marrow and liver. This condition is not as yet chemically characterized. It commonly presents as a conjugated hyperbilirubinaemia in the first six months of life. Jaundice persists for weeks or months, leaving a degree of hepatomegaly and splenomegaly. Histological examination of the liver shows considerable disruption of hepatic structure. Liver function tests commonly return towards normal.

The early sign of neurological involvement is loss of conjugate upward gaze. This is followed by progressive signs of neurological involvement.

Diagnosis

The diagnosis of sphingomyelin storage disorders is based on the finding of decreased sphingomyelinase activity in peripheral blood leucocytes, bone marrow or liver. Histological examination of the tissues shows accumulation of lipids, particularly within reticulo-endothelial cells. The lipid does, however, spread to parenchymal cells. The Niemann–Pick variant is characterized by the presence of such storage material and the presence of sea-blue histiocytes, particularly in the bone marrow and to a lesser extent in the liver.

Wolman's disease (acid esterase deficiency)

This disorder is due to a deficiency of lysosomal acid esterase resulting in an accumulation of cholesterol esters and triglycerides in many organs, particularly the liver and the intestinal mucosa. The liver is large, firm and yellow in colour. The parenchymal cells are engorged by membrane-lined vacuoles of different size. Foamy histiocytes with similar vacuoles are found in clumps, both in the portal areas and between parenchymal cells. There is an increase in portal fibrosis and cirrhosis may develop. There appear to be two main forms which commonly present in the first few months of life with vomiting, diarrhoea, hepatosplenomegaly, steatorrhoea and failure to thrive. Standard tests of liver function are abnormal; radiology of the abdomen shows adrenal calcification.

The clinical course is of progressive deterioration with death usually in the first year of life. In some cases there is very severe liver involvement with jaundice prior to death.

Some patients present in later childhood with hepatomegaly as the only clinical feature, although the biochemical abnormality appears to be similar.

There is, as yet, no specific treatment, although high cholesterol intake may be beneficial (West and Lloyd, 1977).

Hepatic cholesterol ester storage disease

This disorder is associated with a deficiency of acid esterase and results in an accumulation of cholesterol esters in liver, small intestinal mucosa and in the bone marrow. The liver is enlarged and yellow or orange in appearance. It is smooth and soft. All parenchymal cells are filled with lipid droplets which on frozen section stain positive with Sudan 3. Cytoplasm has a lace-work pattern. Rarely fibrosis and cirrhosis develop.

The clinical features are of asymptomatic hepatomegaly sometimes noticed in the first year of life, but in some cases first noticed as late as 19 years. There are no associated symptoms. Laboratory investigations usually show no abnormality but occasionally hyperlipidaemia may be found. Long-term prognosis is as yet uncertain. There is no specific treatment.

A-beta lipoproteinaemia

A-beta lipoproteinaemia is a genetic disorder in which the major defect is absence of plasma beta lipoprotein and complete inability to produce chylomicrons and very low density lipoproteins.

The pathological features are degenerative lesions of the spinal cord and cerebellum involving the spino-cerebellum tract, anterior columns, cerebellum nuclei and the macular area in the retina. Small gut biopsies show foamy changes in the epithelial cells of the villi.

The liver is said to be normal, but in some cases fatty changes have been shown and in one case cirrhosis had developed by the age of 30 months.

Clinical features

The disease is characterized by steatorrhoea, starting in the first months of life, progressive ataxia, and retinitis pigmentosa becoming detectable after the fifth year of life. Patients surviving until adult life may be severely physically and mentally handicapped.

Diagnosis

The diagnosis may be suspected by the finding of acanthocytosis in a fresh, wet, peripheral blood film. Serum cholesterol phospholipid and triglyceride levels are extremely low. Electrophoretic demonstration of lack of beta lipoprotein confirms the diagnosis.

Treatment

A low fat diet eliminates the steatorrhoea. Medium chain triglycerides have been used to improve fat absorption. The appearance of cirrhosis in one case has been speculatively linked with the use of this material.

HEREDITARY TYROSINAEMIA

Definition

This is a genetically determined clinical syndrome characterized by severe liver damage, a renal tubular defect and abnormal tyrosine metabolism. There is a generalized hyperamino-acidaemia with particularly raised levels of tyrosine, phenylalanine and methionine. There is excessive urinary excretion of tyrosine metabolites, particularly para-hydroxy-phenyl lactic acid (pHPLA), and para-hydroxy-phenyl acetic acid (pHPAA). Inheritance is in an autosomal recessive fashion.

Biochemistry

Tyrosine is derived from phenylalanine and dietary and tissue protein. The main metabolic products are shown in *Figure 10.2*. In hereditary tyrosinaemia there is deficient enzymatic acvitity converting para-hydroxy-phenyl pyruvic (pHPPA) acid to homogentistic acid. This may not be the primary abnormality. The exact cause of liver injury in tyrosinosis is not understood. The aromatic derivatives of tyrosine may be toxic to the liver but another suggestion is that the hyper-methioninaemia may be hepatotoxic.

Pathology

The liver is enlarged. Hepatocytes show intense fatty infiltration and hepatocellular necrosis in the acute stage. There is increased hepatic fibrosis which gradually progresses to cirrhosis in chronic cases. Regeneration nodules are prominent. Hepatoma may develop. In the kidney there is tubular degeneration. Islets of Langerhans may show hyperplasia. There may be degenerative changes in the basal ganglia of the brain.

Clinical features

An acute and a chronic form of the disorder are recognized. Both may occur in the same family.

In the acute form the onset is in the first two to six months of life with vomiting, diarrhoea, hepatosplenomegaly, oedema, ascites,

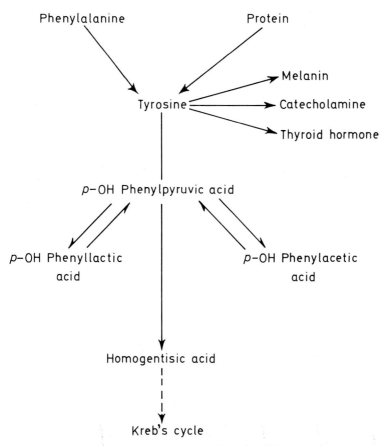

Figure 10.2. Tyrosine in plasma is derived from phenylalanine and tyrosine in dietary and tissue proteins. It is metabolized to melanin catecholamine and thyroid hormone. Catabolism to water and carbon dioxide via the pathway shown is defective in tyrosinaemia possibly due to reduced activity of the enzyme para-hydroxyphenylpyruvic acid oxidase. As a result, para-hydroxyphenylpyruvic para-hydroxyphenyllactic acid and para-hydroxyphenyl acetic acid accumulate in the tissues. These together with tyrosine and phenylalanine are also found in increased concentration in the urine

dyspnoea, a bleeding diathesis and failure to thrive. Jaundice occurs in about one-third of infants. When liver failure develops, deterioration is rapid and unaffected by treatment: 90 per cent of patients die.

The chronic form may continue from the acute illness or may present in later infancy or childhood with features due to cirrhosis and the renal tubular defect. This causes a hyperphosphaturic, hypophosphataemic rickets. Hypoglycaemia may occur in both forms of the disease. In the chronic form hepatic carcinoma can develop.

Laboratory findings

There is a generalized hyperamino-acidaemia with particularly high levels of tyrosine, proline, threonine and phenylalanine.

In the acute form methionine is also raised in most instances. The urine shows a generalized hyperaminoacidaemia but with very high excretion of pHPLA and pHPAA, as well as tyrosine, methionine and hydroxyproline. The urine contains glucose, protein and excessive amounts of phosphate. The serum phosphate is low, calcium normal but alkaline phosphatase elevated if rickets is present. In the acute form, hepatic dysfunction is prominent with all tests of liver function abnormal. Hypoglycaemia may be very severe. The serum albumin may be particularly low and the prothrombin time and partial thromboplastin times and bleeding time grossly prolonged.

Differential diagnosis

There is no specific test for tyrosinaemia. Fructosaemia and galactosaemia must be excluded by specific tests. Primary liver disorders may be complicated by tyrosinaemia but the renal tubular lesions are not evident and it is unusual for excessive urinary pHPLA, pHPAA and pHPPA to be found.

Transient neonatal tyrosinaemia occurs in up to 30 per cent of pre-term infants and in 15 per cent of full term infants, if fed a diet containing more than 3 g protein/kg of bodyweight per day. This starts in the first week of life and persists for a few weeks. The serum tyrosine is elevated to more than three times the normal and the urine contains excessive amounts of pHPLA, pHPAA and pHPPA. The condition can be controlled by reducing the protein intake or by giving ascorbic acid in a dose of 100 mg per day. Although the prognosis is generally considered good, impaired mental development has been recorded.

Treatment

Dietary restriction of phenylalanine and tyrosine is necessary. If hypermethioninaemia is a feature, the dietary intake of this aminoacid too should be restricted. Regular estimation of serum aminoacids while on dietary restriction is necessary. Symptomatic correction of the many metabolic complications, hepatic failure, and the renal tubular defects are required. Hypoglycaemia, hypopotassaemia, alkalosis and bleeding disorders all require appropriate correction. Vitamin D and phosphate are required to control the rickets.

The response to treatment is unpredictable but may be almost complete in the acute form. Relapses may occur with recurrent infection and the prognosis must be guarded. In the chronic form it is usually possible to control the renal lesion but the hepatic disease may progress. Dietary treatment probably has to be continued indefinitely.

GENETICALLY DETERMINED ENZYMATIC DEFECTS IN THE UREA CYCLE

Genetically determined enzymatic defects in the urea cycle produce a high blood ammonia and often orotic aciduria. It seems likely that all defects are inherited in an autosomal recessive fashion but ornithine transcarbamylase deficiency may be inherited in a X-linked fashion. The liver is believed to be the only organ in which this cycle is complete. In severe hepatocellular liver disease and in Reye's syndrome there is an acquired defect in the functioning of this cycle.

Pathology

The principal pathological abnormalities at autopsy are cerebral, cerebellar and basal ganglia degeneration and atrophy. The liver is usually reported as showing some increase in fat and glycogen with no other histological abnormality, except in carbamyl phosphate synthetase deficiency in which there is minimal fibrosis in the portal tract with minor inflammatory cell infiltrate.

Biochemistry

The urea cycle converts large excesses of ammonia into urea. Hyperammoniaemia is a constant feature in all of these disorders but the

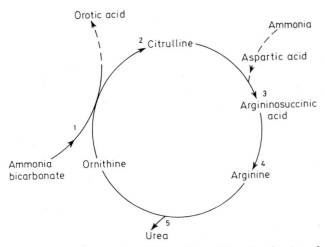

Figure 10.3. The urea cycle. The positions of the site of action of the 5 known enzymatic defects detailed in Table 10.6 are indicated by the numbers in the diagram

degree depends on the protein intake. Ornithine, citrulline, arginosuccinic acid or arginine accumulate in the tissues, depending on the site of the metabolic block (*Table 10.6* and *Figure 10.3*). Blood urea concentration is usually normal as is the urinary urea excretion. Orotic aciduria rises from the diversion of carbamyl phosphate to pyrimidines.

TABLE 10.6
Urea Cycle Disorders

Disorder	Enzyme deficient	Hepatomegaly	Transaminase elevation
(1) Carbamyl phosphate synthetase (CPS) deficiency	CPS	−	−
(2) Ornithine carbamyl transferase (OCT) deficiency	OCT	±	+
(3) Citrullinaemia	Arginosuccinic acid synthetase	+	+
(4) Arginosuccinic aciduria	Arginosuccinase	+	+
(5) Hyperargininaemia	Arginase	−	−

Clinical features

These are rare disorders which show a wide range in severity. Symptoms usually start in the newborn period but may be delayed until late in childhood. Cases starting in the neonatal period are often rapidly fatal.

A feature common to all is a dislike of protein-containing foods. Vomiting frequently follows the ingestion of these. Irritability, lethargy, ataxia, convulsions, coma and mental retardation are common features. The majority of patients fail to thrive. There is commonly hepatomegaly.

Laboratory findings

Hyperammoniaemia and elevated serum and urinary concentrations of the appropriate aminoacids are constant features. Serum aminotransferase concentrations are usually very high. Differential diagnosis includes other inherited disorders causing hyperammoniaemia. These include, hyperornithinaemia, proprionicacidaemia, lysine dehydrogenase deficiency, methylmalonicacidaemia, and familial protein intolerance. Direct assay of the liver enzymes involved may be required to establish the diagnosis.

Treatment

The acutely ill patient often responds within three to ten days to a high carbohydrate, protein-free diet. Exchange transfusion or peritoneal dialysis has been used in infants with severe hyperammoniaemia. Gut sterilization by oral antibiotics may also be useful. A low protein intake of between 0.5 and 1.5 g protein/kg of bodyweight per day supplying minimum requirements of essential aminoacids often controls the symptoms.

FAMILIAL PROTEIN INTOLERANCE

This disorder appears to be due to a genetically determined defect in the transport of basic aminoacids, lysine and arginine. It is inherited in an autosomal recessive fashion. The enzymatic abnormality underlying this defect has not been identified. Pathological changes are limited to the liver in which there is some lymphocyte and macrophage infiltrate in the portal tract with increased fibrosis. In older patients this progresses to early cirrhosis.

Clinical features are vomiting, diarrhoea and aversion to protein-rich foods following weaning. There is growth failure, hepatomegaly and splenomegaly.

The blood ammonia is normal when fasting but increases to above normal when milk is taken. The blood urea is typically low. Serum lysine and arginine are low while alanine and citrulline are high. There is excessively lysine and arginine in the urine.

Treatment consists of a low protein intake.

RARE DISORDERS WITH DISTURBED AMINOACID METABOLISM AND HEPATIC DYSFUNCTION

In two mentally retarded siblings with giant cell hepatitis and cirrhosis, *hyperornithinaemia* and reduced hepatic ornithine ketoacid amino-transferase were found. These children had abnormal liver function tests, mild hyperammoniaemia and a renal tubular defect of the Fanconi type.

In *hyperlysinaemia* the main clinical features are mental retardation, convulsions and lax joint ligaments. No enzymatic abnormality has been demonstrated except in one case in which hepatic lysine dehydrogenase activity was deficient. The aspartate transaminase is frequently elevated but pathological changes within the liver are limited to mild fatty change. The diagnosis is established by the symptomatic deterioration following a loading dose of L-lysine. The symptoms improve on a low protein diet.

PORPHYRIAS

Porphyrias form a rare group of incompletely understood disorders of haem synthesis. They are characterized by an excessive production and excretion of porphyrins and their precursors. They may be classified according to whether an excess of porphyrin production takes place in the liver or bone marrow. These two major groups can be further sub-divided on biochemical grounds.

In attempting to understand the bizarre, sometimes life-threatening clinical manifestations of porphyria, it is important to remember that haem is not confined to haemoglobin but is common also to myoglobin and microsomal cytochromes, catalase and peroxidase.

It appears likely that each of the porphyrias represents a different inborn error of metabolism in haem synthesis. The genetic abnormality may be aggravated by drugs, toxins and neoplasia.

Pathophysiology

The pathophysiology of porphyria remains unclear. Photosensitivity, which occurs particularly in response to exposure of light in the 400—500 nm range, causes erythema, oedema, pruritis and burning. This may be followed by the appearance of vesicular or bullous eruption on the exposed part and healing by deep scarring. There may be extensive ulceration and mutilation of affected areas. It is considered that this may occur because protoporphyrin is changed into an 'excited state' in which they damage both lysosomal and plasma cell membranes. This in turn may release chemical mediators of inflammation.

Some of the porphyrias present with an acute generalized neopathy. In these there is a markedly increased urinary excretion of delta-aminolaevulinic acid. This substance and its metabolite porphobilinogen have been shown to have pharmacological, biochemical, and behavioural effects on the central and peripheral nervous systems.

An important factor in producing symptoms in porphyria is an uncontrolled excessive activity of the enzyme delta aminolaevulinic acid (ALA) synthetase. Normally the activity of this enzyme is controlled by the amount of haem produced. It is the rate-limiting enzyme for the synthesis of haem, being present in much lower concentrations than the enzymes which are involved in later parts of the pathway. The activity of this enzyme can be increased by many drugs, steroids and other chemicals.

Pathological changes in the liver

Although hepatic enzymes are presumably involved in all cases of porphyria, it is only in *erythropoietic porphyria* that marked cellular changes are found within the liver. The usual course of this disease is benign with symptoms restricted to the skin and a mild haemolytic anaemia. There is, however, increasing evidence that liver disease may be a more common feature than has been previously recognized. Light microscopy of the liver shows the appearance of dark brown granules or aggregates in the cytoplasm of hepatocytes, Kupffer cells and portal macrophages. This may be accompanied by bile stasis and varying degrees of portal inflammation, fibrosis and ductular proliferation. This may proceed to cirrhosis or gradually progressive hepatic failure. Cirrhosis has been recorded by the age of six years. An increased incidence of gallstones has also been reported.

TABLE 10.7

Summary of Main Clinical and Biochemical Features of Porphyrias

	Inheritance	Enzyme defect		Clinical features	Main excretory products	
					Urine	Stools
(1) Acute intermittent porphyria (Swedish type)	Dominant	Porphobilinogen deaminase	Acute	Neurological, Abdominal pain, Vomiting, Constipation	Aminolaevulinic acid (ALA), Porphobilinogen (PBG), Coproporphyrin, PBG ALA	Coproporphyrin
(2) Hereditary coproporphyria	Dominant	Coproporphyrinogen oxidase	Acute	Neurological, Abdominal crises, Photosensitivity	Coproporphyrin, Aminolaevulinic acid, Porphobilinogen	Coproporphyrin, Protoporphyrin
(3) Porphyria variegata (South African genetic porphyria)	Dominant ?	Proloporphyrinogen oxidase	Acute	Photosensitivity, Neurological, Abdominal crises	Uroporphyrin iii	0
(4) Cutaneous hepatic (porphyria cutanea trada)	?	Uroporphyrinogen decarboxylase	Chronic	Photosensitivity, Disturbed liver function, Subacute hepatitis and cirrhosis	0	Protoporphyrin

(Left margin, reading vertically: H E P A T I C)

(5) ERYTH Erythropoietic protoporphyria	? Recessive	Ferrochelatase	Chronic	Photosensitivity Gallstones Hepatitis and cirrhosis Mild anaemia	Uroporphyrin 1	0
(6) ROPOI Congenital erythropoietic porphyria	Recessive	Uroporphyrinogen cosynthetase	Chronic	Photosensitivity Pigmentation of teeth Haemolytic anaemia and splenomegaly	Coproporphrin	Coproporphyrin
(7) ETIC Erythropoietic coproporphyria	Recessive	Uroporphyrinogen cosynthetase	Chronic	Photosensitivity Mild anaemia		

Clinical features

The clinical features, mode of inheritance, and diagnostic features are outlined in *Table 10.7*. In all, except acute intermittent porphyria, photosensitivity may occur. An acute generalized neuropathy may occur, not only in acute intermittent porphyria but also in hereditary coprophyria and variegate porphyria.

Abdominal features include severe pain which may be central and colicky or localized to any part of the abdomen. It may extend to the back. It is usually associated with vomiting and constipation.

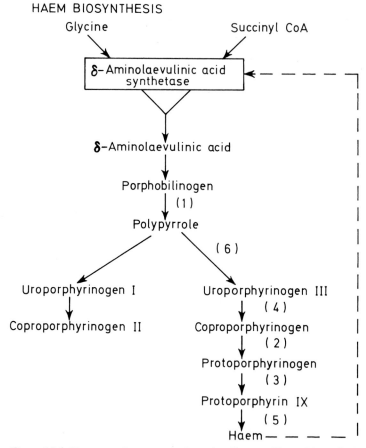

Figure 10.4 Diagrammatic representation of pathways of haem biosynthesis. Delta aminolaevulinic acid synthetase is a rate limiting enzyme. Control of the pathway is by feed-back repression and inhibition of this enzyme by haem. The numbers in the diagram indicate the site of action on the enzyme which is deficient in the biochemically characterized porphyrias detailed in Table 10.7

Pyrexia, tachycardia, and hypertension are occasional features. The disorder may thus mimic any intra-abdominal emergency or renal colic.

Neurological abnormalities include confusion, abnormal behaviour, convulsions or coma. Focal central nervous system involvement may cause a wide and sometimes confusing variety of signs. Peripheral neuropathy is frequent. It may be so severe that respiratory movements are paralysed, or latent, and only demonstrable on testing peripheral nerve conduction.

Hyponatraemia, hypokalaemia, and azotaemia are the most frequent metabolic complications.

Acute symptoms usually start at puberty but they may begin earlier. They are usually intermittent. The duration of attacks ranges from days to months.

Diagnosis

The diagnosis of porphyria may be made on the basis of the patterns of excretion of porphyrins in the urine or stool, but for many of these conditions the specific enzyme defect has been identified in erythrocytes, skin fibroblasts, or liver biopsy specimens.

Treatment of porphyria

Neurological symptoms are best prevented by the avoidance of all drugs which may increase the activity of ALA synthetase. These include barbiturates, sulphonamides, opiates, griseofulvin and steroids (including oral contraceptives). During the acute attacks water and electrolyte disturbances require urgent treatment and a high glucose intake is necessary.

Patients with cutaneous lesions should be protected from direct sunlight; barrier creams are often used to achieve this. Some patients appear to benefit by the administration of beta carotene in a dose of 120 mg per day maintaining a blood level of between 600 and 800 μg/ 100 ml. The effect of this therapy is not evident until two to three months after the initiation.

Patients with anaemia and splenomegaly may benefit from splenectomy.

In patients with evidence of hepatic dysfunction, there is some evidence that the administration of cholestyramine may have a beneficial effect. It is presumed to act by reducing the absorption of protoporphyrins from the intestine.

HAEMOCHROMATOSIS

Definition

Haemochromatosis is characterized by cirrhosis or fibrosis of the liver with increased iron stores, particularly in parenchymal liver cells (*Table 10.8*). Excessive iron storage and characteristic pathological

TABLE 10.8
Classification of Haemochromatosis

Idiopathic (familial)
Associated with chronic anaemia (thalassaemia, pyridoxine-responsive anaemia, hereditary spherocytosis)
Dietary iron overload
Congenital transferrin defect

and functional changes occur also in the heart, pancreas and endocrine organs. The liver iron is increased to between 50 and 100 times the normal.

Pathology

The liver may have a deep rusty brown colour. There is cirrhosis with extensive deposition of iron as haemosiderin in parenchymal cells, Kupffer cells, and in bile duct cells. Haemosiderosis is found also in the heart, pancreas and endocrine organs where it is associated with degenerative and/or fibrotic changes.

Pathogenesis

The metabolic lesion causing idiopathic haemochromatosis remains unknown. Iron absorption is inappropriately increased in patients and their first-degree relatives. Although there is much evidence of increased incidence in siblings the mode of inheritance is still unknown.

Iron absorption, transport and storage A sensitive, finely controlled regulatory mechanism for iron absorption keeps body iron stores in equilibrium if dietary iron intake is sufficient. The precise factors regulating this are still not completely understood. Iron is transported from the intestinal lumen into the mucosal cell on a protein resembling transferrin. Within the mucosal cell it is bound to ferritin. A rate-limiting step transfers some of this iron in the ferric state to plasma. Caeruloplasmin catalyses this step. The transfer into plasma requires transferrin. In plasma the iron is bound largely to transferrin which transports two atoms of ferric iron to the reticulo-endothelial system or tissue stores. Transferrin levels decrease as the iron stores increase. Within tissues iron is stored in a large protein, ferritin. Iron may comprise up to 20 per cent of this molecule. Haemosiderin is probably multiple aggregates of ferritin.

Clinical features

Skin pigmentation, diabetes mellitus and hepatomegaly are the classical features. Cardiac failure and failure of endocrine organs, particularly the pituitary, are frequent features. A specific arthropathy, with joint distribution similar to that of rheumatoid arthritis, has been described. Hepatomata are frequent complications.

Diagnosis

The diagnosis of haemochromatosis is made on the basis of the classical clinical features, together with liver biopsy evidence of cirrhosis or widespread fibrosis and laboratory investigations indicative of excessive iron stores. A high serum iron concentration, saturation of the total iron-binding capacity, increased hepatic iron concentration, provide firm evidence for these.

Recently, increased serum ferritin concentrations have been taken as indicative of high body iron stores. A 24-hour urinary iron in excess of 2.1 mg following intravenous desferrioxamine (0.5 g) is indicative of excessive parenchymal iron stores.

Treatment

The therapy of idiopathic haemochromatosis is repeated venesection until the iron stores have been depleted. Insulin will be required for the diabetes mellitus. The endocrine complications may require specific hormone replacement.

In the haemochromatosis arising secondary to chronic anaemia, venesection is contra-indicated. For such patients chelating agents must be used. Desferrioxamine in a dose of 25 mg/kg per day by intramuscular injection, and oral ascorbic acid 200 mg per day, will increase iron excretion to a level which exceeds absorption in most instances.

BETA THALASSAEMIA

Thalassaemias are genetically determined disorders in which there is
failure of production of the alpha or beta polypeptide chain in haemoglobin molecules. This causes severe anaemia for which blood transfusion is the only treatment. No abnormal haemoglobin is formed but
there is compensatory over-production of other haemoglobins. Much

TABLE 10.9
Thalassaemias/Haemoglobinopathies

Disease	Haemoglobin type	Sickling
Beta thalassaemia major	F A2 ± A	
Beta thalassaemia minor	A2 + A + F	
Alpha thalassaemia	H + A	
Sickle cell/thalassaemia	S + F ± A	+
Haemoglobin C thalassaemia	C + A + F	
Haemoglobin E thalassaemia	E + F + A	+

ineffective erythropoiesis occurs causing marrow hyperplasia. Homozy-
gous and heterozygous states of beta and alpha thalassaemia may be
recognized. Mixed haemoglobinopathy/thalassaemia syndromes occur
and may be recognized by haemoglobin electrophoresis (*Table 10.9*).
Hepatic involvement is a major component in beta thalassaemia.

Pathology

The essential pathological features are those of chronic anaemia and
of progressive haemosiderosis due to increased iron absorption and to
the iron load from blood transfusions. Cardiac muscle, pancreas, liver
and endocrine glands, particularly the pituitary, adrenal and parathyroid, are involved. There are secondary effects of failure of these
organs. The exact mode of liver injury is still speculative. Iron clearly
plays a major role. It first accumulates in the Kupffer cells where it
is associated with some fibrosis. As the child becomes older, the Kupffer
cells appear to become saturated with iron, and iron appears in the
parenchymal cells. Hepatocellular necrosis is often seen in association
with this.

Other important hepatotoxic factors which may be important
include chronic hypoxia, stasis due to cardiac involvement, and nutritional deficiencies. Repeated blood transfusion may expose the child to
blood-borne viral infections, particularly hepatitis type B. In two series
of cases reported from Northern Italy and Greece, 7–10 per cent of

the children were positive for hepatitis B surface antigen, and 32 per cent had antibody to hepatitis B surface antigen (Kattamis *et al*, 1974; Masera *et al.*, 1976). In the Milan study, 14 of 26 biopsied cases had histological features of chronic persistent hepatitis while nine had histological features of chronic active hepatitis. Two-thirds of the total series had biochemical evidence of hepatocellular necrosis.

Splenomegaly is frequently complicated by hypersplenism. The development of cirrhosis and portal hypertension aggravate this tendency.

Clinical features

Beta thalassaemia presents at the age of five to seven months with progressive pallor and poor feeding. There is invariably splenomegaly. Gradually, the child develops a characteristic facial appearance. This consists of frontal bossing, prominence of the malar eminences, sunken bridge of nose, a mongoloid slant to the eyes and exposure of the upper central teeth. Hepatomegaly is usually evidenced by the age of three or four years and becomes progressively more marked with age in most instances. Growth retardation is common by the age of eight years. Puberty is usually delayed, particularly in boys. Gradually features of haemochromatosis develop with the maximum impact on the heart, liver and endocrine organs. Death usually occurs at between the ages of 16 and 24 years due to a failure of these organs. Death may occur much earlier during acute infections.

Laboratory findings

Chronic anaemia with a high reticulocyte count and the presence of target cells is a constant feature. The red cells are frequently hypochromic and microcytic. The precise diagnosis depends on the identification and estimation of concentration of the haemoglobin types identified by haemoglobin electrophoresis.

Liver function tests are frequently deranged with raised serum transaminases. Jaundice is rare. Chest radiography frequently shows cardiomegaly and there may be minor ECG abnormalities. When pancreatic involvement is marked, blood sugar may be high and the glucose tolerance test diabetic. Hypocalcaemia is a feature of parathyroid involvement.

Treatment

The basis of current treatment is frequent blood transfusions to maintain the haemoglobin at a level of around 11.5g/100 ml. This requires the patient to be transfused when haemoglobin drops to 9 g, aiming to increase it to 14 g/100 ml. This regimen, together with folic acid, 5 mg per day, should be started as soon as the diagnosis is made. To prevent the toxic effects of iron overload, desferrioxamine should be commenced at the age of 3 years, with a dose of 25 mg/kg per day by intramuscular injection. It has been shown that a dose of up to 500 mg per day throughout childhood, protects the liver against iron toxicity. It is argued that higher doses or the same dose given by continuous subcutaneous infusion would be even more effective. Vitamin C supplements of 100–200 mg per day should be commenced one month after starting desferrioxamine.

One of the difficult clinical decisions in affected children is to assess the extent of hypersplenism. It is likely that this is present to a significant extent when the blood transfusion requirements exceed 450 ml/kg per year. Severe thrombocytopenia with a bleeding tendency is an absolute indication for splenectomy. Removing the spleen could have an adverse affect, in that it removes a tissue in which the effects of iron overload are relatively benign, but when the above criteria are fulfilled the decreased transfusion requirement outweighs this risk. Splenectomy may expose the child to an increased risk of infection. Penicillin V, 125 mg twice daily, is therefore recommended for an indefinite period following splenectomy.

ZELLWEGER'S SYNDROME
(cerebro-hepato-renal syndrome)

Definition

Zellweger's syndrome (ZS) is characterized by profound psychomotor retardation, marked hypotonia, absent tendon reflexes, abnormal facies, feeding difficulty, usually siezures and multiple congenital abnormalities. It is invariably fatal.

The condition is recessively inherited. The pathogenesis of the abnormality is unknown. High serum iron levels, abnormal increased hepatic uptake of iron, and cirrhosis are variable features. Mitochondrial and peroxisomal abnormalities in hepatocytes have been reported. Urinary excretion of pipecolic acid is increased.

Pathology

The brain shows gyral disorders with non-sclerotic polymicrogyri and smooth areas with shallow convolutions (lissencephaly).

The most prominent hepatic feature is lobular disarray with lack of normal hepatocyte plates and irregular relationship between portal tracts and central veins. In parts of the liver, central veins or portal tracts are grouped together. There is a minor increase in fibrosis in the first ten weeks but thereafter fibrosis becomes marked and cirrhosis develops. There is excessive iron deposition in the liver in the first five to eight weeks of life, thereafter it clears. Splenomegaly is found at post-mortem in the majority of patients. Major cardiovascular anomalies, hypoplastic lungs, and hyperplasia of the islets of Langerhans are commonly found.

Clinical features

Hypotonia and its sequelae are the main neurological features. The majority of infants do have siezures, and nystagmus may occur. Craniofacial features may allow a diagnosis. The forehead is high, the external ears frequently abnormal, there is a large fontanelle. Shallow supraorbital ridge, epichanthic folds, cataracts, peri-orbital oedema and short upper lip are inconstant features.

Failure to thrive is almost invariable and hepatomegaly occurs in the majority of cases, but there is no clinical evidence of hepatic dysfunction in the majority other than spontaneous haemorrhage which can be corrected by vitamin K.

The course is of continuing failure to thrive, with grossly delayed neuromotor development. The majority of cases die by the age of six months.

Laboratory findings

Prothrombin time is frequently prolonged, standard tests of liver function show only minor abnormalities. Jaundice is rare. Elevated serum iron with saturated serum iron-binding capacity has been found in approximately 50 per cent of cases. Excess urinary excretion of pipecolic acid is found, Radiographs show chondriodysplasia punctata in 40 per cent.

MUCOPOLYSACCHARIDOSIS

The mucopolysaccharidoses are a group of related disorders in which skeletal changes, progressive mental deterioration, visceral enlargement and corneal clouding are manifest to varying degrees. Mucopoly-saccharides are deposited in abnormal concentrations in tissue and are excreted in the urine.

Mucopolysaccharides are complex structures containing aminoacids, amino sugars, uronic acids and sulphates. The main disease groups causing hepatomegaly are shown in *Table 10.3*. All are believed to be inherited in an autosomal recessive fashion, except for Hunter's syndrome which is inherited in an X-linked fashion.

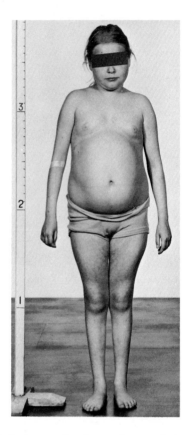

Figure 10.5. Clinical photograph of a patient aged 14 years with Mauriac syndrome. Diabetes mellitus developed at 20 months. Throughout childhood diabetic control had been very difficult with blood sugar levels of from 40 to 500 mg/dl within 24 hours. There is severe growth retardation, massive hepato-megaly (soft liver edge palpable 10cm below costal margin) and marked obesity. Liver biopsy showed excessive glycogen in all hepatocytes but no other abnormality

TABLE 10.10
Disorders Causing Hepatomegally/Hepatic Dysfunction and Frequently
Neurological Abnormalities or Developmental Delay

Chronic hepatic encephalopathy
Fulminant hepatic failure
Reye's syndrome

Infective disorders:	
Intrauterine:	e.g. Rubella, CMV, syphilis, toxoplasmosis
Neonatal:	e.g. Listeriosis, herpes simplex virus infection
Childhood:	e.g. Weil's disease
Inborn errors of metabolism:	
Carbohydrate:	Galactosaemia Fructosaemia Glycogen storage disease *(Table 10.1)* Manonsidosis
Aminoacids:	Urea cycle disorders *(Table 10.4)* Hyperammoniaemias Homocystic-uria Tyrosinosis
Lipids:	Gaucher's disease Neimann—Pick disease Generalized gangliosidosis Wolman's disease A—beta lipoprotein deficiency Alpha—lipoprotein deficiency Fucosidosis
Mucopolysaccharidosis:	*See Table 10.3*
Haem metabolism:	Crigler—Najjar syndrome Porphyria
Mineral disorders:	Wilson's disease Haemochromatosis Zellweger's syndrome
Rare disorders of uncertain cause:	Biliary hypoplasia with characteristic phenotype (Alagille syndrome) Infantile diffuse cerebral degeneration with hepatic cirrhosis Lissencephaly syndrome Lipodystrophy Familial haemophagocytic reticulosis Congenital hepatic fibrosis and polycystic disease of the kidneys and brain malformations

See appropriate Bibliography at the end of the Chapter.

DISORDERS CAUSING HEPATOMEGALY OR HEPATIC DYSFUNCTION AND NEUROLOGICAL ABNORMALITIES OR DEVELOPMENTAL DELAY

Many acquired or genetically determined disorders affect both the liver and the nervous system. The purpose of this section is simply to bring together the range of such disorders. These include various forms of hepatic encephalopathies, infective disorders affecting both the liver and brain and well-defined inborn errors of metabolism. In addition, miscellaneous rare disorders with a putative familial or genetic basis and distinct clinical or pathological features are added. The list (*Table 10.10*) aims to be comprehensive but with already over 2800 separate genetic disorders described, I apologize in advance for inevitable oversights at the time of writing and for inadequacies before the book comes to press.

Neurological syndromes range from delayed neurological development, gradual progressive global loss of brain function, acute coma to specific syndromes such as the extrapyramidal lesion in Wilson's disease or acute peripheral neuropathy in porphyria.

Chronic hepatic encephalopathy (page 263), fulminant hepatic failure (page 126) and Reye's syndrome (page 138) have been described in detail elsewhere. The diagnosis and management of the treatable inborn errors of metabolism, galactosaemia, fructosaemia, tyrosinosis (page 54), glycogen storage disease (page 162), and Wilson's disease (page 233) have been considered in detail elsewhere.

Other rare but currently untreatable disorders such as Zellweger's syndrome which introduced new ideas on pathogenesis of liver disease, and have been the subject of many recent research reports, are dealt with elsewhere in this chapter. The remaining disorders are indicated by name only but the references chosen do provide useful further reading.

BIBLIOGRAPHY AND REFERENCES

Glycogen storage disease

Greene, H.L., Slonim, A.E., O'Neill, J.A. and Barr, R.M. (1976). Nocturnal nasogastric feeding for management of Type 1 glycogen storage disease. *New Engl. J. Med.* **294**, 423

Hug, G. (1976). Glycogen storage disease. Birth defects. *Original Article Series,* Vol. 12, No. 6, p. 145. Baltimore: Williams and Wilkins

McAdams, A.J., Hug, G. and Bove, K.E. (1974). Glycogen storage disease Types 1–X. Criteria for morphologic diagnosis. *Hum. Path.* **5**, 463

Spencer-Peet, J., Norman, M.E., Lake, B.D., McNamara, A.J. and Patrick, D. (1971). Glycogen storage disease in laboratory findings in 23 cases. *Q.Jl Med.* **40**, 95

Starzl, T.E. *et al.* (1973). Portal diversion in the treatment of glycogen storage disease in humans. *Ann.Surg.* **178**, 525

Diabetes mellitus

Court, S. (1978). A study of growth in diabetes. *Archs Dis. Childh.* **53**, 691

Craig, O. (1977). Hepatomegaly and dwarfism. In *Childhood Diabetes and its Management:* p. 226. London: Butterworths

Mandell, F. and Berenberg, W. (1974). Mauriac syndrome. *Am.J.Dis.Childh.* **127**, 900

Aminoacid disorders

Hill, A., Nordin, P.M. and Zaleski, W.A. (1970). Dietary treatment of tyrosinosis. *J.Am.diet.Ass.* **56**, 308

Kekomaki, M.P., Visakorpi, J.K., Perhanentupa, J. and Saxen, L. (1967). Familial protein intolerance with deficient transport of basic aminoacids. *Acta paediat. Scand.* **56**, 617

Levin, B. (1971). Hereditary disorders of the urea cycle. *Adv. clin. Chem.* **14**, 65

Menkes, J.H., Welcher, D.W., Levi, H.F., Dallas, J. and Gretsky, N.E. (1972). Relationship of elevated blood tyrosine to ultimate intellectual performance of premature infants. *Pediatrics* **49**, 218

Palmer, T., Oberholtzer, B.G., Burgess, E.A., Butler, L.J. and Levin B. (1974). Hyperammoniaemia in 20 families. *Archs Dis.Childh.* **49**, 443

Scriver, C.R. and Rosenberg, L.E., (1973). Urea cycle and ammonia in aminoacid metabolism and its disorders. In *Major Problems in Clinical Paediatrics*, p. 234, Chapt. 12, Vol. 10. Philadelphia: Saunders

Scriver, C.R. and Rosenberg, L.E. (1973). Tyrosine in aminoacid metabolism and its disorders. In *Major Problems in Clinical Paediatrics*, p. 338, Chapt. 16, Vol. 10. Philadelphia: Saunders

Yu, J.S., Walker-Smith, J.A. and Burnard, D. (1971). Neonatal Hepatitis in premature infants, simulating hereditary tyrosinosis. *Archs Dis.Childh.* **46**, 306

Rare aminoacidaemias

Bickel, H., Faist, D., Muller, H. and Quadbeck, G. (1962). Ornithinasmal eine weiter Aminosaurenstaffen wechselstroring mit Hirnschadigung, *Dt.med. Wschr.* **47**, 2247

Ghadimi, H. (1972). *The Hyperlysinemias in the Metabolic Basis of Inherited Disease*, 3rd ed. p. 393. Ed. by Stanbury, J.B., Wyngaarden, J.B. and Fredrickson, D.S. New York: McGraw-Hill

Lipid disorders

Fredrickson, D.S. and Sloan, S.R. (1972). In *The Metabolic Basis of Inherited Disease*, p. 783. Ed. by Stanbury, J.B., Wyngaarden, J.B. and Fredrickson, D.S. New York: McGraw-Hill

Neville, B.G.R., Lake, B.D., Stephens, R. and Sanders, M.D. (1973). Neuro-visceral storage disorders with vertical supranuclear ophthalmoplegia, and its relationship to Neimann—Pick disease. *Brain* **96**, 97

Partin, J.S., Partin, J.C., Schubert, W.K. and McAdams, J. (1974). Liver ultrastructure and A-beta lipoproteinaemia: evolution of micronodular cirrhosis. *Gastroenterology* 67, 107

Wolman's disease

Lough, J., Fawcett, J. and Wiegenberg, B. (1970). Wolman's disease. An electronmicroscopic, histochemical and biochemical study. *Archs Path. Chicago* 87, 103

Kamalian, N., Dudley, W. and Beroukhim, F. (1973). Wolman's disease with jaundice and subarachnoid haemorrhage. *Am.J.Dis.Child.* 126, 671

Patrick, A.D. and Lake, D.D. (1973). Wolman's disease. In *Lysosomes and Storage Diseases*, Chapt. 20, p. 453. Ed. by Hers, H.G. and van Hoof, F. New York: Academic Press

West, R.J. and Lloyd, J.K. (1977). Wolman's disease. In *Essentials of Paediatric Gastroenterology*, p. 256. Ed. by Harries, J.T. London: Churchill-Livingstone

Porphyria

Bloomer, J.R. (1976). The hepatic porphyrias: pathogenesis, manifestations and management. *Gastroenterology* 71, 689

Brodie, M.J., Moore, M.R. and Goldberg, A. (1977). Enzyme abnormalities in the porphyrias. *Lancet* 2, 699

DeLeo, V.A., Poh-Fitzpatrick, M. Mathews-Roth, M. and Harber, L.C. (1976). Erythropoietic protoporphyria. *Am.J.Med.* 60, 8

Haemochromatosis

Grace, N.D. and Powell, L.W. (1974). Iron storage disorders of the liver. *Gastroenterology* 67, 1257

Weatherhall, D.J., Pippard, M.J. and Callander, S.T. (1977). Iron loading and thalassaemia – experimental successes and practical realities. *New.Engl.J. Med.* 297, 445

Beta thalassaemia

Kattamis, C., Syriopoulou, V., Davri-Karamouzi, Y., Demetriou, D. and Matsaniotis, N. (1974). Prevalence of Au-Ag and Au-Ab in transfused children with thalassaemia in Greece. *Archs Dis. Childh.* 49, 450

Masera, G., Jean, G., Gazzola, G. and Novakova, M. (1976). Role of chronic hepatitis in the development of thalassaemic liver disease. *Archs Dis. Childh.* 51, 680

Modell, B. (1977). Total management of thalassaemia major. *Archs Dis.Childh.* 52, 489

References for Table 10.10

Alagille, D., Odievre, M., Gautier, M. and Dommergues, J.P. (1975). Hepatic ductular hypoplasia associated with characteristic facies, vertebral malformations, retarded physical, mental and sexual development and cardiac murmur. *J.Pediat.* **86**, 63

Bell, R.J.M., Bradfield, A.J.E., Barnes, N.D. and France, M.E. (1968). Familial haemophagocytic reticulosis. *Archs Dis.Childh.* **43**, 601

Dieker, H., Edwards, R.H., Zurhein, G., Chou, S.M., Hartman, H.A. and Opitz, J.M. (1969). The lissencephaly syndrome; birth defects. *Original Article Series*, Vol. 5. No. 2. p. 53. Baltimore: Williams and Wilkins

Fried, K. *et al.* (1971). Polycystic kidneys associated with malformation of the brain. Polydactily and other birth defects. *J. med. Genet.* **8**, 285

Huttenlocher, P.R., Solitaire, J.B. and Adams, G. (1976). Infantile diffuse cerebral degeneration with hepatic cirrhosis. *Archs Neurol.* **53**, 186

Senior, B. and Gellis, S.S. (1964). The syndromes of total lipodystrophy and partial lipodystrophy. *Pediatrics* **33**, 593

Tay, C.H., Ragagopalan, K., McEvoy, Bowe, E., Kock, C. and Costa, J.L.D. (1974). A recessive disorder with growth and mental retardation, peculiar facies, abnormal pigmentation, hepatic cirrhosis and aminoaciduria. *Acta Pediat.Scand.* **63**, 777

CHAPTER 11

Familial and Genetic Structural Abnormalities of the Liver and Biliary System

INFANTILE POLYCYSTIC DISEASE OF THE KIDNEYS AND LIVER

Infantile polycystic disease of the kidneys and liver (IPCD) is characterized by renal and hepatic enlargement due to replacement of the renal parenchyma by cysts and fibrous tissue, and periportal hepatic fibrosis with dilatation of the bile ducts. The disorder is inherited in an autosomal recessive fashion. It has thus been distinguished from the 'adult' type of polycystic disease which is inherited in an autosomal dominant fashion, usually with a high degree of penetrance. In the adult variety hepatic involvement is rare. The designation 'infantile' is inappropriate since the disorder may cause death *in utero* or present in late childhood, as well as in infancy (Blyth and Ockenden, 1971).

Pathology

In the kidney, the essential lesion appears to be cystic transformation of the terminal collecting tubules, while in the liver the lesion is at the level of the junction of the canals of Hering and adjacent intralobular bile ducts. What causes these lesions is not known. Both are associated with marked increase in fibrous tissue. In the kidney, there is also a loss of functioning nephrones.

The renal weight and size may be increased to as much as ten times normal but the shape is usually preserved. Cysts lined by cuboidal or cylindrical epithelium are distributed radially in both cortex and medulla. In infancy these tend to be less than 1 cm in size but with increasing age the cysts tend to become larger, up to 2 cm. The interstices around the cysts contain much fibrous tissue, immature in infancy, but mature later in childhood. It is only late in childhood that enlarged cysts and increasing fibrosis start to deform the capsule and compress the calyces. With age there is increasing fibrous tissue and loss of renal parenchyma. In the majority of cases renal failure develops early in infancy. The secondary pathological effects are those of renal failure and systemic hypertension. In early infancy abdominal distension and pulmonary oedema cause marked respiratory distress. Pneumonia is a frequent complication.

The liver is enlarged but to a much less extent than the kidneys. There are no macroscopic abnormalities. The microscopic lesions are in the portal tract which show increased deposition of fibrous tissue and an abundance of dilated bile ductules lined by cuboidal epithelium. The hepatic lobular architecture is unchanged and the liver cells are normal. Portal vein branches are distorted, but this is considered to be a secondary phenomenon. The intrahepatic fibrosis causes portal hypertension with the clinically important consequences of oesophageal and gastric varices, splenomegaly and hypersplenism.

In individual cases there is considerable variability in the degree of renal and hepatic involvement. In some instances, renal involvement appears to be focal rather than diffuse. Because of the different ages of presentation of cases in individual families, Blyth and Ockenden (1971) have suggested that four or even five distinct genetic varieties of IPCD may exist. However, no unique pathological differences have as yet been discerned in these groups.

Clinical features

In the newborn period, IPCD may present as a difficulty in delivery because of marked abdominal distension, caused by the gross enlargement of the kidneys. There are no features then of liver involvement.

In the neonatal period and early infancy the clinical features are those of renal involvement (*Table 11.1*). There is marked abdominal distension often causing respiratory embarrassment. Renal failure, systemic hypertension, congestive cardiac failure, respiratory tract infection and failure to thrive are the main problems. The diagnosis may be suspected by the finding of bilateral huge renal masses with or without hepatomegaly and splenomegaly. Death often occurs from pneumonia or congestive cardiac failure. If congestive cardiac failure can be controlled, however, this feature gradually settles with increasing

TABLE 11.1
Features of Infantile Polycystic Kidneys

Fetal	Neonatal	Infancy	Childhood
Oligohydramnios	Marked abdominal distension	Renal failure	Splenomegaly
Potter's facies	Bilateral renal en-	Failure to thrive	Hypersplenism
Dystocia	largement	Hepatomegaly	Alimentary bleeding
	Renal failure	Splenomegaly	Abnormal IVP
	Hypertension		
	Congestive cardiac failure		
	Respiratory distress		
	Histological evidence of liver involvement		

TABLE 11.2
Investigations of Suspected Polycystic Disease in Liver and Kidneys

Excretory urography	Full blood count
Ultrasonic scan of kidneys	Standard tests of liver function
Renal function tests (blood urea, serum creatinine, creatinine clearance tests)	Chest radiography
	Barium meal

In selected cases:

Aortoportgraphy	Kidney biopsy
Splenic venography	ECG
Liver biopsy	Radiology of wrists and hands to exclude renal osteodystrophy

TABLE 11.3
IVP Abnormalities in Infantile Polycystic Disease of the Kidneys

Bilateral, massively enlarged kidneys	A persistent nephrogram (hours or days)
Alternating radio-dense radio-translucent streaks on the nephrogram	Blunted, shortened, indistinct calyces
Homogeneous nephrogram	Rarely, collections of contrast medium in renal papillae indistinguishable from medullary sponge kidney

age and it is often possible to stop digitalization around the age of two years. The failure may, however, relapse with intercurrent infection.

Where renal cyst formation is less widespread, the disease may not present until later infancy or early childhood, with features of renal failure such as polyuria and failure to thrive. In both groups features of progressive renal failure inevitably occur, often requiring support by dialysis or renal transplantation by the age of 5–10 years. Cases present in later childhood with asymptomatic splenomegaly or with alimentary bleeding from portal hypertension. This arises where renal enlargement insufficiency is less severe than in the previous groups.

Investigative findings

Tests of liver function are typically normal although occasionally the alkaline phosphatase may be elevated. There is evidence of renal impairment such as polyuria, biliary/urinary osmolarity, raised blood urea and creatinine and reduced creatinine clearance tests. The most

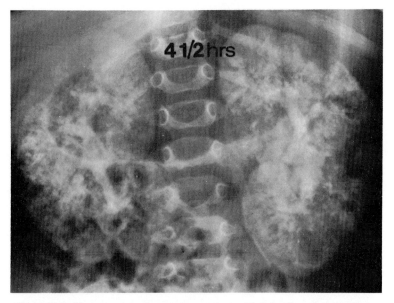

Figure 11.1. Intravenous pyelogram in a patient with infantile polycystic disease of the kidney and liver. Four and a half hours after injection of Urographin a clear nephrogram persists. The kidneys are massively enlarged. There are alternating radio-dense and radiolucent streaks in the cortex. The main calyces are normal but the extremeties are blunted and indistinct

useful investigation is plain radiography of the abdomen and excretory urography. The typical findings are illustrated in *Figure 11.1*. If the blood urea is too high to permit excretory urography, ultrasonic scanning of the kidneys may be helpful in excluding large cysts or obstructive nephropathy.

In rare instances it will be necessary to perform kidney or liver biopsy so that firm genetic guidance can be given. If alimentary bleeding has occurred, endoscopy or barium meal may be necessary to demonstrate varices. *Table 11.2* lists the investigative procedures for suspected polycystic disease of the liver and kidneys.

Treatment and prognosis

Death in infancy usually arises from renal failure, fluid retention or bronchopneumonia. In later childhood death is likely to arise from progressive renal failure. In late childhood or adult life the features of portal hypertension may become more important.

Treatment is thus directed at controlling infection and congestive cardiac failure in infancy, symptomatic treatment of disturbances in fluid electrolyte balance induced by renal failure and systemic hypertension. Renal dialysis and, ultimately, transplantation, may have to be considered.

Surgical relief of portal hypertension (page 315) by portocaval shunting is well tolerated by these patients.

CONGENITAL HEPATIC FIBROSIS

Definition

Congenital hepatic fibrosis is a condition defined pathologically by the presence within the liver of bands of fibrous tissue which often contain linear or circular spaces lined by bile duct cells. The bands of fibrous tissue join all portal tracts. It is commonly associated with intrahepatic portal hypertension but hepatocellular function is almost always preserved. It is not a single entity but in clinical usage the term is usually reserved for a syndrome in which portal hypertension occurs without significant impairment of renal or hepatic function. Pathologically it is most commonly associated with significant renal disease, such as infantile polycystic disease. It must be distinguished from cirrhosis and other causes of portal hypertension in childhood since management and prognosis are different.

Pathology

The unique pathological feature of this condition is the presence throughout the liver of bands of fibrous tissue which are clearly demarcated from hepatic parenchyma (*Figure 11.2*). Portal tracts are

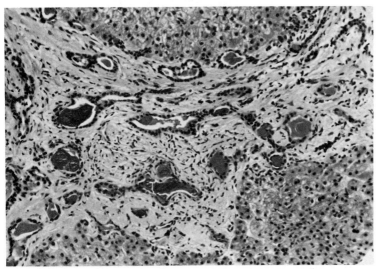

Figure 11.2 Congenital hepatic fibrosis. A wide band of fibrous tissue is seen separating two areas of hepatic parenchyma. Within the fibrous tissue a conspicuous features is the variously shaped spaces lined by bile duct epithelial cells. Some spaces contain densely staining material. No portal vein branches can be seen. There is no inflammatory cell infiltrate. The hepatic parenchyma is normal (percutaneous liver biopsy, haematoxylin and eosin × 100, reduced to seven-eighths in reproduction)

widened. All are linked by these bands of fibrous tissue. The width of the bands vary from case to case, and may increase with age. Most frequently the bands contain many irregularly shaped, narrow, elongated spaces lined by bile duct epithelial cells. In some instances such spaces are very rare, while in others they are frequent, dilated and almost circular. It is uncertain whether these two varieties are different disease entities. Portal vein branches are small and sparse. The liver is enlarged, smooth and hard. Hepatic parenchyma is almost always normal. The histological changes within the liver are indistinguishable from those seen in infantile polycystic disease. Outwith the liver there is splenomegaly and other features of portal hypertension.

Associated disorders

Conditions associated with congenital hepatic fibrosis are as follows.

(1) Infantile polycystic disease (*q.v.*). In some children with this syndrome only 10 per cent of the renal tubules may be involved.

Renal failure and hypertension occur late, by which time the effects of hepatic fibrosis are manifest. In many reports on congenital hepatic fibrosis cases of infantile polycystic disease are excluded since the renal manifestations of this disorder are so prominent.

(2) Ivemark's familial dysplasia. This is a familial disorder characterized by hepatomegaly with features of congenital hepatic fibrosis. There is, in addition, localized renal dysplasia with primitive collecting tubules and much interstitial fibrosis. Renal changes often lead to renal failure in infancy. Increased fibrosis and cystic change is seen also in the pancreas (Ivemark, Oldfelt and Zetterstrom, 1959; Nathan and Batsakis, 1969).

(3) Meckel's syndrome. This is a disorder in which encephalocoele, or anencephaly, cysts in the kidney, polydactyly, and other anomalies may occur. General hepatic fibrosis may also be present (Fried *et al.*, 1971).

(4) Adult type polycystic disease.

(5) Without renal disease, rarely (Murray-Lyon, Ockenden and Williams, 1973).

(6) Nephronophthisis. This is a familial disorder characterized by numerous glomerular cysts marked periglomerular fibrosis, tubular dilatation and interstitial fibrosis, all leading to renal failure at varying ages. It is uncertain whether this arises from a number of discrete entities inherited in a genetic fashion or as a spectrum of disease (Boichis *et al*, 1973).

(7) Medullary sponge kidney (Kerr, Warwick and Hart-Mercer, 1962).

(8) With cortical and medullary renal cysts. Lieberman *et al.* (1971) described five cases of congenital hepatic fibrosis in which the renal parenchyma contain cysts within the cortex and medulla apparently arising in the distal and collecting tubules. The cysts were not radially orientated but were lined by columnar epithelium: four out of the five patients described had renal impairment. Distinction of these cases from infantile polycystic disease may be difficult.

Clinical features

The principal clinical features are abdominal distension, firm hepatomegaly, splenomegaly, hypersplenism and haematemesis or melaena due to alimentary bleeding secondary to portal hypertension. Other features include: abdominal pain, which in some instances may be very prominent; fever due to cholangitis in dilated bile ductules; the hepatitis syndrome of infancy; and features of associated conditions, particularly the renal disorders.

This is a disorder of childhood or early adult life. Where congenital hepatic fibrosis does not complicate infantile polycystic disease, or the other rare syndromes described above, it usually presents at the age of one to two years with abdominal distension due to hepatosplenomegaly. In this age group haematemesis has also been a presenting feature.

In later childhood and in adult life, typical presentation is alimentary bleeding. The time of initial bleed, however, has varied from 8 months to 60 years. It is in late childhood and adult life that abdominal pain and cholangitis most frequently occur. Another cause for abdominal pain is splenic infarction.

Cases come to light when medical examination for some other reason reveals hepatosplenomegaly. Hypersplenism is rarely a problem in early infancy but may be evident by the age of five years. With less than 50 cases of congenital hepatic fibrosis without some renal impairment described in the world literature, the natural history of this condition is still poorly documented.

Diagnosis

Standard tests of liver function such as serum bilirubin, transaminase, albumin, serum proteins, prothrombin time and BSP clearance are typically normal. Alkaline phosphatase, however, may be slightly elevated. Even if there is no urea retention or elevation of the blood pressure, the intravenous pyelogram may be abnormal in up to 30 per cent of cases, showing renal enlargement or distortion of the calyces. Barium meal or endoscopy may show varices.

Liver scan will show marked splenomegaly and hepatomegaly but with the normal isotope uptake.

A definitive investigation is percutaneous liver biopsy, using a Trucut needle. The Menghini technique will not reveal the true extent of the fibrosis.

Odievre, Chaumont and Oiry (1976) described seven patients with congenital hepatic fibrosis and portal hypertension in whom splenic portography showed duplication of the intrahepatic portal vein branches, typically one branch being two to three times that of the other. Similar findings could not be found in 100 splenic venograms in children with other hepatic diagnoses. They suggest that this may be a useful diagnostic investigation where liver biopsy or renograms are inconclusive.

Treatment

The main problem in clinical management is portal hypertension causing alimentary bleeding. Since there is no associated hepatocellular necrosis, hepatic encephalopathy does not complicate bleeding and has not been recorded after portocaval anastomosis. This has led Kerr *et al.* (1961) and Sokhi *et al.* (1975) to advocate early portocaval anastomosis in this condition. It should be noted, however, that such patients may have many years free of bleeding if they avoid aspirin. The former group noted that liver function tests are more frequently abnormal after shunting than before. At least one patient is reported to have died of liver failure after surgery, and other cases have developed portal hypertension and alimentary bleeding after apparently successful surgery. Thus, while it is true that surgery is generally more satisfactory in this form of liver disease than in cirrhosis – 12 of 22

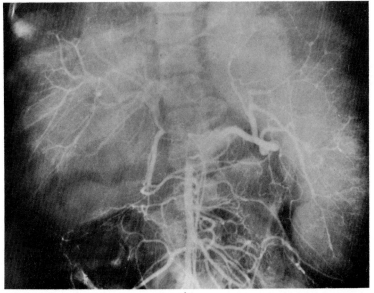

(a)

Figure 11.3 Selective splenic and superior mesenteric angiograms in a patient aged 13 years with congenital infantile polycystic disease and congenital hepatic fibrosis. Symptoms had started at the age of 4 years with alimentary bleeding due to portal hypertension. This had never been a severe problem, however, but hypersplenism now is marked. For the last 4 years she has had significant urea retention. Angiography has been performed by placing a catheter through the femoral artery into the splenic and superior mesenteric artery. (a) Showing marked splenomegaly with numerous small aneurysms in the branches of the splenic artery (cont.)

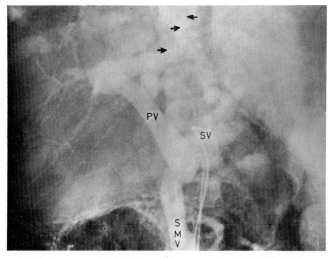

(b)

Figure 11.3 (cont.). (b) The portal (PV) and superior mesenteric (SMV) veins are large and patent. The splenic vein (SV) is not well shown. Much of the splenic outflow appears to run into large gastric and oesophageal collateral veins (→). The right branch of the portal vein and its intrahepatic branches are small. The left portal vein is large and its branches probably normal, suggesting that the right lobe of the liver is more effective than the left. In the capillary and venous phase it is seen that the hepatogram is slightly mottled but there are no clear filling defects in it

reported cases surviving surgery — it should be stressed that the natural history of congenital hepatic fibrosis with or without shunting is as yet poorly recorded. Portosystemic anastomosis, therefore, should be reserved for instances in which marked alimentary bleeding has occurred without aspirin administration and where other causes of alimentary bleeding have been excluded by endoscopy. If the shunt procedure includes splenectomy, it must be remembered that there is an increased risk of severe bacterial infection. If it is followed by thrombosis of the shunt other parts of the portovenous system may also thrombose.

Elective surgery should not be undertaken without full assessment which should include standard tests of liver function, liver biopsy, demonstration of the portosplenic venous system (*Figure 11.3*) by selective arteriography with, in addition in some instances, splenic portography.

Abdominal pain should be treated with analgesics. Cholangitis requires vigorous treatment with systemic antibiotics, such as kanamycin or gentamycin with, however, regular checks on serum levels since there may be renal impairment. Surgery on the biliary tree should be avoided.

FOCAL DILATATION OF INTRAHEPATIC BILE DUCTS

This very rare condition is characterized by a non-obstructive dilatation of intrahepatic bile ducts. Only a portion or the whole of the liver may be involved. The dilated segments are frequently the site of cholangitis. The hepatic parenchyma is normal apart from inflammation and fibrosis around dilated segments which have become infected.

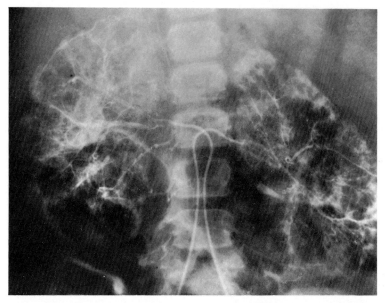

Figure 11.4 Bilateral selective renal angiogram showing large kidneys containing a multitude of cysts all of which are less than 1cm in size. There is a considerable reduction in functioning renal tissue. The appearances are typical of polycystic disease at this age

The condition may occur as a single isolated abnormality (Caroli's disease) and also in association with congenital hepatic fibrosis. Saccular or cylindrical dilatations of the main right and left hepatic ducts and of the common hepatic duct may also occur. Diverticuli may arise from the right and left hepatic ducts. Either of these abnormalities may occur in isolation, or be associated with choledochal cysts.

Clinical and laboratory features

The patients present with abdominal pain, fever and jaundice due to cholangitis or with features of Gram-negative septicaemia. Symptoms may occur at any time in life. There may also be symptoms attributable to the development of biliary calculi, for example, biliary colic. If the lesion is associated with congenital hepatic fibrosis, portal hypertension is likely to be present.

The clinical picture may suggest cholecystitis or cholangitis. Liver function test results would be in keeping with such diagnosis. If the patient is not jaundiced at the time of investigation, the dilated bile ducts may be demonstrated by intravenous cholangiography. They can also be demonstrated by ultrasonic scanning. Invasive techniques such as percutaneous cholangiography or operative cholangiography, must be avoided unless there are strong grounds for suspecting the presence of biliary calculi. Most surgical procedures are liable to be followed by an exacerbation of the cholangitis.

Treatment

Treatment consists of antibiotics to control cholangitis, but it is rarely possible to produce complete sterility of the bile. Since there is no mechanical obstruction, surgery is contra-indicated unless there is very clear evidence of secondary bile duct obstruction due to calculi.

BIBLIOGRAPHY AND REFERENCES

Infantile polycystic disease

Anand, S.K., Chan, J.C. and Lieberman, E. (1975). Polycystic disease and hepatic fibrosis in children. *Am.J.Dis.Child.* 129, 810
Blyth, H. and Ockenden, B.G. (1971). Polycystic disease in the kidneys and liver presenting in childhood. *J.med.Genet.* 8, 257
Lieberman, E. *et al.* (1971). Infantile polycystic disease in kidneys and liver. *Medicine, Baltimore* 50, 277
Osathanondh, V. and Potter, E.L. (1964). Pathogenesis of polycystic kidneys. *Archs Path.* 77, 459

Congenital hepatic fibrosis

Blyth, H. and Ockenden, B.G. (1971). Polycystic disease in the kidneys and liver presenting in childhood. *J.med.Genet.* 8, 257
Boichis, H., Passwell, J., David, R. and Miller, H. (1973). Congenital hepatic fibrosis and nephronophthisis. *Q.Jl.Med.* 42, 221
Fried, K. *et al.* (1971). Polycystic kidneys associated with malformation of the brain, polydactyly and other birth defects. *J. med. Genet.* 8, 285
Ivemark, B.I., Oldfelt, V. and Zetterstrom, R.I. (1959). Familial dysplasia of kidneys, liver and pancreas, A probably genetically determined syndrome. *Acta paediat. Scand.* 48, 1

Keir, D.N.S. *et al.* (1961). Congenital hepatic fibrosis. *Q.Jl.Med.* **30**, 91

Keir, D.N.S., Warrick, C.K. and Hart-Mercer, J. (1962). A lesion resembling medullary sponge in patients with congenital hepatic fibrosis. *Clin.Radiol.* **13**, 85

Lieberman, E. *et al.* (1971). Infantile polycystic disease in kidneys and liver. *Medicine, Baltimore* **50**, 277

Murray-Lyon, I.M., Ockenden, B.G. and Williams, R. (1973). Congenital hepatic fibrosis — is it a single clinical entity? *Gastroenterology* **64**, 653

Nathan, M. and Batsakis, J.G. (1969). Congenital hepatic fibrosis. *Surgery Gynec. Obstet.* **128**, 1033

Odievre, M., Chaumont, P. and Oiry, P. (1976). Roentgenographic abnormalities of the intrahepatic portal system in congenital hepatic fibrosis. *Radiology* **122**, 427

Sokhi, G.S., Morrice, G.J., McGee, J. and Blumgart, L. (1975). Congenital hepatic fibrosis: aspects of diagnosis and surgical management. *Br.J.Surg.* **62**, 621

Sommerchild, H.C., Langmark, F. and Maursath, K. (1973). Congenital hepatic fibrosis: report of 2 new cases and review of the literature. *Surgury* **73**, 53

Intrahepatic bile duct dilatation

Caroli, J. and Corcos, V. (1964). La Dilatation congenitale des voies biliaires intra-hépatiques. *Rev.Méd.Chir.Mal.du Foie*, **39**, 1

Murray-Lyon, I.M., Schilkin, K.B., Laws, J.W., Illing, R.C. and Williams, R. (1972). Non-obstructive dilatation of intrahepatic biliary tree with cholangitis. *Q.Jl.Med.* **41**, 477

CHAPTER 12

Chronic Hepatitis

The concept of chronic hepatitis is an important one. As opposed to acute hepatitis in which complete clinical and histological recovery in a short time is the rule, untreated chronic hepatitis frequently leads to progressive morbidity and irreparable liver damage. The disorder was first described in adults only in 1947. Although intensively studied and described in the adult literature since then, it still presents many diagnostic, aetiological and therapeutic difficulties. Early clinical identification is still a problem.

Definition

In adult patients, chronic hepatitis is defined as an inflammation of the liver, continuing without improvement for at least six months. The inflammatory reaction is demonstrated by persistently abnormal liver function tests and by histological changes. In children this definition is not entirely helpful since progressive inflammatory liver disease may be diagnosed when symptoms have been present for as little as three to four weeks. Conversely, liver biopsy may show features of acute hepatitis after years of continuous or relapsing clinical and biochemical evidence of hepatitis. The nature of the intrahepatic histological change is thus crucial.

In acute hepatitis, the changes are predominantly parenchymal. In chronic hepatitis there are, in addition, inflammatory changes in the portal tract with proliferation of portal tract structures and fibrous tissue. Unfortunately, cirrhosis may often be found at the time of initial biopsy. In children, therefore, definition requires consideration both of the clinical and biochemical features, and of the liver biopsy findings.

Clinical features suggesting chronicity

Chronic hepatitis should be suspected in a patient with hepatitis in the following circumstances.

(1) When clinical and biochemical abnormalities in apparent acute hepatitis persist beyond two to three months.
(2) In an acute hepatitis associated with hypergammaglobulinaemia, positive antinuclear factor, or prolonged prothrombin time.
(3) In an apparent relapse of acute hepatitis.
(4) If hepatitis follows cholestatic jaundice in early infancy.
(5) Associated with low serum alpha-1 antitrypsin concentration.
(6) Associated with low caeruloplasmin.
(7) If serum positive for hepatitis B surface antigen for more than one month.

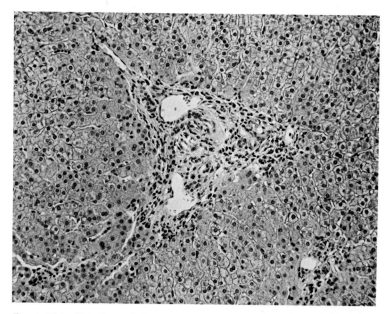

Figure 12.1. Chronic persistent hepatitis. There is a mononuclear inflammatory cell infiltrate in the slightly swollen portal tract. The limiting plate at the junction of the portal tract and the hepatic parenchyma is virtually intact. The cells with elongated nuclei in the portal tract are fibroblasts which are present in a slight excess. A few inflammatory cells are seen in the hepatic parenchyma – in the lower left corner. No other abnormalities are seen in the hepatic parenchyma (percutaneous liver biopsy, haematoxylin and eosin × 125, reduced to two-thirds in reproduction)

TABLE 12.1
Pathological Features in Liver Biopsy

Chronic persistent hepatitis	Chronic active hepatitis
Chronic inflammatory cell infiltrate in widened portal tracts sharply demarcated from hepatic parenchyma	Chronic inflammatory cell infiltrate in portal tracts with marked perilobular hepatitis and 'piecemeal' hepatocellular necrosis
Minimal erosion of limiting plate	Marked fibroblastic proliferation
Normal hepatic parenchyma	Distortion of hepatic lobular architecture
± Slight fibrosis of portal tracts	Inflammatory cell infiltrate in parenchyma
Fine fibrous septa in parenchyma	± Signs of acute hepatitis
Areas of liver cell necrosis with inflammatory cell infiltrate	Liver cell 'rosettes' at the periphery of lobules
Kupffer cell prominence	Inflamed intralobular fibrous septa

Liver biopsy

Percutaneous liver biopsy is essential in all cases to confirm the diagnosis and assess the need for treatment. In some cases, there may be a temporary contra-indication to biopsy because of the prolonged prothrombin time. Treatment is required to correct coagulation abnormalities before biopsy can be safely performed. The major pathological categories are chronic persistent hepatitis and chronic aggressive hepatitis. (*Table 12.1*).

Chronic persistent hepatitis

Chronic persistent hepatitis (*Figure 12.1*) is characterized by an inflammatory infiltrate, mainly of mononuclear cells which may include a few plasma cells, virtually confined to widened portal tracts. There may be small fibrous septa extending out from the tracts but the liver architecture is preserved. There is minimal erosion of the limiting plate where hepatic parenchyma meets the portal tract. There may be small infrequent foci of liver cell necrosis with inflammatory cells in the parenchyma and prominent Kupffer cells.

The differential diagnosis includes non-specific reactive hepatitis due to systemic illness or gastrointestinal disease; in this the liver cells are likely to show variation in cell size with increased Kupffer cell proliferation and some intralobular inflammation, residual viral hepatitis, malignancy, leukaemia and lymphosarcoma. In malignancy there is commonly inflammation in the portal triads but it is usually less dense than in chronic persistent hepatitis. In leukaemia and lymphosarcoma the cellular infiltrate is extremely dense. Biliary tract disease may show very similar inflammatory infiltrate but there are usually some polymorphonuclear leucocytes present and more marked bile duct proliferation.

Chronic aggressive hepatitis

Chronic aggressive hepatitis (*Figure 12.2* and *12.3*) is characterized by the presence of a perilobular hepatitis extending into the hepatic parenchyma adjacent to the portal tracts and causing hepatocellular

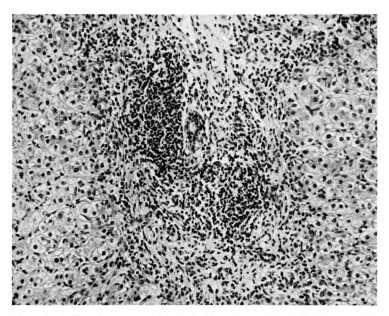

Figure 12.2 Chronic aggressive hepatitis. There is considerable widening of the portal tracts with an intense mononuclear cell infiltrate. The junction between the portal tract and hepatic parenchyma is irregular and inflammatory cells extend from the portal tract out into the parenchyma. In the upper part of the portal tract there is increased fibrosis. The hepatocytes show some vacuolation and there is patchy inflammatory cell infiltrate throughout the parenchyma (percutaneous liver biopsy, haematoxylin and eosin × 125, reduced to two-thirds in reproduction)

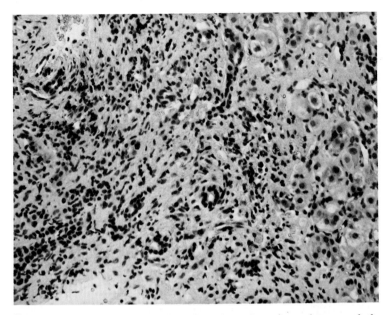

Figure 12.3. Chronic aggressive hepatitis. A section of portal tract and the adjacent hepatic parenchyma is shown from another portal tract in the same biopsy. There is typical piecemeal necrosis of the hepatic parenchyma on the right. The interface between the portal tract and hepatic parenchyma is almost completely lost. Hepatocytes are swollen and have assumed abnormal configurations, such as rosettes. They are surrounded by lymphocytes and some groups of hepatocytes are isolated from other parts of the hepatic lobule. Within the portal tract the elongated nuclei or fibroblasts can be seen. These represent an integral part of the hepatic reaction in chronic aggressive hepatitis (percutaneous liver biopsy, haematoxylin and eosin × 320, reduced to two-thirds in reproduction)

necrosis, giving rise to the term 'piecemeal necrosis'. The liver cells are swollen and may assume pseudo-ductular arrangements. This process is associated with marked proliferation of fibroblasts and collagen deposition. These changes disturb the lobular architecture but true cirrhosis is, by definition, absent. The presence of so-called 'bridging' lesions, in which proliferative fibroblasts and inflammatory cell aggregates link the portal tracts to each other or to hepatic vein, is a further pathological feature indicating chronicity. The liver cells are often swollen and pale staining. There may be parenchymal cellular infiltrate similar to acute hepatitis. The liver cell plates may appear as glandular structures termed 'rosettes', sometimes with a central lumen and often surrounded by compressed sinusoids and inflammatory cells.

The histological findings in the liver may vary from lobule to lobule and from time to time. It is often difficult to discern whether or not cirrhosis is present. In the late stages cirrhosis, with or without the features of chronic aggressive hepatitis is an invariable finding. If, however, the disease is controlled by drugs or undergoes complete spontaneous resolution, only residual scarring may be found. It is important to appreciate that these histological changes which are commonly associated with the syndrome of chronic active hepatitis may also be found in Wilson's disease and in chronic liver damage due to drugs such as methyldopa.

Chronic lobular hepatitis

Chronic lobular hepatitis is a poorly studied entity in which there are within the hepatic parenchyma, histological changes similar to those seen in acute viral hepatitis; namely, liver cell degeneration and necrosis maximal around the central veins with infiltration by inflammatory cells and Kupffer cell proliferation. Occasionally, such features may be present months or years after the onset of an acute hepatitis or may be found in the presence of relapsing hepatitis. Occasionally, these histological features are also found in association with the perilobular changes characteristic of chronic aggressive hepatitis. This is an entity which requires further study.

CHRONIC PERSISTENT HEPATITIS

The diagnosis of this condition is based on the histological findings described above.

Clinical aspects

The patient may present following a mild or moderately severe hepatitis. Most frequently there are no gastrointestinal or hepatic symptoms but the diagnosis may be suspected when the serum transaminase values fail to return to normal. On occasions the condition may present without any previous evidence of liver disease and be detected as a result of the persistent abnormality in biochemical tests of liver function performed as part of the routine medical examination, or in the investigation of some unrelated complaint. Physical examination may show no abnormality or there may be slight hepatomegaly without any features suggestive of chronic liver disease.

Characteristically, the serum bilirubin is normal but the transaminase elevated to between two and five times normal. Such abnormalities may persist for many years. The serum alkaline phosphatase is usually normal, as are the serum immunoglobulins. The hepatitis B surface antigen may be found in the serum.

Differential diagnosis

In such patients it is absolutely essential to exclude Wilson's disease by appropriate tests (page 239). Serum alpha-1 antitrypsin should be determined by protease inhibitor phenotyping and consideration given

TABLE 12.2
Causes of Chronic Hepatitis in Childhood

Chronic active hepatitis	Sequelae of hepatitis in infancy –
Chronic persistent hepatitis	metabolic, familial idiopathic, and
Wilson's disease	idiopathic
Liver disease associated with alpha–1	Bile duct lesions – choledochal cyst
antitrypsin deficiency	(see cirrhosis)
Drug therapy – isoniazid, methyldopa,	Parasitic infections – schistosomiasis
antimitotic agents, oxyphenisatin	Inflammatory disease of large bowel

to the possibility of other forms of chronic liver disease, such as cystic fibrosis, or ulcerative colitis. A careful history should be taken with special attention given to drug exposure and exposure to possible hepatotoxins (*Tables 9.1 and 9.2*).

Prognosis

In the absence of any such additional factors, an excellent prognosis can be given. It should be noted, however, that in occasional patients serial liver biopsies show progression from chronic persistent hepatitis to chronic aggressive hepatitis. Such changes may represent those of sampling error rather than a true progression of the disease. It seems prudent to advise that patients with chronic persistent hepatitis should be reviewed to determine that no new clinical abnormality has occurred and that the liver function tests have returned completely to normal. No drug treatment is required. The patients should be encouraged to live a full active life without dietary restrictions.

CHRONIC ACTIVE HEPATITIS

This is defined as a continuing inflammatory lesion of the liver with a potential to progress to more severe liver disease (including cirrhosis), to continue unchanged or to subside spontaneously or with treatment.

Clinically there are features of progressive or recurrent hepatocellular dysfunction and often features of portal hypertension if the disease is severe.

Clinical features

Chronic hepatitis may present with features of an acute hepatitis, namely, anorexia, nausea and vomiting proceeding to jaundice with hepatomegaly, dark urine and pale stools. Ascites, marked splenomegaly, and the finding of extrahepatic manifestations of liver disease, such as spider angiomata, should suggest the diagnosis even when the duration of symptoms is short (*Table 12.3*). In other patients, presenting as acute hepatitis, it is only where jaundice persists beyond four weeks that the possibility of chronic liver disease is considered.

TABLE 12.3
Extrahepatic Manifestations of Chronic Active Hepatitis

Site	Manifestation
Skin	Spider angiomata, malar flush, acne, inflammatory papules, striae gravidarum, urticaria, lupus erythematosus
Locomotor system	Arthralgia, arthritis
Renal system	Albuminuria, haematuria, glomerulonephritis, renal tubular acidosis
Pulmonary system	Pleurisy, pleural effusion, multiple pulmonary arteriovenous anastomosis, fibrosing alveolitis
Endocrine system	Cushinoid features, gynaecomastia in males, amenorrhoea, thyroiditis
Haemopoietic system	Coomb's positive haemolytic anaemia
Ocular system	Iridocyclitis

More frequently the presentation is insidious with such non-specific symptoms as lethargy and anorexia, and the diagnosis is suggested by hepatomegaly, present in over 95 per cent of cases reported, or by the finding of strikingly abnormal biochemical liver function tests. In such patients it is impossible to know the duration of the illness. Often the pathological changes are much more advanced, with considerable fibrous tissue deposition, than would be suggested by the history. Half the cases have splenomegaly, and approximately 25 per cent of cases will have some of the extrahepatic features listed in *Table 12.3*.

The disease has been recorded from the age of 2 to 75 years. In the paediatric age group it occurs rarely before the age of six years but increases in frequency thereafter. The maximum age incidence is probably between 10 and 30 years. Seventy per cent of cases in adult series are female, and this has been similar in most paediatric series reported.

Some patients at presentation are acutely ill with anorexia, weight-loss and fever as well as specific features of hepatocellular failure. Others are surprisingly active, well grown and well nourished. Epistaxis, bleeding gums and bruising with minimal trauma are frequent complaints. Acne is often prominent. Spider naevi are virtually constant. Amenorrhoea is usual, the menses returning as improvement occurs. Very rarely, a cholestatic picture is seen. Ascites, oedema, and hepatic encephalopathy are late features.

Our knowledge of the natural history is not complete, and even in adult patients recognition of this disorder came at a time when corticosteroids were already established as a powerful panacea for all kinds of conditions, and few patients with chronic active hepatitis have been observed without any steroid therapy. It seems that with no treatment the course is very variable, but is likely to be punctuated by periods of exacerbation with symptoms of acute hepatocellular dysfunction and increased jaundice. Pathologically, there is increased necrosis involving either a limited perilobular area, the entire lobule or even consecutive lobules.

Increased fibrous tissue accumulation leading to cirrhosis is the inevitable sequel. In the late stages of the disease, hepatic inflammation is less evident and the final features may be that of a quiescent cirrhosis.

Laboratory investigations

Serum transaminases are raised to values of between 2 and 30 times normal; in most paediatric series the majority of values lying between 4 and 10 times normal. In contrast, the serum alkaline phosphatase is only modestly elevated by 20–50 per cent or may be normal. Hyperbilirubinaemia is reported rarely in cases of insidious onset, but does occur during exacerbations. The serum albumin is usually normal early in the course. The prothrombin time is frequently prolonged by three to four seconds at an early stage, with more marked prolongation occurring later. When the BSP uptake from serum has been estimated it is invariably found to be delayed.

A characteristic abnormality is hypergammaglobulinaemia with values almost invariably greater than 30 g/litre and often values greater than 36 g/litre being found. The serum immunoglobulins are elevated, with the IgG being greater than 1,800 mg/dl. In approximately 50 per cent of cases, tissue autoantibodies, particularly antinuclear factor and smooth muscle antibody are found in significant titres. Antimitochondrial antibodies occur less frequently. A few cases show positive rheumatoid factor, Coomb's positive haemolytic anaemia and thyroid autoantibodies. Rarely, liver-kidney microsomal autoantibody may be the sole marker.

Some patients will be found to be hepatitis B surface antigen positive. In these, the biochemical abnormalities are often less marked than in the hepatitis B surface antigen negative cases and the total elevation of gammaglobulins less. These patients may have an elevated IgM, as well as IgC.

Aetiology and pathogenesis

The aetiology of chronic active hepatitis is unknown. Since in about 25 per cent of cases the disease seems to start as an acute hepatitis, research interest has concentrated on possible disorders of immune mechanisms which normally eliminate such acute infection. Present hypotheses are based largely on research done in adult patients, but supported by limited date obtained from studies in children with this condition.

Genetic predisposition

First-degree relatives of patients with chronic active hepatitis have raised serum gammaglobulins. More than 60 per cent of patients with chronic active hepatitis have the same histo-compatibility antigen, HLA, B8. Subjects who have the B8 antigen reject renal transplant and clear the hepatitis B virus more rapidly than those with other histo-compatibility antigens. High antibody titres to measles, rubella, smooth muscle and *E.coli*, are more frequently found in such patients.

Immunological abnormalities

Considerable recent research has been directed towards investigations of abnormalities of *the immune system* in the pathogenesis of this condition. An autoimmune basis for this disease is suggested by its association with other autoimmune conditions such as thyroiditis, and renal tubular acidosis, and the frequent finding in the serum of autoimmune markers. In most adult series between 30 and 50 per cent have antinuclear antibodies, while up to 25 per cent have anti-mitochondrial antibodies and a larger percentage smooth muscle anti-bodies. In paediatric series, antinuclear antibodies are found with a similar frequency, but the other markers have been infrequently deter-mined. The marked lymphocytic infiltration in the liver has been considered to be part of an immunological attack on the liver, perhaps directed against liver cell components rendered antigenic by viral or toxic injury.

Liver specific autoimmunity has yet to be convincingly demon-strated but the recent isolation by Meyer zum Buschenfelde of two human liver specific lipoproteins, one a normal constituent of the hepatocyte membrane and the other a soluble cytoplasmic protein, has given a new stimulus to the search for an autoimmune basis in chronic active hepatitis (Meyer zum Buschenfelde *et al.*, 1976). The injection of these two antigens into rabbits produces an inflammatory cell lesion in the liver similar to chronic active hepatitis. By means of *in vitro* inhibition of leucocyte migration, sensitization to this protein can be demonstrated in the leucocytes of 90 per cent of patients with untreated chronic active hepatitis. Leucocyte sensitization to such a hepatocyte surface antigen might be expected to damage hepatocytes. Further evidence to implicate liver specific lipoprotein in the patho-genesis of continuing liver damage in chronic active hepatitis, is provided by a recent research investigation using an *in vitro* system in which isolated rabbit hepatocytes are incubated with lymphocytes from patients with and without liver disease (Smith *et al.*, 1977).

Lymphocytes from patients with untreated chronic active hepatitis kill a large percentage of the hepatocytes in this test system. The percentage killed can be considerably reduced by the addition of very small amounts of liver specific protein to the test system. It is suggested that the antigen binding sites on the lymphocytes are saturated by this liver specific protein and therefore are unable to react with liver specific lipoprotein on the hepatocyte cell membrane. The hepatocyte is thus spared. While this mechanism may not be involved in initiating liver damage, it may be important in maintaining it.

Hepatitis viruses

Infection with hepatitis viruses may be important in initiating liver injury. In adults with chronic active hepatitis, sera from between 3 and 51 per cent of patients is persistently positive to hepatitis B surface antigen.

In most paediatric series only a minority of cases are hepatitis B surface antigen positive, but in the series reported by Meyer zum Buschenfelde *et al.* (1976), 14 of 21 cases were positive. However, a percentage of the population varying from 0.1 per cent in Western Europe to more than 10 per cent in S.E. Asia has persistently hepatitis B surface antigen in the serum without clinical, biochemical or pathological evidence of liver disease. The exact mechanisms which determine whether hepatitis B virus will produce an acute self-limiting hepatitis, a symptomatic carrier state or chronic aggressive hepatitis are at present unknown. Some of the difficulties in understanding the immune responses may be caused by the use of tests of variable sensitivity, and particularly with tests of cell mediated immunity by the influence of ill-understood and therefore uncontrolled factors in the test system.

In typical cases of acute hepatitis, hepatitis B surface antigen is present in the serum for 10–14 days before liver disease can be detected. Specific antibody to hepatitis B surface antigen and cell mediated immunity to the antigen, demonstrated by leucocyte migration inhibition, appears coincidentally with the onset of liver disease. The antigen becomes undetectable shortly thereafter.

Subjects who become persistent carriers of HBsAg, have demonstrable HBsAg in the cytoplasm of their hepatocytes and develop no antibodies to the HBsAg whether liver disease is present or not. It is thus suggested that viral infection may persist because of a quantitative (or qualitative?) defect in the production of neutralizing antibody allowing the virus to penetrate previously uninfected liver cells. In the carrier there is no biochemical or histological evidence of progressive liver disease, leucocyte migration inhibition to HBsAg is present in a minority (13 per cent). In contrast, 47 per cent of carriers who have biochemical and histological evidence of ongoing liver disease do show leucocyte migration inhibition, as did 63 per cent of patients with chronic aggressive hepatitis. These findings would appear to support the hypothesis that liver damage in chronic HBsAg carriers is due to a cellular immune response, perhaps directed at a viral antigen.

Ineffective 'supressor' T-cell hypothesis

To link these recent research observations with the observed auto-immunity to liver specific protein, and possible hepatocyte cell surface antigens the hypothesis of T-cell and B-cell interaction proposed by Allison, Denman and Barnes (1971) is invoked. In brief, T-cells are held to recognize and react to new virus associated antigens on the hepatocyte cell surface, not only by attacking and killing the hepatocyte, but also by activating B-cells to become responsive to hepatocyte cell surface antigens (*Figure 12.4*).

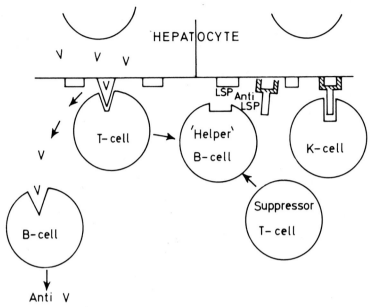

Figure 12.4. Virus (V) replicates within the hepatocyte. It causes virus-related antigen (▽) to appear on the hepatocyte surface. T lymphocytes (T-cell), which are considered to be the cells involved in cell mediated immunity, react with these antigens causing cell death. Virus is released from the hepatocyte and reacts with B-cells (lymphocytes which produce antibody) and anti-viral antibody is produced. The interaction of T-cells and virus-related antigen on the hepatocyte surface is thought to cause 'helper' B-cells to react to form antibodies to normal components of the hepatocyte plasma membrane, such as liver-specific lipoprotein. (LSP). Antibodies to liver specific lipoprotein (anti-LSP) attaches itself to the hepatocyte cell membrane. Cell lysis follows. This may be caused by a third immunocyte, the K-cell which reacts with the non-antibody (Fc) portion of the antibody molecule. This reaction should cease as soon as all virus infected cells are killed. In some patients it is thought that this continues, either because the virus is not cleared completely from the hepatocyte, for example, HBV, or because the so-called suppressor T-cell has a genetically determined defect in its action in controlling autoimmune antibody production

Damaging autoantibodies are thus produced which attach themselves to the cell surface antigen, following which necrosis occurs. The necrosis may be due to complement fixation but could also be due to the action of yet another 'immunocyte', the K-cell, which reacts with the Fc portion of antibody molecules (the portion which does not react with antigen). In the hepatocyte cytotoxicity system referred to above, cytotoxicity is abolished if K-cells and B-cells are removed from the system, but persists if T-cells only are removed. A continuing production of damaging autoantibodies, clearly crucial in this hypothesis of pathogenesis, is thought to be controlled by so-called 'suppressor' T-cells, which are functioning inefficiently, due either to a continuous T-cell activation by infective agents, or by an intrinsic, perhaps genetically determined defect in suppressor T-cell activity. Support for this latter hypothesis comes from the association of defective T-cell function and increased immune responsiveness with the histocompatibility antigen HLA B8.

Management

Depending on the degree of hepatocellular failure the patient may require therapy such as bed-rest, sodium and fluid restriction for oedema, infusions of albumin, fresh frozen plasma or vitamin K. While the diagnosis is being established the patient should be investigated for latent infections such as tuberculosis, peritonitis, urinary tract infection and should be nursed in a cubicle to minimize the risks of exposure to illnesses such as measles which can cause prolonged ill-health in the immunosuppressed patient.

Drug treatment (Figure 12.5a,b)

For treatment to be effective it must be started before cirrhosis has developed. Corticosteroids, in spite of their many side-effects, are the drug of choice. In a controlled trial in adult patients, steroids produced such a favourable response in the treated group that continuation in the trial became unjustifiable. Nevertheless, 3 of the 22 patients died (Cook, Mulligan and Sherlock, 1971). A well planned, double-blind trial from the Mayo Clinic showed a significant beneficial effect,

Figure 12.5. (a) Chronic aggressive hepatitis suppressed by drug therapy. A widened portal tract with intense fibrosis and patchy mononuclear cell infiltrate is shown. The junction between hepatic parenchyma and portal tract is now clear-cut (percutaneous liver biopsy, haematoxylin and eosin × 125, reduced to two-thirds in reproduction). (b) A reticulin stained biopsy (× 80, reduced to two-thirds in reproduction) shows distortion of the hepatic parenchyma by fibrous septa. Widened portal tract is shown with islets of hepatocytes without hepatic veins surrounded by fibrous tissue, cirrhosis having supervened. These biopsies are from a girl aged 12 years who had had two episodes of jaundice between the age of eight and ten years when investigations showed she had the full syndrome of chronic active hepatitis. Symptoms and liver function tests returned to normal within one year of commencing treatment and had been normal for one year prior to the above biopsies. Unfortunately, cirrhosis is now present

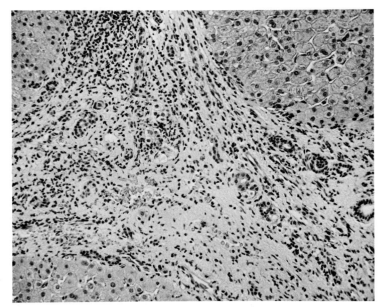

Figure 12.5 (a)

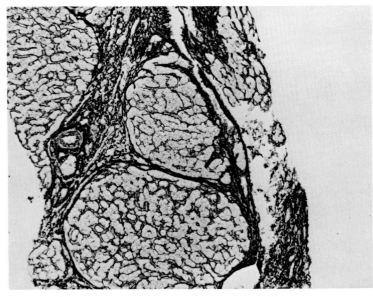

Figure 12.5 (b)

particularly in the decrease of transaminase, bilirubin and gamma-globulin, but again 20 per cent failed to respond and died with hepato-cellular failure. (Soloway *et al.*, 1972). Although no controlled trials have been reported in children, available evidence suggests that in them the prognosis is at least as good, if not better (Dubois and Silverman, 1974).

Prednisolone in a dose of 1—1.5 mg/kg per day should be given at the time of diagnosis, even before a histological diagnosis is confirmed, if a prolonged prothrombin time precludes safe biopsy. The aim of treatment is to induce a complete biochemical control of the hepatitis, while avoiding side-effects from the steroids. Full doses are usually required for the first four weeks of treatment, but thereafter it may be possible to reduce the dose gradually over the course of three to four months. It is rarely possible to adopt an alternate day regimen. Experience with adult patients suggests that in the disease associated with HBsAg in the serum, higher doses may be required for longer, but no controlled trials have been reported.

Excessive weight-gain in the first weeks of treatment occurs almost inevitably, but serious side-effects can often be avoided. In a minority of cases complete biochemical remission cannot be achieved without producing significant side-effects from the steroids. In these circum-stances reduction of the steroid dose and the addition of azathioprine (1 mg/kg per day) often results in biochemical control of the hepatitis. 6-Mercaptopurine has been reported to control chronic aggressive hepatitis in childhood, as has azathioprine as a single drug used in adults. The majority of adult studies suggests that a combination of prednisolone and azathioprine may be better. Azathioprine is perhaps best used when the disease has been brought partially under control by steroids.

D penicillamine appears to be as effective as corticosteroids in controlling chronic active hepatitis in adults, but the incidence of side-effects is such that its use can only be justified as an adjunct to steroid therapy when this is creating difficulties because of side-effects.

When biochemical abnormalities have been controlled, it is advisable that the patient stays on the same treatment for at least one year. If the liver biopsy at this stage shows no evidence of continuing histolo-gical activity, therapy could be safely discontinued. If there is still histological activity, therapy should be maintained. Careful follow-up is required after therapy is stopped.

Prognosis

The severity of chronic active hepatitis, its course and prognosis are extremely variable. Untreated continuing aggressive hepatitis will lead inevitably to cirrhosis: 34 per cent have cirrhosis by six months, 90 per cent by two years (Mistilis and Blackburn, 1970). In a few patients the disease will eventually become quiescent with little symptomatic upset but with established cirrhosis.

Where the disease has had an acute onset and treatment is instituted early in the course, a reversal to normal histology does occur. Where the disease is of greater chronicity at the time of diagnosis, and there is already a marked increase of intrahepatic fibrosis or even an already established cirrhosis, reversal is less likely. A very guarded prognosis should therefore be given initially and the patient's course followed carefully. In such patients it is likely that corticosteroids will produce a feeling of well-being and an improvement in liver function tests. Immunosuppressants are usually poorly tolerated, causing marked marrow depression. Although the immune reaction in the liver may be depressed and the rate of hepatocellular necrosis decreased, there is little evidence that the progression of collagen deposition and fibrosis is altered by treatment.

BIBLIOGRAPHY AND REFERENCES

Alagille, D., Gautier, M., Herouin, C. and Hadchouel, M. (1973). Chronic hepatitis in children. *Acta paediat. Scand.* **62**, 566

Allison, A.C. Denman, A.M. and Barnes, R.D. (1971). Co-operating and controlling functions of thymus-derived lymphocytes in relation to autoimmunity. *Lancet* **2**, 135

Becker, M.D., Scheuer, P.J., Baptista, A. and Sherlock, S. (1970). Prognosis of persistant hepatitis. *Lancet* **1**, 53

Cook, G.E., Mulligan, R. and Sherlock, S. (1971). Controlled prospective trial of corticosteroid therapy in active chronic hepatitis. *Q.Jl.Med.* **40**, 159

DeGroote, J. *et al.* (1968). A classification of chronic hepatitis. *Lancet* **2**, 626

Dubois, R.S. and Silverman, A. (1974). Treatment of chronic active hepatitis in children. *Postgrad.med.J.* **50**, 386

Eddleston, A.L.W.F. (1976). Aetiological factors in immune-mediated liver disease. In *Immunological Aspects of the Liver and Gastrointestinal Tract*, p. 291. Ed. by Ferguson, A. and MacSween, R.N.M. Lancaster, England: M.T.P. Press

Grossman, A., Rosenthal, F.M. and Szanto, P.B. (1962). Chronic active hepatitis with hypergammaglobulinaemia in childhood. A report of 8 cases. *Pediatrics* **29**, 933

Lawton, A.R., Persky, W.V., Schofield, L.M. and Cooper, M.D. (1973). Chronic active hepatitis in childhood: favourable response to intensive immunosuppressive therapy. *Paediat. Res.* **7**, 364

Meyer zum Buschenfelde, K.H., Baumann, W., Arnold, W. and Fraudenberg, J. (1976). Immunological aspects of chronic active hepatitis. In *INSERM, Paris* **49**, 15

Mistilis, S.P. and Blackburn, C.R.B. (1970). Active chronic hepatitis, *Am.J. Pediat.* **48**, 484

Page, A.R., Good, R.A. and Pollara, B. (1970). Long-term results of therapy in patients with chronic liver disease associated with hypergammaglobulinaemia. *Am.J.Med.* **47**, 765

Sherlock, S. (1974). Progress report: chronic hepatitis. *Gut* **15**, 581

Smith, A.L., Cochran, A.M.G., Mowat, A.P., Eddleston, A.L.W.F. and Williams, R. (1977). Cytotoxicity to isolated rabbit hepatocytes by lymphocytes from children with liver disease. *J.Paediat.* **91**, 584

Soloway, R.D. *et al.* (1972). Clinical, biochemical and histological remission of severe chronic active liver disease: a controlled study of treatment and early prognosis. *Gastroenterology* **63**, 820

Tolantino, P. (1976). Chronic active hepatitis in childhood. *Paediatrician* **5**, 67

CHAPTER 13

Wilson's Disease

Wilson's disease in childhood may mimic any form of parenchymal hepatic disorder. More than 50 per cent of cases present before puberty with no neurological abnormality. Without treatment there is progressive damage to the liver and brain, and premature death occurs. Early treatment is relatively safe and very effective. Wilson's disease with all its protean presentations must be considered in all children with unexplained hepatic disorders, general ill-health or deteriorating school performance. Equally important is the recognition and treatment of asymptomatic siblings of identified cases.

Definition

Wilson's disease is an inborn error of metabolism associated with the accumulation of toxic amounts of copper in the liver, brain, kidneys and corneas. It is inherited in an autosomal recessive fashion. The basic genetic defect is unknown.

Pathogenesis

An abnormality in the transport and storage of copper resulting in copper accumulation is thought to be important in pathogenesis. High concentrations of copper are found in the liver, brain, corneas and renal tubules in patients dying with this disease. Two major abnormalities in copper metabolism have been confirmed in research work in the last ten years: diminished biliary excretion of copper and impaired caeruloplasmin production. A positive copper balance is present in patients with Wilson's disease in spite of increased urinary copper excretion. Early in the disease intestinal absorption of copper is normal, as is hepatic clearance of albumin-bound absorbed copper. As the liver copper binding proteins become saturated, there is first slowing down of hepatic uptake followed by biochemical and then clinical evidence of liver damage.

One recent investigation has suggested that the synthesis of an abnormal copper binding protein may be important in pathogenesis, while another has suggested that deficient lysosomal incorporation of copper may be a more important defect in copper storage. With hepatocellular death, there is release of copper, which accumulates in and damages other tissues. When the cerebral copper binding proteins are saturated, a characteristic pattern of brain damage develops. Manifestations of renal tubular injury usually appears simultaneously. Very rapid copper release is thought to cause the haemolytic anaemia sometimes seen early in the clinical course of Wilson's disease.

An abnormally low serum concentration of caeruloplasmin is the most constant biochemical abnormality in Wilson's disease, being found in over 90 per cent of patients. In one paediatric series 23 per cent had a normal caeruloplasmin in spite of active disease. Similarly, low caeruloplasmin values are found, however, in some heterozygotes. Caeruloplasmin is a blue, copper-containing serum alpha-2 globulin which transports copper. Copper incorporation into caeruloplasmin is deficient in Wilson's disease. In adult life, serum caeruloplasmin levels are relatively constant at between 0.2 and 0.45 g/litre. In cord blood the levels are much lower, usually being less than 0.1 g/litre. By the age of two months, adult levels are reached and early in infancy the levels are often higher, declining to the adult range by the age of 10−12 years. The newborn liver has a much higher concentration of copper than the adult, the concentrations varying up to 63 μg/g dry weight, as opposed to the usual adult range of 15−50 μg/g dry weight. In the newborn, 60 per cent of the copper is in the liver cell cytoplasm, the remainder being associated with a copper-binding protein, mitochondrocuprein which is present in concentrations more than 80 times that of the adult values. In Wilson's disease the concentration is increased in the cytoplasm and in the mitochondria early in the disease, but late in the disease much is sequestrated in lysosomes.

Pathology

Hepatic From asymptomatic patients investigated because of an affected relative, knowledge of the early hepatic pathology is available. Characteristically, there is marked fatty infiltration of the hepatocytes, often with prominent glycogen containing vacuoles in the nuclei.

By electronmicroscopy, hepatic mitochondria are seen to be bizarre in shape with electron dense vacuoles which sometimes contain granular or crystalloid material. Microbodies are frequent. Such changes are thought to be characteristic. Unfortunately, these hepatocellular changes are often associated with mesenchymal reaction, increased fibrosis, and occasionally, even cirrhosis. Early in the disease, specific stains for copper using rubeanic acid are negative, even though the liver copper determined chemically is between 3 and 30 times normal.

In symptomatic patients, the liver may be enlarged but is commonly normal in size, or even shrunken due to multilobular cirrhosis. In addition to the features noted above, chronic aggressive hepatitis and Mallory's cytoplasmic hyalin as seen in alcoholic liver disease, may also be present. In advanced disease the appearances are those of cirrhosis with no specific features although a few hepatocytes may show fatty change and glycogen-containing nuclei. Pigmented granules are frequent. Rubeanic acid stains for copper are at this stage positive, although liver copper concentration may be lower in the early stages of the disease. There are commonly features of secondary portal hypertension and often of hypersplenism.

Cerebral The cerebral changes are found mainly in the corpus striatum which shows shrinkage, cavitation, decrease in the number of neurones and in myelinated nerve fibres and increased astrocytosis. Similar, but less severe changes are seen in the cerebellum, the thalamus and the cortex.

Other sites Copper is found deposited also in the deep layers of the cornea just within the limbus, extending in a ring around the cornea. It may be deposited also in the lens to give a 'sunflower' cataract. Copper can be found deposited also in the renal tubular cells.

Clinical features

The classic form of this disease, progressive lenticular degeneration with tremor, increasing muscular rigidity, asymptomatic cirrhosis, Kayser–Fleischer rings in the cornea and functional renal disturbances, commonly has its onset in the second decade of life. It is infrequently found in childhood and may only develop in those in whom hepatic injury is not lethal.

Paediatric presentation In childhood, the vast majority of patients have a hepatic onset. The mode of presentation is, however, *very variable, mimicking all forms of liver disease in childhood* (*Table 13.1*). Symptomatic liver disorder due to Wilson's disease has not been

TABLE 13.1
Hepatic Presentations of Wilson's Disease

Asymptomatic hepatomegaly	Asymptomatic cirrhosis
Hepatosplenomegaly with vague gastrointestinal symptoms	Gastrointestinal haemorrhage due to portal hypertension
Jaundice with oedema and ascites	Chronic aggressive hepatitis
Subacute hapatitis (presumed viral)	?Cholestatic liver disease of infancy
Fulminant hepatitis	

diagnosed before the age of four years, but two of ten children described by Odievere *et al.* (1974) had hepatic symptoms by the age of three years. The majority present in the second or third decade but the onset may be as late as the fifth decade. Early symptoms may be totally non-specific but examination may reveal clinical and biochemical features of significant liver disease.

Wilson's disease may present with *neurological abnormalities*, such as clumsiness, slurring of speech, difficulties with fine movements or behaviour problems (*Table 13.2*).

TABLE 13.2
Non-hepatic Presentations of Wilson's Disease

Acute haemolytic anaemia	Kayser–Fleischer rings
Neurological disorders	Melanin hyperpigmentation of legs and scars
Behaviour disturbances	Arthralgia
Renal tubular abnormalities	
Vitamin D resistant rickets	

In children, in particular, a *haemolytic crisis* may be the first manifestation of the disease. Rarely, *vitamin D resistant rickets*, renal rickets or the Fanconi syndrome may be the first indication of disease. On occasions, it has been diagnosed by finding Kayser–Fleischer rings on routine ophthalmogical examination in which the slit lamp was used.

Laboratory findings (*Figures 13.1* and *13.2 a,b*)

Liver function tests indicate a variable degree of hepatocellular necrosis with or without hypoalbuminaemia. Although peripheral blood may show features of haemolytic anaemia, these changes are usually transient but there may be features of hypersplenism. Urinary abnormalities secondary to excess copper deposition include haematuria, proteinuria, glycosuria and hyperaminoaciduria. Phosphaturia and uricosuria associated with low serum concentrations of phosphate and uric acid may be found. Defects in acidification of the urine have also been reported. These abnormalities are not specific for Wilson's disease and show no diagnostic pattern.

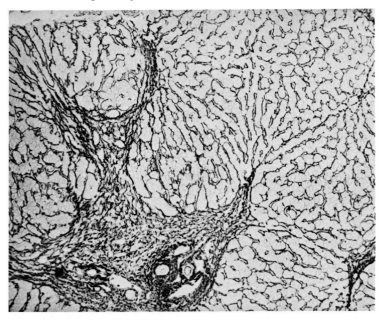

Figure 13.1. Wilson's disease. Percutaneous liver biopsy (reticulin X 150, reduced to seven-tenths in reproduction) from a girl aged nine years. It shows extensive fibrosis around an enlarged portal tract with wide fibrous septa extending out into the hepatic parenchyma. The reticulin framework for the hepatocytes within the hepatic parenchyma is normally orientated. A hepatic vein branch is seen in the upper right-hand corner. The patient presented five months previously with malaise and tiredness. The mucosae were pale but there were no other abnormalities on examination. The haemoglobin was 8.0 g/dl with slightly hypochromic red cells. The reticulocyte count ranged from 7 to 14 per cent. There was no occult blood loss and extensive investigations uncovered no cause for haemolysis. Because the serum aminotransferase level was elevated on one occasion, she was referred for further hepatic investigations. There were no clinical features of liver disease. Wilson's disease was diagnosed on the basis of Keyser–Fleischer rings, very low serum caeruloplasmin, high urinary copper and a high copper content in the liver biopsy. A low copper diet, penicillamine and pyridoxine were recommended. Liver function tests have remained normal, the patient is no longer anaemic. There have been no neurological abnormalities

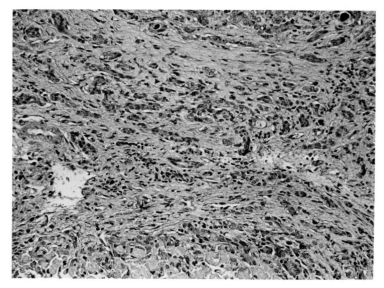

Figure 13.2 (a)

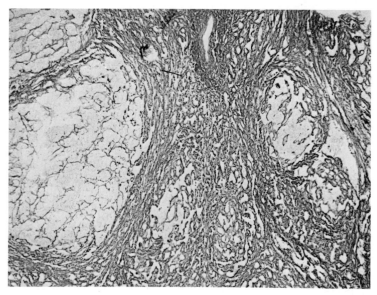

Figure 13.2 (b)

Course

The subsequent course of Wilson's disease is variable. Usually there is gradual progression of the hepatic disease with involvement of other systems. There may be spontaneous remission of symptoms with exacerbation by intercurrent infection. Haemolytic episodes may recur over one to two years, to be followed by an asymptomatic period of some years. Untreated, there is progressive liver disease, leading to cirrhosis and hepatic encephalopathy with death usually in a few years, but sometimes within weeks of the first onset of symptoms. Neurological features may never appear but when they do, they may be mistaken for those of portosystemic shunting.

Diagnosis

Wilson's disease is very rare, with an estimated incidence in the range of 1/100,000 to 1/200,000. Its clinical features are non-specific in the early treatable stages. A high level of suspicion in all forms of unexplained hepatic disorder in childhood is necessary to make the diagnosis. Consanguinity of parents, unexplained liver or neurological disease in siblings, previous history of haemolytic anaemia or clinical evidence of neurological abnormality should be additional prompts to exclude this disorder by the following specific investigations.

Figure 13.2. Wilson's disease. Post-mortem liver specimen from a boy aged 11 years. ((a) Haematoxylin and eosin × 150; (b) Reticulin × 150, both reduced to seven-tenths in reproduction.) The features are those of cirrhosis. (a) Showing an area of fibrous tissue with many bile ducts, presumably due to collapse of hepatic lobules. There is much fibrous tissue but little inflammatory cell reaction. (b) Showing regenerative nodules with hepatocytes of varying size surrounded by abnormally orientated reticulin and without hepatic vein branches. These are surrounded by dense bands of fibrous tissue. Twelve months previously the parents had become concerned because of deteriorating school performance and lethargy. After seven months some abdominal discomfort and abdominal distension was noted. Liver disease was suspected eight weeks before his death when he became anorexic, vomited, and developed jaundice. A clinical diagnosis of infectious hepatitis was made at that time but when it was found the prothrombin time was prolonged by 15 seconds and albumin 24 g/litre, chronic underlying liver disease was suspected. The serum caeruloplasmin was 10mg/dl, slit-lamp examination of the cornea showed typical Kayser–Fleischer rings. Purpura and alimentary haemorrhage, generalized oedema, ascites, and encephalopathy rapidly developed. Penicillamine and steroids as well as full supportive therapy as for fulminant hepatitis, did not arrest the downhill course. Unfortunately, the patient is just one of a number of children and young adults in whom the diagnosis of Wilson's disease had not been made until decompensated cirrhosis was present. In none has therapy arrested the progression of the disease

Ophthalmoscopic examination by slit lamp

Kayser–Fleischer rings must be sought by an experienced examiner using a slit lamp. They appear as brown or greenish-brown deposits of copper just within the limbus. They are always bilateral and usually complete but occasionally they may be absent at the medial and lateral aspects. They may be seen by the naked eye especially if viewed with a light directed from the side, but most frequently they can only be demonstrated with a slit lamp. Although in children this sign is pathognomic of Wilson's disease the rings are rarely found below the age of seven. Their absence, therefore does not exclude the diagnosis.

Serum caeruloplasmin determination

A low caeruloplasmin of less than 20 mg/dl (0.2g/litre) is suggestive of Wilson's disease, in the absence of nephrotic syndrome, severe malabsorption, or protein-losing enteropathy. In most forms of liver disease the caeruloplasmin is high, but in fulminant hepatitis, chronic active hepatitis and tyrosinosis low values may be obtained. Low values are unfortunately found also in 10–20 per cent of heterozygotes, who have no evidence of disease.

Between 4 and 20 per cent of patients with Wilson's disease may have a normal caeruloplasmin. Pregnancy, oestrogens and oral contraceptives cause elevation of caeruoplasmin, even when it is low. In spite of these reservations, caeruloplasmin determination is the single most useful investigation in suspected Wilson's disease (*Table 13.3*), over 80 per cent of cases having levels of less than 0.1 g/litre.

Urinary copper determination

Increased urinary copper excretion is regularly found in Wilson's disease with more than 100 μg per day being excreted as opposed to the normal rate of less than 40 μg per day. Frequently, in Wilson's disease, the values are up to 1,000 μg per day. In this and other liver disorders associated with abnormal copper retention, such as biliary cirrhosis, the ingestion of 0.5 g penicillamine twice a day increases urinary copper to greater than 1,000 μg and frequently to levels as high as 3,000 μg. Normal individuals and heterozygotes for Wilson's disease, excrete less than 800 μg per day.

High urinary copper values have been found in such long-standing biliary disorders as biliary atresia, liver disease complicating cystic fibrosis, subacute sclerosing cholangitis, but in these the urinary concentration is usually less than 300 µg per day, except when there is much hepatocellular necrosis (*Table 13.4*).

Serum copper determinations are not helpful in the diagnosis of Wilson's disease since very low, normal or high values may be found.

TABLE 13.3
Serum Caeruloplasmin (g/litre)

	Range	*M ± S.D.*	
Normal			
Newborn	0.018–0.13	0.065	
Child	0.22–0.53	0.46 ±	0.52
Adult	0.18–0.65	0.30 ±	0.03
Wilson's disease			
Heterozygote	0.1 –0.51	0.28 ±	0.08
Asymptomatic	0.0 –0.19	0.056 ±	0.07
Symptomatic	0.0 –0.43	0.036 ±	0.053
Other liver disease			
Cirrhosis		0.39 ±	0.12
Chronic active hepatitis		0.28 ±	0.06
Primary biliary cirrhosis		0.54 ±	0.17
Biliary tract lesion		0.49 ±	0.19

(From Sternlieb and Scheinberg, 1968; Sass-Kortsak, 1975; and Ritland, Steinnes and Skrede, 1977)

TABLE 13.4
Urinary Copper Concentrations in Children and Adults with and without Wilson's Disease: Effect of Penicillamine

Urinary Cu µg/24 hours	
Normal children	8–30 µg per day
Adults	10–40 µg per day
Wilson's disease	
Heterozygote	<50
Asymptomatic	>30
Symptomatic	
+ Penicillamine 0·5g/bd	
Normal adult	< 800
Heterozygote	< 850
Wilson's disease	>1,000

(From Sternlieb and Scheinberg, 1968; Sass-Kortsak, 1975)

Copper content of liver biopsy

The normal liver copper is usually between 20 and 40 μg/g dry weight and levels of greater than 40 μg are unusual. In Wilson's disease the liver copper is commonly greater than 250 μg/g dry weight, although levels as low as 90 μg may be found in some patients. Heterozygotes have levels of between 40 and 210 μg/g dry weight. In chronic cholestatic states, very high liver coppers may be found (*Table 13.5*).

Radioactive copper studies

Studies using radioactive isotopes of copper are rarely necessary for diagnosis, but in patients with equivocal copper studies, in whom liver biopsy is contra-indicated, the rate of copper incorporation into caeruloplasmin may help in the diagnosis. This test involves the intravenous injection of copper-64 (^{64}Cu) (half-life 12.8 hours) or ^{67}Cu (half-life 68 hours) followed by the determination of total serum copper and that bound to caeruloplasmin at 12-hourly intervals in the subsequent three days.

In Wilson's disease, practically no copper is incorporated into caeruloplasmin but it does occur to an appreciable extent in heterozygotes and in patients with other forms of liver disease causing hypocaeruloplasminaemia and occurs to a greater extent in normal individuals. Such investigations should only be undertaken in referral units with the necessary expertise.

Treatment

Untreated Wilson's disease is invariably fatal. Except in the terminal stages of the illness, treatment will reverse features of hepatocellular injury and may cause some improvement in the neurological state. It makes no attempt to correct the genetic abnormality, but uses drugs to deplete the excessive body store of copper. A *diet* containing less than 0.6 mg of copper per day as opposed to normal dietary copper of 1–5 mg per day, is necessary in patients with Wilson's disease to prevent positive copper balance. Chocolate, nuts, mushrooms, cocoa and shellfish should be avoided.

D-penicillamine, introduced in 1956, is the most effective agent available at present for diminishing copper stores. If therapy is started in the pre-symptomatic phase, the development of the disease can be prevented. If given in the presence of early liver or neurological disease there is gradual clinical and biochemical improvement and even a return

TABLE 13.5
Liver Copper Content in Normal Subjects, Wilson's Disease and other
Hepatic Disorders

	μg/g dry weight	M ± S.D.
Normal		
Adults	15–57	
Newborn	15–65	
Wilson's disease		
Heterozygote	39–213	117 ± 51
Asymptomatic	152–1828	983 ± 365
Symptomatic	94–1360	588 ± 304
Other liver disease		
Cirrhosis	17–136	39
Chronic active hepatitis	15–80	40 ± 22
Primary biliary cirrhosis	80–940	411 ± 261
Biliary tract lesion	120–350	203 ± 77

(From Sternlieb and Scheinberg, 1968; Sass-Kortsak, 1975; and Ritland, Steinnes and Skrede, 1977)

to normal over the course of some months or years. If cirrhosis has already developed, or there is neural loss or advanced gliosis, permanent sequelae will remain. In adults, doses of 500 mg twice a day increasing to 1g/twice a day after six months if improvement is slow, are recommended. In children aged less than 12 years, a dose of 50–75 per cent of the adult dose is recommended. *Pyridoxine*, 5–10 mg per day should be given to combat the antipyridoxine effects of penicillamine.

Side-effects

Serious toxic effects of penicillamine which can occur at high dose levels include the nephrotic syndrome, Goodbaster's syndrome, lupus erythematosus, agranulocytosis and optic neuritis (preventable by pyridoxine.) Long-term treatment may cause desquamation and friability of the skin. Hypersensitivity reactions such as urticaria, fever, lymph gland enlargement and depression of the total white blood count and platelet count occur in 10–20 per cent of cases, usually early in the course of the disease. These stop when the drug is discontinued but may require treatment with antihistamines or corticosteroids. If penicillamine is re-introduced in doses of 10–50 mg per day and gradually increased, the drug can be tolerated in most cases.

Alternative therapy

If serious side-effects occur and penicillamine has to be stopped, therapy with tetraethylene tetraamine hydrochloride in a dose of 400 mg three times a day should be used. It is an effective drug but is in very limited supply.

The degree of de-coppering should be ascertained by periodic measurements of 24-hour urinary excretion of copper. This is best done by interrupting treatment for a few days and then administering a standard dose of penicillamine, for example 0.5 g every 12 hours. When successfully de-coppered, the urinary copper excretion is close to normal and usually less than 80 µg per day. When penicillamine is given excretion increases to between 500 and 800 µg per day.

It has been shown that liver transplantation can reverse a number of the clinical and metabolic abnormalities found in patients with liver disease. Such a measure should not be necessary, however, if Wilson's disease is diagnosed early before irreparable organ damage has occurred. Patients with Wilson's disease may require the symptomatic therapy necessary for patients with cirrhosis. Surgical procedures are poorly tolerated. Portosystemic shunts should not be produced since these are almost invariably followed by progressive encephalopathy.

Investigation of siblings of patients with Wilson's disease

Siblings of a patient have a 1:4 chance of having the disease. Absence of symptoms of abnormalities on clinical examination does not exclude the possibility that the individual is affected by the disease. Appropriate treatment before clinical features are evident prevent the development of the disease.

TABLE 13.6
Investigation of Siblings of Patients with Wilson's Disease

(1)	Clinical examination for evidence of hepatic or neural disease
(2)	Ophthalmic examination for Kayser–Fleischer rings
(3)	Biochemical studies for evidence of liver or renal disease
(4)	Serum caeruloplasmin determination
(5)	Urinary Cu determination with and without penicillamine 0.5 g twice a day
(6)	If not contra-indicated, percutaneous liver biopsy for Cu determination and routine histological examination
(7)	If biopsy is not indicated and investigations 2–5 are not diagnostic, intravenous radioactive infusion followed by determination of total and caeruloplasmin bound copper over three days

It is mandatory to carry out procedures 1–5 listed in *Table 13.6*. If these are normal, it may be presumed that the individual does not have Wilson's disease. If they show any abnormality, the usual course would be to proceed to percutaneous liver biopsy for determination of the copper content. This should establish the presence or absence of Wilson's disease.

If liver biopsy is contra-indicated, it is necessary to measure the rate of incorporation of radioactive copper into the caeruloplasmin.

If the investigation indicates Wilson's disease, a low copper diet and penicillamine therapy should be instituted. If Wilson's disease has been excluded by these tests it would seem prudent to advise a repeat of procedures 1–4 at two-yearly intervals, lest the clinical course of Wilson's disease in a particular family be atypical.

BIBLIOGRAPHY AND REFERENCES

Buchanan, G.R. (1975). Acute haemolytic anaemia as a presenting manifestation of Wilson's disease. *J.Pediat.* **86**, 245

Evans, G.W., Dubois, R.S. and Hambridge, K.M. (1973). Wilson's disease, identification of an abnormal copper-binding protein. *Science* **181**, 1175

Iser, J.H. *et al.* (1974). Haemolytic anaemia of Wilson's disease. *Gastroenterology* **67**, 290

Odievere, M., Vedrene, J., Landrieu, P. and Alagille, D. (1974). Les Fromes Hepatiques 'Pures' de la Maladie de Wilson Chez L'Enfant. *Archs fr. Pediat.* **31**, 215

Reed, G.B., Butt, E.M. and Landing, B.H. (1972). Copper in childhood liver disease – a histologic, histochemical and chemical survey. *Archs Path.* **93**, 249

Ritland, S., Steinnes, E. and Skrede, S. (1977). Hepatic copper content, urinary copper excretion and serum caeruloplasmin in liver disease. *Scand. J. Gastroent.* **12**, 81

Sass-Kortsak, A. (1975). Wilson's disease. A treatable liver disease in children. *Pediat. Clin. N. Am.* **22**, 963

Sass-Kortsak, A. and Sarkar, B. (1973). Age related changes in copper and biological transport of copper. A commentary. *J.Pediat.* **82**, 905

Sternlieb, I. and Scheinberg, I.H., (1968). Prevention of Wilson's disease in asymptomatic patients. *New Engl.J.Med.* **278**, 352

Sternlieb, I. (1972). Evolution of hepatic lesion in Wilson's disease. In *Progress in Liver Diseases*, p. 511. Vol. 4. Ed. by Popper, H. and Schaffner, F. New York: Grune and Stratton

Sternlieb, I. *et al.* (1973). Lysosomal defect in hepatic copper excretion in Wilson's disease (hepato-lenticular degeneration). *Gastroenterology* **64**, 99

CHAPTER 14

Cirrhosis and its Complications

Cirrhosis is the end-stage of many forms of liver injury. The main patho-physiological effects are impaired hepatic function, due to loss of hepatocytes, and portal hypertension. It may be complicated by the development of hepatocellular carcinoma.

Definition

Cirrhosis is defined pathologically as a replacement of the normal hepatic structure by 'regenerative' nodules which are surrounded by prominent fibrous tissue. The fibrous tissue frequently contains anastomosis between efferent and afferent vascular systems causing portosystemic shunting. These fibrous and vascular changes cause further hepatocellular necrosis leading to further collagen deposition and to yet more liver cell damage; thus a vicious circle is established.

In regenerative nodules hepatocytes are not arranged in single plates, with a regular distribution of portal tract and hepatic veins, but as clumps of hepatocytes plates two, three or four cells in thickness with irregularly placed or inconspicuous hepatic vein tributaries. The hepatocytes, even in a single nodule, often show considerable pleomorphism, some cells appearing normal, others having both cellular and nuclear enlargement. Although the diagnosis of cirrhosis implies an irreversible or even progressive pathological change, it is still compatible with growth and normal activity for many years.

Classification

There are many classifications of cirrhosis, depending on aetiology or

TABLE 14.1
Classification of Cirrhosis

Pathological	*Aetiological and clinical*
Micronodular	Post-necrotic cirrhosis
Macronodular	Biliary cirrhosis
Incomplete septal cirrhosis	
Biliary cirrhosis	

Clinical classification	
Compensated, inactive	Decompensated, inactive
Compensated, active	Decompensated, active

pathogenesis, the stage of development and the amount of hepatocellular necrosis, as well as on the clinical effects and necessity for treatment. An awareness of the pathological classification of micronodular, macronodular and incomplete septal cirrhosis is important in the interpretation of material obtained by liver biopsy. In defining aetiology and clinical management a division into two main groups is more helpful: they are post-necrotic cirrhosis which follows any form of hepatocellular damage, and biliary cirrhosis, in which the primary abnormality is in the biliary tree.

Cirrhosis may also be divided clinically into compensated and decompensated stages (*Table 14.1*). In compensated cirrhosis there are no symptoms attributable to hepatocellular failure, but in the decompensated stage these are present. It may be further subdivided into inactive cirrhosis in which there is no biochemical evidence of hepatocellular necrosis, or active cirrhosis, in which there may be evidence of hepatocellular necrosis with or without abnormalities in non-organ specific immunological tests.

Pathological classification

Micronodular cirrhosis is characterized by nodules of approximately equal size of up to 1cm in diameter, surrounded by bands of fibrous tissue of equal width. Very few hepatic veins and portal tracts are seen.

Macronodular cirrhosis is characterized by nodules of various size up to 5 cm in diameter, many being multilobular. Broad, fibrous septa surround these nodules. The liver may be shrunken and deformed.

Incomplete septal cirrhosis has elements of both macronodular and micronodular cirrhosis but the regeneration is not conspicuous, hepatic veins and portal tracts are frequently seen but rarely in the appropriate position relative to one another. Fibrous bands are seen traversing the parenchyma.

Biliary cirrhosis

In chronic bile duct obstruction, increasing fibrosis develops within the portal tracts, growing out into the parenchyma and linking adjacent portal tracts. Concentric fibrosis develops around the bile ducts. The hepatic parenchyma is relatively unchanged initially, and central (hepatic) veins persist. Eventually, true regeneration nodules develop and gradually the distinguishing features of this form of cirrhosis may be obliterated.

Liver biopsy appearances

In wedge biopsies of liver taken at laparotomy, the above features can readily be demonstrated. In percutaneous needle liver biopsy, it is frequently difficult to demonstrate all these features, particularly if the specimen is taken from a large macronodule or if a fragmented specimen is obtained.

The following features are often observed in cirrhosis and suggest the diagnosis:

(1) The liver feels hard.
(2) The specimen fragments in the needle or during processing in spite of good techniques.
(3) A core of tissue of unequal width is obtained.
(4) Biopsy consists of nodules of liver tissue without discernable hepatic veins or portal tracts but having a thin layer of connective tissue surrounding them. This is often best seen with a reticulum stain. These nodules may sometimes have attached fragments of fibrous tissue containing an excessive number of portal tracts.
(5) A relative excess of hepatic vein branches.
(6) Thickening of liver cell plate.
(7) Hyperplasia of hepatocytes.
(8) Abnormal hepatocytes with enlarged nuclei or enlarged cytoplasm.

Pathogenesis

Following severe hepatic injury due to infection, toxins such as paracetamol, or following hepatic resection, liver is capable of phenomenal regrowth with persistence of normal hepatic architecture. Why an apparently similar insult in one patient will be followed by return to functional and structural integrity while in others it is followed by cirrhosis, is uncertain.

An important element is the accumulation of abnormal amounts of fibrous tissue. This is important at two levels. Pericellular fibrosis may interfere with the nutrition of individual hepatocytes. The larger fibrous tissue septa which dissect lobular architecture carry vascular anastomosis which alter hepatic haemodynamics. Both processes may lead to hepatocyte death which itself may stimulate more fibrosis. Fibrosis also appears to be promoted by the development of bile duct reduplication in the portal tracts, the proliferating bile ducts appearing to form a template on which collagen is deposited.

The importance of hepatocellular necrosis in perpetuating the changes that lead to cirrhosis is uncertain. It may occur as a result of continuing action of the initial infection or noxious agent. It would appear that when the necrosis occurs in the liver cells near the portal tracts, cirrhosis is most likely to develop. It is impossible to say whether the observed changes in these hepatocytes occur primarily or secondarily. The factors that control hepatic regeneration are poorly understood. Hepatocellular regeneration normally occurs to an extent that is critically controlled so that the apparent total hepatocyte mass does not exceed a certain amount. Normally it occurs within a well-defined reticulin framework.

Whatever the primary abnormality, these three processes are followed by abnormal blood flow within the liver. Blood may flow directly from the hepatic artery to portal vein, or to the hepatic vein branches without traversing sinusoids. There may thus be hypoxic damage to liver cells aggravating the hepatocellular necrosis and leading to ever more fibrosis and vascular changes.

Clinical features of cirrhosis

Compensated disease

The specific clinical features of cirrhosis are those of chronic hepatocellular failure and portal hypertension. In well compensated cirrhosis the principal features will be those of the underlying cause. Where, for example, cirrhosis has followed chronic active hepatitis, cutaneous features such as striae or acne may be present, while if it has followed a genetic abnormality, specific markers of this disease may be present; for example, Kayser–Fleischer rings in Wilson's disease, or chronic respiratory tract infection and pancreatic insufficiency in cystic fibrosis. Where jaundice has followed a bile duct obstruction, pruritus, jaundice, xanthelasma (*Figure 14.1*), malabsorption and deficiency of fat-soluble vitamins (particularly vitamin D and K) may be prominent features.

Malnutrition and/or failure to thrive may be presenting features in chronic hepatocellular failure in childhood. Many factors contribute to this. There may be poor calorie intake secondary to anorexia. Absorption, particularly of fats, may be deficient due to the effects of poor bile salt secretion. Portal hypertension may, in itself, also cause malabsorption. If steatorrhoea is marked, there may be a deficiency of fat-soluble vitamins, such as A, D and K.

Circulatory and respiratory changes

The main vascular abnormality associated with cirrhosis is portal hypertension. This is associated with the development of collateral vessels which by-pass the liver, and by a reduction in effective hepatic blood flow. Cirrhosis may also be associated with changes in systemic pulmonary and visceral circulation. A hyperkinetic circulatory state commonly exists. There is an increased cardiac output and commonly a decreased peripheral resistance. The blood volume is also elevated. The mechanisms of these changes are not fully understood.

The most prominent change in the peripheral circulation is the development of so-called vascular spiders. These contain a central

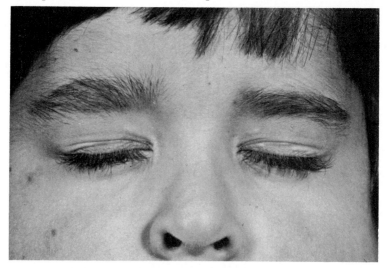

Figure 14.1. Xanthelasma in a boy with chronic obstructive liver disease progressing to biliary type cirrhosis. The xanthelasma regressed when he was treated with cholestyramine

arteriole from which radiates numerous fine vessels superficially resembling spiders legs. They range in size from a pin-head up to 0.5 cm in diameter. Pressure on the centre of the lesion with a pin causes blanching of the whole lesion. They are found commonly in the vasculatory territory of the superior vena cava. They disappear if the blood pressure falls due to shock or haemorrhage. The appearance of new spiders is suggestive of progressive liver damage. Spiders occur also in normal persons, particularly children, and unless more than ten are present these should not be taken as indicative of liver disease. The development of many, and the increasing size of older ones, is suggestive. White spots which, when examined with a lens, show in the centre the beginnings of a spider, are also typical of cirrhosis. These are most prominent on the buttocks and arms.

Palmar erythema, an exaggeration of the ordinary speckled mottling of the palm, may also be found in cirrhosis. It is quite frequently seen in normal children and in children with chronic febrile illnesses.

Clubbing of the fingers may be found, particularly in patients with biliary cirrhosis. White nails are a prominent feature of cirrhosis, but this is less frequently seen in children than in adults. Pulmonary arteriovenous anastomoses also occur. These lead to intrapulmonary shunting and oxygen desaturation in the peripheral blood. Pulmonary hypertension is a rare complication.

For these reasons, and for others which are not understood, patients with cirrhosis are prone to bacterial infection, which may take the form of respiratory tract infection with bronchitis or pneumonia. Spontaneous peritonitis may also occur.

Abdominal findings

These are variable and depend on the underlying cause of the cirrhosis. There may be marked abdominal distension, which may be caused by enlargement of the liver and spleen and by the accumulation of ascites. Commonly the liver is small in size and impalpable. Hepatic dullness is reduced to a small area in the right antero-lateral chest wall, above the costal margin. The liver is likely to be enlarged in biliary cirrhosis. If palpable it is firm and it may be possible to discern nodules on the edge or on the anterior surface. The spleen is likely to be palpable, often reducing in size if prodded. Free fluid is best demonstrated by shifting dullness rather than eliciting a fluid wave. Portal blood may be deviated via the para-umbilical veins to the umbilicus, and prominent collateral veins may radiate from the umbilicus towards the systemic circulation.

Features indicating decompensation

Development of peripheral oedema and ascites indicates diminished hepatocellular function and decompensation. Another important sign is the development of hepatic encephalopathy and a characteristic sweetish slightly faecal smell of fetor hepaticus on the exhaled breath.

The appearance of jaundice in a patient with post-necrotic cirrhosis is also indicative of very advanced disease and decompensation. Spontaneous bruising and epistaxis, caused by both deficiency of platelets due to hypersplenism and by impaired hepatic production of clotting factors, is also a grave sign. In advanced disease, patients may often run a low grade fever without associated infection. However, many patients will develop blood-borne infection and/or peritonitis caused by both Gram-positive and Gram-negative bacteria. Septicaemia is often a terminal event in patients with hepatocellular failure. Particularly in patients receiving corticosteroids, fever may be inconspicuous and there may be little leucocytosis.

Laboratory investigations

Routine laboratory tests of liver function may be entirely normal in a patient with cirrhosis. Often, however, tests of liver function do show abnormalities (*Table 14.2*). Of tests which are routinely performed, perhaps the most useful is the serum protein electrophoresis. This may show a low albumin level with normal or increased gammaglobulins.

TABLE 14.2
Abnormalities of Liver Function Tests in Cirrhosis

Test	Post-necrotic cirrhosis	Biliary cirrhosis	Decompensated cirrhosis
Albumin	Normal or decreased	Normal or decreased	Decreased
Globulin	Normal	Normal	Normal
Prothrombin time after vitamin K	Normal or prolonged by 2–3 seconds	Normal	Prolonged by more than 5 seconds
AST	Normal or increased to × 2 normal	Normal or slightly increased	Increased × 2–6 normal
Alkaline phosphatase	Usually increased to × 1½ normal	Increased × 2–3 normal	Normal or increased
BSP clearance at 45 minutes	>5 per cent	>5 per cent	>20 per cent
Bilirubin contents	Normal	Normal or slightly increased	Increased

Serum alkaline phosphatase is often elevated, particularly in biliary cirrhosis. In this condition, the total cholesterol in the serum is elevated but the ester concentration is reduced. The prothrombin time is frequently prolonged. The serum transaminases may be increased but often to a value of only 50 per cent above the upper limit of normal. In many instances it will be normal. The most sensitive, easily available test of liver function is the Bromsulphalein clearance test which shows abnormal serum retention greater than 5 per cent of the injected doses of Bromsulphalein 45 minutes after its intraveous injection. The term active applied to cirrhosis indicates that there is clinical, biochemical or histological evidence of progressive liver disease. In an inactive cirrhosis these features are absent.

The peripheral blood count will often show a modest decrease in the haemoglobin concentration with levels of 2–3g below normal. Red cells are frequently normochromic and normocytic. The total white blood count is frequently decreased to a level of less than 5,000/mm^3 and the platelet count, too, is frequently low, often with levels of less than 100,000/mm^3. In advanced disease the red blood cells show marked acanthocytosis (Burr cells).

A respiratory alkalosis may develop in cirrhosis. In addition, potassium depletion caused by hyperaldosteronism may also cause a metabolic alkalosis.

Radiological, endoscopic and scintiscan investigations

A barium meal may show varices in the oesophagus, stomach or duodenum. If the varices are small they may only be visible using a double contrast technique. Peptic ulceration is said to be more common in adults with cirrhosis and it should certainly be looked for in children, particularly if they have alimentary bleeding. Endoscopy, using a flexible fibre-optic endoscope, may be necessary to confirm varices and is invaluable in identifying the site of bleeding.

Liver scintiscans, following the intravenous injection of isotope, such as technetium-99m, confirms the normal or small liver size. The pattern of isotope uptake is mottled with a reduced peak count rate. Splenic enlargement can be identified and the isotope uptake by the spleen is often greater than that of the liver.

Ultrasonic scanning is also a useful extension of physical examination confirming the degree of hepatosplenomegaly. It also can show enlargement of the portal or splenic veins if there is significant portal hypertension. If there are associated gallstones, dense echoes may be seen from the biliary tree.

Diagnosis

The diagnosis will ultimately rest with the biopsy findings. The principal difficulty in diagnosis will be confusion with congenital hepatic fibrosis, or problems in interpretation arising from an unrepresentative sample of liver tissue being obtained. Such difficulties are less likely to arise if a Trucut needle is used to obtain the biopsy.

Laparoscopy, allowing visualization of the upper and lower surfaces of the liver, is frequently used in the assessment of cirrhosis in adults. It is particularly valuable where malignant change is suspected, in that the biopsy needle can be directed visually to the suspicious lesion. The investigation does cause considerable discomfort and can only be done in children under a general anaesthetic. It rarely needs to be performed.

The diagnosis of cirrhosis is a two-step process, aiming for an assessment of the degree of liver injury and the determination of its cause (*Tables 14.3–14.5*). The provisional diagnosis of cirrhosis may frequently be made on the basis of the history of past liver damage and the physical findings, without recourse to any laboratory investigations. Typical biochemical changes and the presence of varices on an upper gastrointestinal tract radiograph provide valuable supporting evidence. The investigations referred to above may also give a guide to further investigations.

Differential diagnosis

Three conditions still cause diagnostic difficulties at this stage.

In extrahepatic portal hypertension, liver function tests are typically normal but very frequently there is some prolongation of the prothrombin time, often by four to five seconds, and the bromsulfophthalein sodium uptake may be decreased.

Infiltrative disorders such as reticuloses may also cause difficulties since the peripheral blood count is in no way diagnostic and they may be complicated by portal hypertension.

Another difficulty arises in constrictive pericarditis in which abdominal manifestations may greatly exceed those in the chest, and the raised jugular venous pressure is either overlooked or its significance not appreciated.

Aetiological diagnosis

Ultimately, confirmation of the diagnosis requires liver biopsy. Before this is undertaken, however, an attempt must be made to try to

TABLE 14.3
Causes of Biliary Cirrhosis

Extrahepatic biliary atresia	Bile duct stenosis or obstruction
Intrahepatic biliary hypoplasia	Choledocholithiasis
Choledochal cyst	Cystic fibrosis
Ascending pyogenic cholangitis	Ulcerative colitis
Cholangitis due to Fasciola,	Byler's disease
Clonorchis sinensis , Ascaris	Familial intrahepatic cholestasis

TABLE 14.4
Post-necrotic Cirrhosis

Post-hepatitic	Hepatitis in infancy, especially if alpha-1-antitrypsin deficient
	Chronic active hepatitis
	Acute viral hepatitis
	Hepatitis due to drugs – actinomycin D, methotrexate
	Toxins – aflatoxin
	Radiation
Venous congestion	Constrictive pericarditis
	Ebstein's anomaly
	Budd–Chiari syndrome
	Congestive cardiac failure
	Venacaval webs

Veno-occlusive disease (Jamaican)

Indian childhood cirrhosis

Ulcerative colitis

TABLE 14.5
Genetic Causes of Cirrhosis

Wilson's disease	Gaucher's disease
Galactosaemia	Wolman's disease
Fructosaemia	A beta lipoproteinaemia
Glycogen storage disease Type IV	Sickle cell disease
Glycogen storage disease Type III	Thalassaemia
Hurler's syndrome	Hepatic porphyria
Cystic fibrosis	Haemochromatosis, idiopathic
Alpha-1 antitrypsin deficiency	Haemochromatosis secondary to chronic
Tyrosinosis	haemolytic disease
Cystinosis	Zellweger's syndrome
Niemann–Pick disease	Byler's disease
Cholesterol ester storage disease	Coprostanic acidaemia

determine which of the many causes of liver damage may have been responsible, so that the liver tissue may be subjected to appropriate histological, biochemical analysis to determine the cause. This is particularly important in those genetic metabolic disorders such as fructosaemia, in which liver biopsy is the only means by which a definite diagnosis may be established (*Tables 14.6, 14.7*).

In many instances the cause of the liver damage will be evident on the basis of the past history and examination findings. This is particularly so with biliary type cirrhosis, but there are exceptions. In some patients with ulcerative colitis the liver damage is out of all proportion to the gastrointestinal symptoms; in such patients barium enema or sigmoidoscopy may reveal quite marked changes in the colonic mucosa, with very few symptoms. Rarely, cirrhosis may be a presenting feature in cystic fibrosis. Patients with both choledochal cyst and tumours of the biliary tree may present with few of the classical features and have advanced liver disease when first coming to medical attention.

In considering the genetic disorders, principal consideration must be given to those conditions in which treatment if started early is effective, for example, Wilson's disease, galactosaemia, fructosaemia, glycogen storage disease and tyrosinosis. Unfortunately, in all of these conditions, therapy at best will only have an ameliorating effect if cirrhosis is already established at the time of diagnosis. In other genetic disorders, for example, thalassaemia, precise diagnosis may have therapeutic implications, such as the administration of desferrioxamine. Unfortunately, for many genetic disorders, such as alpha-1 antitrypsin deficiency, precise diagnosis is important only in that it allows appropriate genetic advice to be given and, to a lesser extent, some guide to prognosis.

In post-necrotic cirrhosis reversal of the features is of course impossible. Where it has followed chronic active hepatitis, this process may continue and considerable symptomatic improvement may occur if the disease process if controlled by immuno-suppressants. Similarly, if liver damage is caused by drugs (page 151), symptomatic improvement may follow their withdrawal.

Although liver biopsy may show features specific for such conditions as chronic active hepatitis, cystic fibrosis, Wilson's disease, alpha-1 antitrypsin deficiency, frequently there will be no features indicative of what has in the past caused liver damage.

Management

Having made a histological diagnosis of cirrhosis and confirmed the aetiology, the aim of management is to minimize the effect of the cause of liver disease, if this is possible, and to prevent or control the

TABLE 14.6
Investigation of Patients with Suspected Cirrhosis

All cases

Serum proteins including electrophoresis,	Full blood count
	Serum urea
Serum immunoglobulins	Electrolytes and bicarbonate
Bilirubin	Chest radiography
Aspartate transaminase	Barium meal
Alkaline phosphatase	Liver scintiscan
Cholesterol	Liver biopsy
Prothrombin time	

Selected cases

BSP clearance	Intravenous pyelogram
Ultrasonic scan	Laparoscopy
Intravenous cholangiogram	Alphafetoprotein
ECG	Blood gases

TABLE 14.7
Aetiological Investigations in Selected Patients with Cirrhosis

Peripheral blood tests

Alpha 1-antitrypsin phenotype
Caeruloplasmin
Fasting blood sugar, pyruvate and lactate
Red cell glycogen content
Red blood cell galactose-1-phosphate uridyl transferase
Haemoglobin electrophoresis
Serum iron and total iron binding capacity
Serum aminoacids
Serum cholesterol and lipoproteins
Serum bile acids
Hepatitis B surface antigen, antibody to hepatitis BsAg, antibody to hepatitis B core
Antibody to hepatitis A virus
Serum immunoglobulins
Serum tissue autoantibodies

Urine tests

24-hour copper excretion
Porphyrins
Aminoacids
Non-glucose reducing substances
Mucopolysaccharides

Miscellaneous

Sweat electrolytes
ECG
Intravenous pyelogram
Inferior venacavagram
Cardiac catheterization
Catheterization of hepatic veins
Cholangiography

complications (*Table 14.8*). Those occurring in children are similar to those in adult life, but the impact of nutritional deficiencies in the growing child are greater than in the adult.

Nutritional problems

Anorexia is frequently a symptom in cirrhosis. In addition, a degree of fat malabsorption is almost invariable. Deficiency of fat-soluble vitamins A, D and K will develop unless oral vitamin supplements are given at a dose of at least twice normal. If steatorrhoea is marked, it will be necessary to give vitamin K, 5mg intramuscularly weekly, and vitamin D, in a dose sufficient to prevent rickets. A dose of 10,000 units intramuscularly at monthly intervals will often suffice for this, but this must be controlled by regular measurements of the serum calcium phosphate and alkaline phosphatase, since some patients will respond very satisfactorily to such a dose while others will be refractory. In an effort to decrease steatorrhoea and to improve nutrition, medium chain triglycerides should be given since these can be absorbed in the presence of low bile salt secretion. If the serum cholesterol is high, or xanthelasma develops, a low cholesterol diet is advisable. Cholestyramine, in a dose of 4–8 g given four times daily with meals, also helps to prevent and control this complication. This drug is also invaluable in controlling pruritus in biliary cirrhosis. It may also cause some improvement in liver function in patients with post-necrotic cirrhosis. The exact mechanism of its action is not certain, but it should be tried. If features of hepatic encephalopathy develop, dietary protein intake should be reduced to zero and then gradually increased to the maximum tolerated. There is no evidence that avoidance of adherence to any particular type of food has any influence on the progression of established cirrhosis.

Portal hypertension

Portal hypertension causes splenomegaly, ascites and alimentary bleeding. Splenomegaly and hypersplenism rarely require surgical intervention, unless associated with severe alimentary bleeding. Ascites, a major problem, is considered in detail below.

Bleeding from varices in the oesophagus, the stomach or the duodenum, or from associated peptic ulceration or oesophagitis, is a major complication of cirrhosis. Fuller consideration of the management of this problem is given elsewhere (page 308). Portal decompression by portocaval anastomosis in the cirrhotic patient is almost always associated with some deterioration of liver function and may be followed by hepatic encephalopathy. There is a considerable operative mortality. If the patient survives surgery, death from bleeding may be prevented, but death from hepatic failure or hepatic encephalopathy may be precipitated. Only in patients with cystic fibrosis is there some evidence that portocaval anastomosis may prolong a full life.

ASCITES AND OEDEMA IN CHRONIC LIVER DISEASE
(cirrhosis)

The mechanism of formation of ascites and oedema in chronic liver disease is complex and imperfectly understood. Nevertheless, a know-ledge of current understanding of its patho-physiology is essential

TABLE 14.8
Complications of Cirrhosis

Portal hypertension	Bleeding diathesis
Ascites	Increased susceptibility to infection
Hepatic encephalopathy	Impaired fat absorption
Hyperdynamic circulation	Malignant hepatoma
Endocrine changes	Gallstone formation
Impaired hepatic metabolism of drugs and hormones	Renal failure

if rational treatment is to be given. Two distinct but interrelated processes are involved: (a) redistribution of fluid within the body; and (b) increase in water content of the body.

These cause a disturbance of the normal equilibrium between the formation and removal of extracellular fluid.

Fluid redistribution

The exchange of fluid between capillaries and tissue spaces clearing the peritoneal cavity is dependent on the hydrostatic and osmotic pressures inside and outside the blood vessels.

Two factors in liver disease favour the development of ascites: (a) hypoalbuminaemia; and (b) hypertension in the hepatic sinusoids and portal venous system.

Hypoalbuminaemia, due to reduced albumin synthesis in the liver, lowers the intracapillary colloid osmotic force allowing the transfer of fluid into the tissue spaces and hence into the peritoneal cavity. This effect in itself is probably of minor importance compared with the effect of the high hydrostatic pressure in the hepatic sinusoids and the portal venous system. There are important differences in the effect of hypertension in these two parts of the circulation. If hypertension is limited to the portal system, ascites is likely to be minimal unless the albumin concentration drops.

In contrast, where hepatic vein obstruction occurs, for example, in advanced cirrhosis or in the Budd—Chiari syndrome, ascites is severe and often intractable. In cirrhosis the sinusoidal pressure is increased not only by the back pressure effect of hepatic vein obstruction, but also by the direct hepatic artery inflow into the obstructed sinusoidal bed. Much fluid with a high protein content, therefore, exudes into the perisinusoidal spaces to be taken up by the hepatic lymphatics. In cirrhosis dilated lymphatic channels which drain to the portahepatis and hence to the thoracic duct are easily observed. When the carrying capacity of the lymphatic system is saturated, extravascular fluid with a very high protein content weeps from the liver surface. Ascitic fluid, however, rarely has a protein content as high as that found in the thoracic duct, presumably because of dilution by fluid from the serosal surface of the gut. This also arises only when the production of tissue fluid in the intestine exceeds the capacity of the lymphatics to transport it.

Increased fluid retention

The factors which lead to increased fluid retention in cirrhosis are poorly understood. In spite of a normal or increased cardiac output, total renal blood flow is reduced. In part, this may arise because of diversion of much of the cardiac output to the splanchnic bed. Renal vasoconstriction is also a possibility.

Increased sodium reabsorption

There seems to be greater evidence of redistribution of blood flow within the kidney substance. Blood flow to the outer cortex where most of the functioning glomeruli are to be found is reduced. There is increased blood flow to the juxtamedullary nephrons which have an increased capacity for sodium reabsorption. The mechanism of this redistribution of blood within the kidney is not known, but the total effect is to reduce glomerular infiltration and increase sodium reabsorption. What causes the excess sodium reabsorption is not known. It is currently attributed to an unidentified 'third factor' acting on the proximal tubules.

An unidentified cause of increased sodium reabsorption is markedly *increased aldosterone production*. In addition, there is possibly a failure of aldosterone inactivation by the diseased liver. Aldosterone normally appears to act as a fine control of sodium reabsorption through its action on the distal tubules, the major site of sodium reabsorption being in the proximal convuluted tubule.

Adverse effects of ascites

There is a formidable number of possible complications associated with ascites (*Table 14.9*). For some patients, however, it may be a

TABLE 14.9
Complications Associated with Ascites

Increased incidence of haemorrhage from varices	Pulmonary insufficiency, atalectasis and pneumonia
Hepato-renal syndrome	Difficulty in walking or crawling
Spontaneous bacterial peritonitis	Iatrogenic
Anorexia	Azotaemia
Hernia formation	Hypokalaemia
Pleural effusion	Hyponatraemia
	Encephalopathy

benign, concurrent complication. As in all branches of medicine, it is essential to remember the vow: *primum non nocere*, particularly since treatment will not influence the underlying disease process.

Treatment

Sodium restriction In adults, sodium restriction is the keystone of treatment. In children a very low sodium diet is rarely tolerable, particularly if the child is already anorexic. It may be expeditious, therefore, not to demand a strictly low sodium intake but to compromise with a diet of restricted sodium content; for example, not greater than 5 mEq per day in a child aged 1–4 years, not greater than 20 mEq per day in a child aged 5–11 years and not greater than 30 mEq per day in a child aged 12–14 years.

Diuretics Currently available diuretics have revolutionized management. We have powerful drugs, and considerable care is required if they are to be used to best advantage. Their use requires frequent clinical reassessment, together with electrolyte determination in both serum and urine. The diuretic of choice is the aldosterone antagonist spirono-lactone, having the advantage of causing potassium retention which is very desirable in cirrhotic patients, who are usually potassium depleted. Hyperkalaemia rarely occurs but it may do if a patient has urea retention with renal failure. Its disadvantage is that it has no effect for about four days after starting treatment. Different patients have different degrees of hyperaldosteroidism, so a flexible dosage regimen is required. Doses required in cirrhotic patients are considerably greater than in other disorders causing fluid retention.

The following are appropriate initial doses:

Age 1–3 years	12.5 mg four times a day
Age 4–7 years	25 mg four times a day
Age 8–11 years	27.5 mg four times a day
Age 12 years and older	50 mg four times a day

If there is no weight-loss after four days the dose should be doubled. If diuresis still does not occur and sodium excretion in the urine is still low, the dose may be increased by a further 50 per cent and in most instances diuresis will occur. The most serious side-effect of spirono-lactone therapy is hyponatraemia. This may be complicated by hepatic encephalopathy or renal failure.

If spironolactone alone does not control ascites, a kaliuretic diuretic in small doses may be added to the regimen. These diuretics act on the proximal tubules. Thiazide derivatives, frusemide and ethacrynic acid are most commonly used. Their toxicity is largely due to the excessive urinary losses of potassium and chloride which they cause. This is closely related to the diuretic potency. Frusemide and ethacrynic acid have a greater effect on pH and also appear to increase ammonia production, and for that reason their use is more frequently com-plicated by hepatic encephalopathy. It is suggested that chlorothiazide in a dose of 25 per cent of the recommended dose when used alone, should be given initially. This will often produce a very satisfactory diuresis. It is important to try to reduce weight slowly, that is, at a rate equivalent to less than 1kg per day in the adult. Larger doses may produce a much more dramatic fall. Some patients will be refractory to this dosage regimen and it must be increased slowly. When these drugs are being used it is important to frequently measure serum and urinary urea electrolytes, serum urea and creatinine. It may be important to assess the intracellular potassium state by means of an ECG.

Paracentesis Paracentesis should not be performed as a therapeutic measure, except in the following circumstances.

(1) To relieve pain due to abdominal distension caused by ascites.
(2) To relieve severe dyspnoea.
(3) To minimize other complications of ascites which are aggravated by increased abdominal pressure due to ascites: (*a*) variceal haemorrhage; and (*b*) hepato-renal syndrome.
(4) To facilitate diagnostic investigations or surgical procedures.

Paracentesis with reinfusion In adults, aspiration of ascites and re-infusion into a systemic vein has been used as an adjunct to diuretic therapy. If the ascitic fluid is ultrafiltrated complications of vascular overload can be avoided. This form of therapy does result in adult patients being hospitalized for shorter periods than with conventional diuretic therapy, but it does not appear to have increased the total percentage of patients in whom ascites can be controlled. Surprisingly, in some cases, the ascites may remain absent for periods of 6–8 weeks before it reaccumulates. When used in children in our unit it has been a useful adjuvant to diuretics.

Diagnostic paracentesis is an essential procedure in cirrhosis when complicated by unexplained fever, diarrhoea, abdominal pain or encephalopathy.

Portocaval anastomosis Where persistent intractable ascites cannot be controlled by the above forms of therapy consideration should be given to surgical measures. The most effective is decompressed portal hypertension by a side-to-side portocaval anastomosis. Unfortunately, in a patient with intractable ascites, the operative mortality of this procedure is considerable and it can only very rarely be indicated.

CHRONIC HEPATIC ENCEPHALOPATHY

Chronic hepatic encephalopathy is a complex neuropsychiatric syndrome. It occurs classically in cirrhosis with portosystemic shunting but it may occur following shunting for extrahepatic portal hypertension. The acute, severe form occurs in fulminant hepatitis. It is characterized by intellectual impairment, clouding of consciousness which may progress to stupor and coma, and personality change. The speech may be slurred. The most characteristic neurological abnormality is the so-called 'flapping tremor'. This is elicited by asking the patient to attempt maximum dorsiflexion of the wrist with the forearm fixed. A rapid flexion-extension movement at the metacarpal, phalangeal and wrist joint develops, sometimes accompanied by lateral movements of the digits. Tendon reflexes are also increased early but later become reduced. There may be various neurological signs indicating organic cerebral disease. A particularly typical feature is marked variability of the signs.

Pathogenesis

The brain in chronic hepatic encephalopathy may show no abnormality. There may be an increase in the number of protoplasmic astrocytes and rarely neural degeneration and demyelination. It is thought that the neural dysfunction is largely secondary to metabolic changes. The exact nature of these metabolic changes is not completely understood. Clinical observations and studies in experimental models emphasize the importance of nitrogenous products – particularly ammonia – derived from gut content. Cerebral intoxication occurs when such substances are not metabolized by the liver. These speculative toxins are thought to be produced by bacterial action in the bowel since symptoms can often be relieved by oral, wide-spectrum, non-absorbed antibiotics, such as neomycin. As well as ammonia, methionine and some of its derivatives such as methylmarcaptan have been implicated. There is also evidence that short-chain fatty acids may contribute to hepatic coma, at least in some patients. The possibility also exists

TABLE 14.10
Precipitating Causes of Hepatic Encephalopathy

Gastrointestinal haemorrhage	Constipation
Diuretics	Sedatives
Systemic infection	Renal failure
High protein diet	Development of hepatocellular carcinoma
	Pancreatitis

that biogenic amines, such as octopamine or false neuro-transmittants may also have a role. Other factors which have been implicated include a lack of essential substrates for normal brain function, for example, glucose. In addition, changes in intracellular metabolism due to the hypokalaemic alkalosis so often present in cirrhosis, may also contribute.

The *precipitating causes* of hepatoencephalopathy given in *Table 14.10* are thought to potentiate the above mechanisms. Gastrointestinal haemorrhage acts in two ways, it puts more protein for ammonia production into the bowel, and the hypovolaemia may compromise both hepatic and renal function. In infection, increased tissue metabolism leads to an increased endogenous nitrogen load and hence increases ammonia production. Infection may also lead to dehydration.

Treatment

The basis of treatment is to try to improve liver function and to prevent ammonia accumulation. Although ammonia is formed in muscle and kidney, it is the ammonia production by the gut which has to be modified in hepatic encephalopathy. Within the gut the main precursor of ammonia is urea. Urea diffuses through the gastrointestinal and small intestinal mucosa, and in the colon is changed to ammonia by the action of ureases which are mainly bacterial but may also be mucosal. The ammonia is transported to the liver and in health is metabolized back to urea. There are two main methods of reducing ammonia production by the gut: (a) protein restriction; and (b) reducing bowel flora. Protein restriction is of value possibly by reducing the total body urea pool. It may also be beneficial in that it reduces the production of urea and other potential toxic nitrogenous metabolites within the gut. Broad-spectrum antibiotics act by reducing the amount of bacterial urease available by partial sterilization of the bowel. Neomycin is the antibiotic most commonly used.

Lactulose, a non-absorbable synthetic disaccharide (beta-14 galactoside fructose) is also effective in preventing or treating recurrent encephalopathy. It produces an osmotic fermentative diarrhoea with lactic and acetic acid production which causes a drop in pH in the colon and hence a reduction in ammonia reabsorption. Some patients will respond more satisfactorily to the administration of neomycin, while others respond more satisfactorily to lactulose. If coma occurs, colonic lavage will rapidly reduce ammonia production and absorption.

In adults, other methods have been used. These include colonic by-pass – a major surgical procedure, which does ameliorate encephalopathy but the attendant morbidity and mortality is severe. Antibodies to urease, the urease inhibitor acetohydroxamide and colonization of the bowel by Lactobacillus, have not been proven to be effective in adult patients and have not been systematically evaluated in children.

Hypokalaemia, particularly if associated with alkalosis, must be corrected. It causes increased ammonia concentration by its effect on the kidney. Not only is ammonia formation by the kidney increased, but the ability of the kidney to excrete ammonia is also decreased.

The other measures which are essential are the identification, correction and future avoidance of precipitating causes. Alimentary bleeding is the most frequent and most serious. The essence of management is to stop the bleeding if possible, to remove the blood from the gut as rapidly as possible by gastric aspiration, purgation and enema, and to replace the blood by transfusion to prevent hypoperfusion of both brain and liver. All sedatives are potentially dangerous and best avoided. The safest is perhaps diazepam. The dose should be from 25–50 per cent of the dose normally required for a child of that weight. The dose must not be repeated until the effects of the previous dose have disappeared. In unexplained coma, latent infections such as urinary tract infection, septicaemia or peritonitis must be excluded.

ANAEMIA

A refractory, normocytic anaemia commonly develops in cirrhosis. There may be many contributory factors. There may be iron deficiency secondary to blood loss from oesophageal varices, poor iron absorption and low transferrin levels. Thrombocytopenia and deficiency of other clotting factors may aggravate blood loss. Other factors causing low haemoglobin concentrations include shortened red cell survival due to splenomegaly or haemolysis. Rarely, the haemolysis may be associated with a positive Coomb's test. In biliary cirrhosis, vitamin E deficiency may be a factor. Erythropoietic activity in the bone marrow may be decreased. This is commonly attributed to hypersplenism but indeed the mechanism is not understood. Finally, the blood volume may be increased giving a low haemoglobin concentration although the total red blood cell mass is not decreased.

Treatment

Most of the above factors cannot be modified by therapy. If the serum iron is low and the total iron binding capacity elevated, oral iron will be helpful, but often the total iron binding capacity is within normal range and iron therapy is not beneficial. Vitamin E may help in biliary cirrhosis. Steroids should be considered in haemolytic anaemia if the anaemia is contributing to symptoms. Portocaval anastomosis without splenectomy rarely increases the haemoglobin concentration but if the spleen is removed and the bleeding stops the haemoglobin is likely to rise. It is rarely necessary to remove a spleen in a patient with cirrhosis because of hypersplenism.

RENAL FAILURE

Oliguric renal failure without structural abnormalities in the kidney is frequently the cause of death in advanced cirrhosis. Typically there is a slow spontaneous development of azotaemia, oliguria, dilutional hyponatraemia and a low urinary sodium excretion.

The cause of the renal failure is not understood. Pathogenic factors which are currently thought to be of importance are: (a) renal arterial construction; (b) diminished effective extracellular fluid volume; and (c) increased renal venous pressure.

There is a substantial reduction of glomerular filtration rate and of effective renal plasma flow. The exact mechanism which eventually leads to impaired water excretion remains to be clarified.

Renal failure may on occasions follow the development of ascites, vigorous diuretic treatment, paracentesis, or gastrointestinal haemorrhage. In many instances, however, these factors cannot be incriminated.

There is no effective treatment but the condition must be distinguished from other causes of renal failure in cirrhotic patients such as plasma volume depletion and hypertension, electrolyte depletion secondary to diuretic therapy and neomycin nephrotoxicity. It may be easily distinguished from acute tubular necrosis by measuring the urinary osmolarity. In acute tubular necrosis this is low and fixed, while in renal failure complicating cirrhosis this is increased to a level greater than plasma.

SPONTANEOUS BACTERIAL PERITONITIS

This complication occurs in patients in whom cirrhosis is complicated by ascites. Characteristically, the patient has fever, abdominal pain, reduced or absent bowel sounds and, often, features of hepatic encephalopathy. Occasionally, abdominal pain is absent and no rebound tenderness may be found. The offending organism is likely to be a Gram-negative Bacillus or Pneumococcus. The diagnosis is made by means of a diagnostic ascitic tap which reveals a cloudy, ascitic fluid with a white count of around $1,000/mm^3$ or more. The cells are predominantly polymorphonuclear neutrophil leucocytes. The protein concentration is frequently low, less than 20 g/litre. Often the same organism may be recovered from the blood culture.

Vigorous treatment with broad-spectrum antibiotics such as gentamycin and ampicillin is advocated.

BIBLIOGRAPHY

Cohen, N. and Mendelow, H. (1965). Concurrent active juvenile cirrhosis and primary pulmonary hypertension. *Am.J.Med.* **39**, 127
Conn, H.O. (1972). The rational management of ascites. In *Progress in Liver Diseases*, p. 269 Vol. 4. Ed. by Popper, H. and Schaffner, F. New York: Grune and Stratton

Kravath, R.E., Scarpelli, A.M. and Bernstein, J. (1971). Hepatogenic cyanosis: arterio-venous shunts in chronic active hepatitis. *J.Pediat.* **78**, 238

Martini, G.A., Baltzer, G. and Arndt, H. (1972). Some aspects of circulatory disturbances in cirrhosis of the liver. In *Progress in Liver Diseases*, p. 231. Vol. 4. Ed. by Popper, H. and Schaffner, F. New York: Grune and Stratton

Rubin, E. and Popper, H. (1967). The evolution of human cirrhosis deduced from observations in experimental animals. *Medicine, Baltimore* **46**, 163

Schauer, P.J. (1970). Liver biopsy in the diagnosis of cirrhosis. *Gut* **11**, 257

Scott, H.W. and Foster, J.H. (1967). Surgical experience in the management of cirrhosis of the liver in children. *Am.J.Surg.* **113**, 102

Sherlock, S. (1975). Hepatic cirrhosis. In *Diseases of the Liver and Biliary System*. 5th ed., p. 425. Oxford: Blackwell

CHAPTER 15

Hepato-biliary Lesions in Cystic Fibrosis

Introduction

Cystic fibrosis is a disorder of exocrine secretory glands throughout
the body. It is inherited in an autosomal recessive fashion. The biochemical basis of the condition is unknown. Mucus-producing glands
throughout the body produce an abnormally tenacious viscid secretion.
Increased sodium and chloride concentrations are found in the
secretions of the serous glands, such as sweat or saliva. Both abnormalities contribute to the pathological effects of the disorder. An unexplained feature of the condition is the variable severity of pathological change in different organs. Principal changes occur in the respiratory system, intestinal canal and pancreas. Affected males are
usually sterile due to absence of the vas deferens. Nasal polyps are
common. Heat prostration due to salt loss occurs in warm environ-
ments.

Full consideration of the pathological and clinical effects of involvement of these organs would be inappropriate in this text. Pancreatic
exocrine insufficiency can largely be corrected by oral pancreatic
supplements. In the last decade, regular physiotherapy and antibiotics
have helped to minimize and control respiratory involvement.

Prognosis

Recent surveys show that over 70 per cent of children diagnosed in
infancy survive beyond the age of 12 years and that 50 per cent of
these will have minimal or no respiratory insufficiency. In the Cystic
Fibrosis Clinic at The Boston Children's Hospital the mean age at
death was 1.5 years in the period between 1940 and 1948, but had

been extended to 16 years by the period 1968–1970. The Boston group currently follow 95 patients who are over the age of 25 years. With such prolonged survival, it is now evident that as many as 20 per cent of adolescents with cystic fibrosis have cirrhosis and its complications.

HEPATO-BILIARY DISEASE

Pathology and pathogenesis

Many factors may contribute to the development of *cirrhosis* and its complications (*Table 15.1*). A major cause is thought to be the involvement of mucus-producing glands which drain into the biliary system. The most prominent of these are at the portohepatis. Hyperviscid bile is produced obstructing bile flow. The portal tracts show bile duct

TABLE 15.1
Hepato-biliary Lesions in Cystic Fibrosis

Focal biliary fibrosis ⟶ Cirrhosis
Prolonged neonatal intrahepatic cholestasis
Small gallbladder (35–50%)
Gallstones
Cholangiolitis
Cardiac cirrhosis
Drug-induced hepatitis
Fatty metamorphosis
Haemosiderosis
Viral hepatitis A, B; Cytomegalovirus

reduplication, increased fibrosis, inflammatory cell infiltrate and a gradual destruction of periportal liver cells. This process of focal biliary fibrosis may begin in fetal life. It proceeds without clinical manifestation. Gradually more and more parts of the liver are involved, with destruction of hepatocytes and their replacement by fibrous tissue. Ultimately, the normal hepatic architecture becomes distorted and deranged and a biliary type of cirrhosis with regenerative nodules develops. Cirrhosis has been documented histologically at the early age of four years and is present at autopsy in between 9 and 25 per cent of cases (Bodian, 1953; di Sant'Agnese and Blanc, 1956; and Mearns, 1974).

In keeping with the unequal degree of injury to different organs, there is no constant rate or severity of liver damage. It has been suggested, however, that there is a familial predilection to severe liver damage.

In infancy, jaundice with conjugated hyperbilirubinaemia may occur in association with cystic fibrosis due to obstruction of the extrahepatic bile ducts. At autopsy or laparotomy the bile ducts and gallbladder contain thick or even solid bile which may completely block the common hepatic duct. It may be so hard that it has to be picked out rather than washed out. The intrahepatic pathological changes range from a reversible increase in portal tract infiltration, and cholestasis with bile in the hepatocytes and Kupffer cells to an obstructive biliary cirrhosis, established by the age of five months.

GALLBLADDER LESIONS

Gallbladder abnormalities are very common in cystic fibrosis. They are particularly commonly found in association with cirrhosis. Seven out of eight patients with cirrhosis had such abnormalities as compared with 17 of 49 patients without cirrhosis (Feigelson *et al.,* 1975). Approximately 20 per cent have very small gallbladders. A further 20 per cent have gallbladders which do not concentrate cholecystographic agents. Gallstones are found in up to 8 per cent of cases (Warwick *et al.,* 1976), and cholecystitis may complicate such cases. The mechanism of these abnormalities is uncertain.

The incidence of very small gallbladders does not appear to rise with age, and may thus represent an associated lesion similar to the absence of the vas deferens rather than an effect of the hyperviscid secretion. The importance of possible reductions in bile acid pool secondary to the high faecal bile acid loss seen in cystic fibrosis is unknown.

The pathophysiological consequences of these abnormalities are uncertain. Such gallbladders clearly do not concentrate bile. Normal post-prandial gallbladder contraction mediated by the gut hormone cholecystokinin, which causes discharge of bile into the duodenum at the optimum time for digestion, cannot occur. This may aggravate malabsorption caused by pancreatic exocrine insufficiency. These abnormalities in the biliary system with the potential for bile stasis will increase the risks of cholangitis. They may thus play a part in producing cirrhosis.

HEPATOCYTE ABNORMALITIES

Liver biopsy in patients with cystic fibrosis frequently shows the accumulation of fat within the hepatocytes. On some occasions this may be sufficiently severe to cause massive hepatomegaly (Stern *et al.,* 1976). The causes of fatty liver include acute starvation, of both carbohydrate and protein, prolonged under-nutrition, kwashiorkor and obesity. Fatty liver is caused also by toxins such as carbon tetrachloride, and drugs such as ethanol and tetracycline. It can also be a prominent feature in metabolic liver disease such as Wilson's disease and fructosaemia.

In these various conditions the fatty liver may revert to normal, and proceed to acute hepatic necrosis or to cirrhosis. The presence of excessive hepatic fat in cystic fibrosis does raise the possibility of a toxic or dietary cause of liver damage with potential chronicity. No specific toxin or dietary cause has as yet been identified. Tetracycline is a drug which was frequently used in cystic fibrosis in the past and does cause fatty deposition in hepatocytes, but not necessarily chronic liver damage. Other possible contributory causes for liver injury, indicated in *Table 15.1*, include drug-induced hepatitis, excessive iron absorption secondary to pancreatic exocrin insuffiency, resulting in haemosiderosis, endotoxin injury from chronic respiratory tract infection, and perhaps an element of congestive hepatic injury secondary to increased intrathoracic pressure or right ventricular failure. The importance of viral hepatitis in causing liver injury is unknown. Where acute viral hepatitis has been recognized, it has usually followed an uneventful course.

LIVER DISEASE IN INFANCY

Clinical features

Obstructive jaundice appears to be a rare complication of cystic fibrosis in the newborn period. Eleven cases have been reported in the English literature. Out of a group of 126 infants with hepatitis seen in our unit, two had cystic fibrosis.

Jaundice starts in the immediate post-natal period or up to the age of four weeks. In 50 per cent of patients there is a history of meconium ileus. Jaundice is associated with dark urine and pale stools. Hepatosplenomegaly is not evident. Liver function tests show a conjugated hyperbilirubinaemia with moderate AST elevation to between two and three times normal, but the alkaline phosphatase levels are near the upper limit of normal for the child's age. Jaundice is recorded as lasting from 4 to 52 weeks. Death from liver failure may occur as early as 20 days. Four of ten reported cases died of liver disease by the age of three years. Some infants make a complete recovery, and in the short term do not develop further liver disease, but follow-up to adult life has not been reported.

Diagnosis is suspected from the history of meconium ileus or on the previous detection of excessive albumin in the meconium. In the absence of such a history the features are indistinguishable from idiopathic neonatal hepatitis and only the determination of electrolytes in sweat will confirm or refute the diagnosis.

Management

Milder cases resolve spontaneously. An expectant attitude in supportive care, as detailed for infantile cholestasis, is indicated. If there is persistent complete cholestasis, laparotomy should be undertaken and cholecystography attempted. Solid bile may have to be picked from the gallbladder. If the common hepatic duct is obstructed it should not be opened, but an attempt made to flush it out with saline solution injected via the gallbladder. The tube may be left *in situ* to allow this to continue post-operatively. Complete recovery following such management has been recorded.

An even rarer hepatic complication occurring in early childhood is massive hepatomegaly, due to severe fatty infiltration of the liver. Only two such cases have been reported, both had severe pulmonary symptoms. In neither was cirrhosis evident at post mortem.

LIVER DISEASE IN LATER CHILDHOOD AND ADOLESCENCE

Incidence and age at onset of symptoms

The frequency of liver disease in cystic fibrosis is extremely difficult to assess and, indeed, in a disease with such variable manifestations no precise answer may be possible. In *Table 15.2* the incidence of hepatic

TABLE 15.2

Criteria	Percentage abnormal		Source
Liver enlargement	0.5		Crozier (1974)
	62		
Abnormal scan	40		Feigelson et al. (1972)
Serum alkaline phosphatase			
$<$ 4 years	0		Boat et al. (1974)
$>$ 16 years	47		
Liver biopsy	50		
Gamma-glutamyl transpeptidase	30–60	90	Isenberg et al. (1974)
Cholecystogram	40		
Elevated aspartate transaminase	10		Mearns (1974)

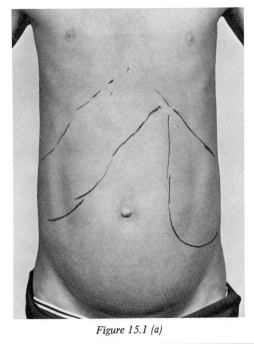

Figure 15.1 (a)

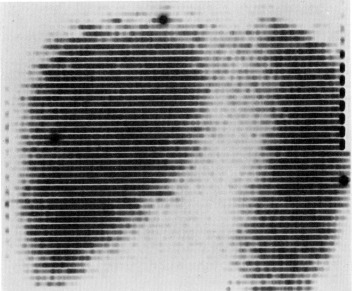

Figure 15.1 (b)

abnormalities assessed in different ways is recorded. The frequency of clinically important liver impairment in cystic fibrosis varies from report to report, as indicated earlier only 2 per cent of the children attending the Boston Children's Hospital with cystic fibrosis had cirrhosis, but in adolescents and older people the incidence was 20 per cent. Four of 104 children aged five years or more, attending a clinic in London, had clinically important liver disease (Mearns, 1974). Twelve of 81 patients observed by Feigelson (1975) in Paris had cirrhosis.

Clinical features

The clinical features (*Figures 15.1* and *15.2*) are those of cirrhosis. In many patients liver disease is asymptomatic. It is suspected only when abdominal examination reveals hepatomegaly with a firm liver edge or splenomegaly. Occasionally, alimentary bleeding from oesophageal varices is the first indication of hepatic involvement. Some patients may present with abdominal distension, due to splenomegaly or ascites. Such is the variability of cystic fibrosis that in some patients hepatic symptoms, including alimentary bleeding, may be the dominant presenting manifestations. Liver function tests may be only mildly abnormal or even normal. Most commonly the transaminases and alkaline phosphatase values are raised to between 1½ and 3 times normal. Jaundice, hypo-albuminaemia and hypoprothrombinaemia are rare except in advanced decompensated disease.

Management

In the majority of patients early signs of hepatic enlargement or spleno-megaly may start by the age of ten years but it is often in adolescence

Figure 15.1. (a) A girl aged eight years who had been found to have cystic fibrosis at the age of three years, when a sibling was born with meconium ileus. The patient had mild respiratory symptoms. Hepatomegaly became evident by the age of five years and splenomegaly by six years. The spleen and liver have subsequently become larger. There are no other clinical features of liver disease. The liver function tests are normal other than the transaminase, elevated at 58 iu/litre. There is moderate hypersplenism, with a platelet count of between 50,000 and 90,000/mm³. (b) The print of the liver scan confirms hepatomegaly and splenomegaly. The black dots represent the costal margin. There is a massive increase in the uptake by the spleen and the isotope uptake by the liver is not homogeneous. Percutaneous liver biopsy showed typical features of cystic fibrosis with early biliary cirrhotic changes

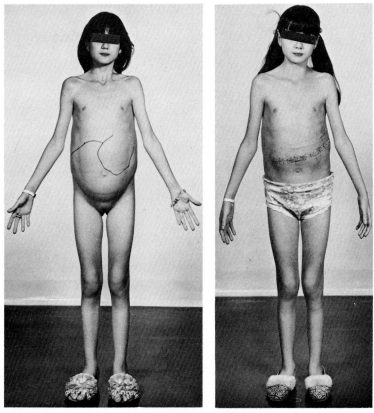

(a)   (b)

Figure 15.2. (a) Clinical photograph of a girl aged 11 years with distended abdomen due to massive splenomegaly and moderate hepatomegaly. Finger clubbing is present. She had three major alimentary bleeds from oesophageal varices during the preceding 18 months. She had only moderate respiratory symptoms having a Schwachman score of 78. Serum albumin was 38 g/litre, aspartate transaminase 57 iu/litre, prothrombin time was prolonged by four seconds. The haemoglobin was 10 g/100 ml, white count 3,800/mm³ and the platelet count 50,000/mm³. (b) Following intensive physiotherapy, a splenectomy and lieno-renal anastomosis was performed. She made an uneventful recovery from surgery. Varices, assessed by barium meal, had disappeared within four months. Two years later she is more active than she was before surgery and there has been no deterioration in her respiratory state

that alimentary bleeding from varices or hypersplenism become trouble-some. The management of these two complications of cirrhosis has been considered in dealing with cirrhosis in general. Some aspects of these problems when complicating cystic fibrosis deserve further con-sideration.

Portosystemic shunt surgery

In other forms of cirrhosis, control trials have shown that porto-systemic shunting may reduce alimentary bleeding but does not prolong survival because of progression of hepatic disease and may cause the development of hepatic encephalopathy. In cystic fibrosis an over-riding factor limiting life expectancy may be the respiratory state. The prognosis for cirrhosis itself in cystic fibrosis may be rather better than for other forms of cirrhosis. Hepatocellular failure appears to occur relatively rarely. The major difficulties which are unresolved include the assessment of the risk of further alimentary bleeding as opposed to the acute and long-term risks of surgery. It has not been shown that portosystemic shunting causes an early deterioration of liver function in patients with cystic fibrosis but the long-term effects are not known. It has not been shown whether or not splenectomy for hypersplenism improves survival. It does cause a rise in the granu-locyte count but whether this influences the rate of progression of respiratory disease has not been resolved.

The results of portosystemic shunting in six patients, five of whom had variceal bleeding, are detailed by Stern et al. (1976). Four had spleno-renal shunts, one had a spleno-renal shunt but subsequently required a portocaval shunt, while one child had a portocaval shunt. Four still survive 1–13 years after surgery. Two died over eight years after surgery. None showed intellectual deterioration. Liver function tests were unchanged by surgery. All patients have good school perfor-mance and an excellent work record.

Schuster et al. (1977) report their experience of surgery in 35 of 48 patients with portal hypertension. Nine patients with a mean age of 14 years died of respiratory or hepatic failure within six months of surgery; four of these had had emergency shunts and the overall clinical status at the time of surgery was poor, the mean clinical score being 59 (Schwarchmann and Kulczyki, 1958). Eight patients who had a mean age at death of 11 years with a clinical score at the time of assessment of only 50 were considered to have disease too far advanced to merit surgery. Sixteen patients with a mean age of 15 years and a clinical score of 70 had portosystemic shunts. Nine had spleno-renal shunt and six portocaval shunts. They survived for between one month and 15 years after surgery, the mean survival being six years and nine months. Eleven patients who had surgery at a mean age of 12 years and 4 months, with a clinical score of 67, died between the ages of 9 months and 11½ years (mean 4 years) following surgery. In five of those who died within two years, 'extraneous factors' were considered responsible. Four patients with a mean age of 20 years and a clinical score of 73 were not offered surgery.

In this report the authors do not document the effects of surgery on intellect or liver function. In presenting their work at scientific meetings they have affirmed that these do not deteriorate and, indeed, life expectancy and the quality of life may be improved. They conclude that in patients with demonstrable varices, a portal pressure of greater than 27 cm of water and pulmonary status, prophylactic shunting should be considered before pulmonary disease is too severe. If hypersplenism is present, splenectomy should be combined with portal decompression.

This is no small undertaking. Such patients require intensive medical therapy pre-operatively with antibiotics, vigorous physiotherapy and adequate psychological preparation. Schuster et al. (1977) advise pre-operative tracheostomies five to seven days before operation to improve tracheal toileting. We have not found this necessary in three patients operated on in our Unit. Detailed supervision is required in the post-operative period. A number of deaths in the Boston series occurred during this time.

At present we would offer surgery to patients fulfilling the criteria indicated by Schuster et al. (1977), but only if the patient has had significant alimentary bleeding unprovoked by aspirin.

HYPERSPLENISM

Hypersplenism may be associated with symptomatic thrombocytopenia and with very low granulocyte counts. Both of these are reversed by splenectomy. There is no documented evidence that the increased granulocyte count favourably affects bacterial growth or modifies the response of the respiratory system to infection. Nor has increased susceptibility to infection been documented following splenectomy. Hypersplenism is not corrected by reducing portal pressure, the spleen has to be removed. The most favoured operation is therefore splenectomy combined with a lieno-renal shunt if the splenic vein is greater than 1 cm in diameter. If it is not, a portocaval anastomosis should be used, but this can be difficult because of retroperitoneal oedema. Splenectomy should not be performed without attempting some form of portosystemic shunt. In the immediate post-operative period, the platelet count may rise to values of greater than 800,000/mm^3, a concentration associated with an increased risk of thrombosis in major blood vessels; these must be prevented. The administration of aspirin in a dose of 300 mg t.d.s. when the platelet count rises to 500,000 appears to be effective.

The other complications of cirrhosis occur relatively infrequently. On some occasions marked hypoprothrombinaemia may occur and can be corrected, often by the administration of vitamin K in a dose of 5, 10 or 15mg daily. The exact dose can be monitored by measuring the prothrombin time. It is rare that it is necessary to use diuretics in liver disease complicating cystic fibrosis.

BIBLIOGRAPHY AND REFERENCES

Boat, T.F., Doerschuk, C.F., Stern, R.C. and Mathews, L.W. (1974). Serum alkaline phosphatase in cystic fibrosis. *Clin.Pediat.* 13, 505

Bodian, D.M. (1953). *Fibrocystic disease of the pancreas*, p. 104. New York: Grune and Stratton

Crozier, M.D. (1974). Cystic fibrosis – a not-so-fatal disease. *Pediat.Clins.N.Am.* 21, 935

Feigelson, J., Pecau, Y., Cathelineau, L. and Navarro, J. (1975). Additional data on hepatic function tests in cystic fibrosis. *Acta pediat.Scand.* 64, 337

Isenberg, J.N., L'heureux, P., Warwick, J.W. and Sharp, H. (1974). Detection of cirrhosis in cystic fibrosis: lack of correlation with gammaglutamyl transpeptidase and biliary tract roentgenograms. *Gastroenterology* 66, 87

Mearns, M.B. (1974). Cystic fibrosis. *Br.J.Hosp.Med.* 12, 497

di Sant'Agnese, P.A. and Blanc, W.A. (1956). A distinctive type of biliary cirrhosis associated with cystic fibrosis of the pancreas. *Pediatrics* 18, 387

Schuster, S.R., Shwachmann, H., Toyama, W.M., Rubino, A. and Taik-Khaw, K. (1977). The management of portal hypertension in cystic fibrosis. *J. pediat.Surg.* 12, 201

Shwachmann, H. (1972). The heterogeneity of cystic fibrosis, in birth defects, *Original Article Series*, 8, 2: 102

Shwachmann, H. and Kulkzycti, L.L. (1958). Long-term study of 105 patients with cystic fibrosis. *J.Am.med.Ass.* 69, 6

Stern, R.C., Stevens, D.P., Boat, T.F., Doerschuk, C.F., Izint, R.J. and Mathews, L.W. (1976). Symptomatic hepatic disease in cystic fibrosis: incidence, course and outcome of portosystemic shunting. *Gastroenterology* 70, 645

Taylor, W.F. and Qaqundah, B.Y. (1972). Neonatal jaundice in cystic fibrosis. *Am.J.Dis.Child.* 123, 161

Tyson, K.R.T., Schuster, S.R. and Shwachmann, H. (1968). Portal hypertension in cystic fibrosis. *J.pediat.Surg.* 3, 271

Valman, H.B., France, N.E. and Wallis, P.G. (1971). Prolonged neonatal jaundice in cystic fibrosis. *Archs Dis.Childh.* 46, 85

Warwick, W.J., L'heureux, P.R., Sharp, H.L. and Isenberg, G.M. (1976). Gallstones in cystic fibrosis. *Proceedings of VII International Cystic Fibrosis Congress.* p. 100

Wilroy, R.S., Crawford, S.E. and Johnson, W.W. (1966). Cystic fibrosis with extensive fatty replacement of the liver. *J.Pediat.* 68, 67

CHAPTER 16

Liver and Gallbladder Disease in Sickle Cell Anaemia

Introduction

Sickle cell anaemia is a severe chronic haemolytic anaemia caused by a genetically determined abnormality in the beta polypeptide chain of haemoglobin. A valine molecule is substituted for a glutamic acid molecule. In affected individuals between 80 and 100 per cent of haemoglobin is of the S variety, the remainder being haemoglobin F. The red cell life is limited to 15—25 days and bilirubin production increased six-fold.

In states of low oxygen saturation haemoglobin S molecules arrange themselves as parallel equidistant particles which stretch the red cell membrane into the typical crescent-shaped sickle cell. These cells are rigid, fragile, and move with difficulty through capillaries. Blood in which sickling occurs shows a marked increase in viscosity. Any circumstance which would lead to an increase in the degree of oxygen desaturation, sets in train a vicious cycle of events of sickling → increased viscosity → stasis → increased hypoxia → and even more sickling leading to tissue hypoxia and cell death.

Clinical features of sickle cell anaemia

Symptoms and signs of sickle cell anaemia are few except during acute episodes termed 'crises' in which occlusion of blood vessels by masses of sickling cells leads to tissue hypoxia. Children with sickle cell disease tend to be slight in appearance with pallor, scleral icterus, thin extremities and a protuberant abdomen. Splenomegaly is common during infancy and in early childhood, but the spleen becomes reduced in size by repeated infarction and is rarely palpable after the age of ten years. A few children go on with presisting splenomegaly.

Hepatomegaly is present in nearly all infants and children, becoming more marked during crisis. The liver is characteristically smooth, of normal consistency and non-tender. The serum bilirubin levels are often between 1 and 4 mg (17–70 μmol/litre) and aspartate transaminase levels elevated to values of between 20 and 50 per cent above the upper limit of normal for the child's age.

In under-developed countries with under-nutrition, a high incidence of parasitic infection and poor health facilities, the mortality in sickle cell anaemia in infancy and childhood is very high. With good nutrition and health care, survival into adult life is usual.

During crisis, infarction may involve any organ of the body. Very frequently abdominal pain, fever and increased jaundice may occur without there being demonstrable hepatobiliary disease.

Patients with sickle cell anaemia do have an increased incidence of both liver and gallbladder disease. Gallstones occur with increasing frequency after the age of ten years. Between 20 and 40 per cent of patients at autopsy have cirrhosis.

Hepatic pathology in sickle cell disease

Six major factors causing hepatic injury are recognized; they are as follows.

(1) Anoxic necrosis of hepatocytes due to stasis in hepatic sinusoids.
(2) Sickling in the hepatic artery (arterioles) causing hepatic infarct (s).
(3) Cholelithiasis.
(4) Viral hepatitis related to transfusions.
(5) Haemosiderosis.
(6) Congestive changes secondary to poor cardiac function.

Portal vein blood during digestion has a low oxygen saturation. Hepatic cells extract more oxygen as the blood traverses the sinusoids. Sickling of red cells occurs within the sinusoids, particularly towards the central vein, and more so, during sickling crises. Few sickled red cells are found in the hepatic veins, being trapped with platelets and fibrin within the sinusoids. These aggregates are ingested by Kupffer cells which swell and appear to distort sinusoids. In addition, there is within the space of Disse deposition of collagen and basement membrane thickening. Anaemia and local circulatory effects due to these cellular changes may further damage hepatocytes. Hepatocytes around the central vein become enlarged and stain less intensely with haematoxylin and eosin.

The cells become depleted of glycogen. Electronmicroscopy shows that the rough endoplasmic reticulum occupies less volume, mitochondria become distorted and vary greatly in shape and size. There will be focal hepatocyte death. Within a few days of remission of the crisis, these hepatocellular changes become less marked and revert to near normal within 10–14 days. Kupffer cell hyperplasia persists.

Hepatic features in sickle cell disease

Jaundice

Jaundice is a frequent feature in patients with haemoglobin S disease. In the stable, healthy state, the amount of haemoglobin destroyed each day and changed into bilirubin is approximately six times that of individuals with haemoglobin A. When the rate of red blood cell destruction exceeds the rate at which bilirubin can be excreted, the serum bilirubin concentration rises. The concentration of serum bilirubin can be loosely correlated with bilirubin production and the reticulocyte count. If 90 per cent of the serum bilirubin is unconjugated, the jaundice may reasonably be attributed to a very rapid rate of haemolysis. If more than 10 per cent of the bilirubin is conjugated, the cause will be some form of hepatocellular damage or an abnormality of the bile ducts or gallbladder. It is rare for the total bilirubin to exceed 6 mg/100 ml (100 μmol/litre) in the absence of any hepatobiliary disease.

Extreme hyperbilirubinaemia

Extremes of hyperbilirubinaemia with serum bilirubin concentrations of between 20 and 60 mg/100 ml (340–1,000 μmol/litre) occasionally occur and are poorly explained. Some may be due to viral hepatitis type A but, in the absence of an easily available marker for this condition, the diagnosis is difficult to sustain. The prodroma and clinical features of acute viral hepatitis are similar in patients with sickle cell disease, and to those with haemoglobin A. The diagnosis may be suggested by transaminase levels of more than 30 times normal. Choledocholithiasis is another possible cause.

Such hyperbilirubinaemia may run a benign course with complete resolution of all abnormalities within four to six weeks of the onset of the jaundice (Buchanan and Glader, 1977). This is in contrast to an earlier report describing five individuals who died of fulminant hepatic failure with hepatocellular necrosis, having presented similarly. The degree of elevation of the serum transaminases would appear to be a better guide to prognosis than bilirubin. If only between four and ten times normal the prognosis would appear to be good.

CHOLELITHIASIS

The persistent high level of bilirubin excretion is complicated by the formation of gallstones. These are typically of the pigment type and are not radioopaque. Many identified stones, however, do contain much calcium bilirubinate and in some reports up to 50 per cent of identified stones are radioopaque. Detection usually requires cholecystography, so that the incidence of gallstones is not well documented. It would appear to be less than 10 per cent below the age of 12 years, rising to over 30 per cent in patients aged 14 years and older. In one series (Barrett-Connor, 1968), 73 per cent of patients over the age of 16 years, had gallstones. With the exception of malignancy, all possible complications of gallstones have been reported in this condition. Choledocholithiasis, perforation of the gallbladder, necrosis of the gallbladder and cholecystitis have all been documented in childhood.

Diagnosis

A major clinical problem is to try to distinguish symptoms and signs due to gallstones from those due to an abdominal crisis and associated intrahepatic stasis. In both conditions there may be ill-localized upper abdominal pain and tenderness, perhaps more marked on the right side. The serum bilirubin is likely to be elevated to values up to between 6 and 10 mg/100 ml (100–170 μmol/litre) with 50 per cent of the bilirubin conjugated. Modest rises of serum alkaline phosphatase to levels 50 per cent above the upper limit of normal and of serum transaminases to three or four times normal, occur in both disorders. The diagnosis rests on radiological studies. As explained elsewhere, these are often unsatisfactory in the acute state. Ultrasonic scanning and excretion of ^{99}Tc pyridoxylline glutamate may give a clue to the diagnosis. More commonly, a plain radiograph of the abdomen showing radioopaque stones, repeated oral cholecystograms or intravenous cholangiograms if the jaundice fades, are required for diagnosis. If jaundice persists a percutaneous cholangiogram may be required.

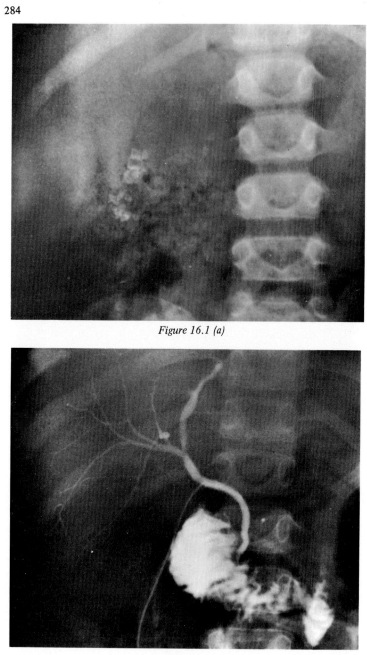

Figure 16.1 (a)

Figure 16.1 (b)

If gallstones are confirmed, it is still difficult to ascribe symptoms to them. The possible risk of stones in the gallbladder must be weighed against the risks of their surgical removal by cholecystectomy. This operation is not without its risk in any child, but carries an even greater risk in sickle cell disease without careful preoperative management. This entails replacement of the patient's haemoglobin S blood in a series of transfusions of group-compatible haemoglobin A blood, sufficient to reduce the percentage of haemoglobin S in the blood to less than 50 per cent. A series of 1–2 unit transfusions at weekly intervals will usually produce this effect over three to four weeks. It is vital to prevent hypoxia during and after surgery.

Indications for cholecystectomy

At present cholecystectomy is recommended for gallstones in children with sickle cell disease who have had complications of their gallstones, or in patients who have repeated abdominal crises which are indistinguishable from gallbladder disease without invasive investigations. In

Figure 16.1. R.C., date of birth 4.2.66, was diagnosed as sickle cell anaemia at the age of 18 months. She was admitted to hospital with a respiratory tract infection. The haemoglobin was 8.4g/dl with a reticulocyte count of 38 per cent. Haemoglobin electrophoresis showed haemoglobin S and A2. In the subsequent year she was admitted to hospital on a number of occasions with respiratory tract infections, sometimes complicated by severe anaemia with haemoglobins of as low as 3.9 g/dl being recorded. Blood transfusion was required on four occasions. Between the age of five and eight years she had episodes of intermittent jaundice associated with anorexia, nausea and right hypochondrial pain. Radiology of the abdomen (a) showed ring shadows in the gallbladder area indicative of gallstones. Her jaundice had never been severe, the highest recorded level being 6.3 mg/dl (108 μmol/litre) but during some of these episodes the serum transaminases had been as elevated as 160 iu/litre (upper limit of normal 40). The case was unusual in that at the age of eight years she had marked splenomegaly, the splenic edge being palpable 6cm below the costal margin. Because her haemoglobin was lower than it had been earlier in life, it was elected to remove her spleen and gallbladder in one operation. When the decision to operate was taken the cells in the peripheral blood showing sickling was 79 per cent. Over a six-week period she was transfused with eight units of blood which resulted in the percentage of sickle cells falling to 9 per cent. At laparotomy she was found to have an enlarged gallbladder which contained ten black pigmented stones up to 0.8cm in diameter. The epithelium of the gallbladder was ulcerated in some areas the cystic duct was cannulated and through the cannula an operative cholangiogram showed free flow into the duodenum with no filling defects and no dilatation of the common bile duct or hepatic ducts. (b) The post-operative course was uneventful. A liver biopsy taken at laparotomy showed no abnormality. Since operation the patient has continued to be anaemic but has had no further attacks of jaundice

these, it is clearly preferable to perform elective surgery for cholecystectomy than to be faced with the risk of subjecting a patient to surgery when the symptoms are due to a sickle cell crisis.

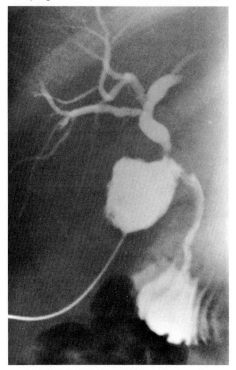

Figure 16.2. Showing the percutaneous cholangiogram of another child with sickle cell anaemia, diagnosed at the age of three years. One year before referral he had had two episodes of jaundice accompanied by abdominal pain. Cholecystectomy which had been followed by an attempt to place a T-tube in the bile duct, had been followed by an increase in jaundice and persistence of abdominal pain. During the eight month period between this operation and referral, jaundice had occurred on five occasions. For six weeks prior to referral, he had had pruritis and abdominal distension. The urine was dark, but the stool colour was normal. On examination there was jaundice, hepatomegaly and ascites. The haemoglobin was 8 g/dl, the total bilirubin 620 μmol/litre, the conjugated bilirubin 420 μmol/ litre. Transfusion with compatible blood without sickle cell haemoglobin was given to reduce the percentage of sickled cells in peripheral blood to less than 30 per cent. The percutaneous cholangiogram shows dilatation of the intrahepatic bile ducts with a marked stricture at the level of the portohepatis. At laparotomy a fibrotic mass was found in the portohepatis. A duct remnant was found within this and an end-to-side choledocho-jejunostomy was performed over a silastic splint. A Roux-en-Y loop of jejunum was fashioned. Following surgery the serum bilirubin fell to 102 μmol/litre, but the long-term prognosis must be very guarded.

ACUTE HEPATITIS

Acute hepatitis occurs rarely in sickle cell disease. When it does the prodroma, clinical and histological features are similar to those in patients with haemoglobin A. The course is generally benign but the high incidence of cirrhosis (16–40 per cent reported at post mortem in patients with sickle cell disease) may be a long-term sequela.

HAEMOSIDEROSIS

A further factor causing possible liver damage is iron deposition within the liver. This arises from both increased iron absorption and from transfusions. Although iron accumulation in the liver in childhood in sickle cell disease is significant, evidence that this causes liver damage is at present tenuous.

Secondary hypersplenism

Very rarely, the spleen remains persistently large in patients with sickle cell disease. Hypersplenism becomes suspected when there is a progressive fall in haemoglobin concentration in the absence of crisis in a patient who previously maintained a constant low haemoglobin. It may be demonstrated more exactly by the reduced survival of normal erythrocytes in the patient's circulation. In such instances, splenectomy will remove the extracellular defect and allow the haemoglobin to return to the higher compensated level.

Treatment

No treatment is available which modifies the underlying defect. The value of blood transfusion in preparing the patient for surgery has already been emphasized. It has a place also in any severe complicating illness, such as severe hepatitis. Hypoxia and acidosis should be prevented. Patients with sickle cell disease are unduly prone to bacterial infection, particularly pneumococcal and haemophilus influenza. Prophylactic antibiotics are indicated.

BIBLIOGRAPHY AND REFERENCES

Ariyan, S., Shessel, F.S. and Pickett, L.K. (1976). Cholecystitis and cholelithiasis masking as abdominal crises in sickle cell disease. *J.Pediat.* 58, 252

Barrett-Connor, E. (1968). Sickle cell disease and viral hepatitis. *Ann.intern.Med.* 69, 517

Buchanan, G.R. and Glader, P.E. (1977). Benign course in extreme hyperbilirubinaemia in sickle cell anaemia: analysis of six cases. *J.Pediat.* 91, 21

Cameron, J.L., Maddrey, W.C. and Zuidema, G.D. (1971). Biliary tract disease in sickle cell anaemia. *Ann.Surg.* 174, 702

Rosenblate, H.J., Eisenstein, R. and Holmes, A.W. (1970). The liver in sickle cell anaemia: a clinical–pathologic study. *Archs Path.* 70, 235

Serjeant, G.R. (1974). *The Clinical Features of Sickle Cell Disease*, p. 87. New York: Elsevier

CHAPTER 17

Indian Childhood Cirrhosis

Indian childhood cirrhosis is considered separately from other forms of cirrhosis since it is the end-product of an idiopathic form of liver disease with unique histological, clinical and biochemical features. It is said to be a significant cause of mortality in the pre-school child in India and to be the fourth most common cause of death in large paediatric centres in that country. It occurs frequently in India, Pakistan, Sri Lanka, Burma and in Indian immigrants in Malaysia. It is rare in Indians living in East Africa or in the United Kingdom.

Pathology

The three unusual histological features in this disorder are the accumulation of hyalin within the hepatocytes, marked fibrous tissue deposition throughout the liver parenchyma and a distinct lack of regeneration nodules.

Early in the disease, there is swelling and vacuolation of hepatocytes with focal inflammatory cell infiltrate around necrotic cells. There is minimal infiltration and inflammation of the portal tracts. Hepatocytes contain so-called Mallory's hyalin bodies which are most commonly associated with alcoholic liver injury but are seen also in Wilson's disease and primary biliary cirrhosis. These appear as distinct bodies with smooth or irregular outlines seen in the perinuclear region of hepatocytes, reddish-purple when stained with haematoxylin and eosin. Electronmicroscopy shows that the hyalin is composed of loose bundles of thin, actin-like cytoplasmic filaments enclosing and surrounded by many free ribosomes. There is no fatty infiltration. The reticulin framework is collapsed in the periportal and pericentral areas with deposition of immature fibrous tissue in these parts of the hepatic lobules.

When the disease is fully established, the hepatocytes become more swollen and contain more marked hyalin accumulations. Hepatocytes appear to merge into large cells and in 10 per cent of cases giant cell transformation is seen. There is marked glycogen depletion. In a preliminary study, Portmann *et al.,* (1978) have observed on orcein staining a marked accumulation of coarse dark-brown granules and aggregates throughout the hepatocytes, similar to those seen in Wilson's disease. The nuclei may be normal or pale and in some instances have very prominant nucleoli giving the so-called 'bird-eye' appearance. Kupffer cells are prominent, containing much iron and lipofusin. There is a marked and aggressive mesenchymal reaction with fibroblasts proliferating throughout the hepatic lobules, isolating small clumps of hepatocytes which become surrounded by bands of active, fibrous tissue. This severe mesenchymal reaction, and its associated vascular effects, aggravate the primary process. There is a striking lack of re-generation, although the final picture may be not unlike micronodular cirrhosis, with marked distortion of the liver architecture. In the late stages there may be hyperplasia of bile ducts with lymphocytic and polymorphonuclear neutrophil leucocyte infiltration in the portal tracts.

Eosinophil and plasma cell infiltration is rarely seen.

Clinical features

In approximately 75 per cent of cases the course moves insiduously through three stages. The early stage is characterized by irritability, anorexia and low-grade fever. On examination there is abdominal distension with an enlarged smooth liver with a sharp 'leaf-like' edge, palpable up to 7 cm below the right costal margin. Splenomegaly may be found in up to 50 per cent of cases.

When cirrhosis is fully established, these features persist, but the liver becomes harder and splenomegaly constant. There is, in addition, ascites and distension of superficial portosystemic venous shunts. In 50 per cent of cases there is persistent jaundice. The progression to cirrhosis takes from one to eight months. The final stage is that of decompensated cirrhosis with a shrinking liver, gastrointestinal bleeding, repeated pulmonary infection, oedema, and eventually hepatic ence-phalopathy.

Approximately 25 per cent of cases run a more rapid course, similar to that of a sub-acute hepatitis, with high fever and persisting jaundice, until death three to four months after the onset. In only a few instances has clinical improvement and regression of histological features been recorded.

Laboratory abnormalities

Standard tests of liver function show changes compatible with hepato-cellular necrosis. There is a generalized aminoaciduria and frequently reducing substances are found also in the urine. There may be excessive urinary losses of zinc and copper, pointing to a renal tubular lesion. The serum albumin concentration gradually falls and the albumin/globulin ratio is reversed. Concentration of the three serum immuno-globulins, IgA, IgG, and IgM are all elevated. Smooth muscle antibodies are present in up to 45 per cent of cases. In younger children, serum alphafetoprotein is frequently elevated. Levels of the serum complement components $C'3$ and $C1q$ are markedly low, possibly being used in antigen/antibody complexes. Cell mediated immunity is depressed as assessed by both the phytohaemoagglutinin response of lymphocytes *in vitro* and also by depressed cutaneous hypersensitivity. The hepatitis B surface antigen is present in the serum of 15 per cent of patients as compared with 1 per cent of control patients, when assessed by rapid counter immune electrophoresis.

Epidemiological considerations

The goegraphical distribution is considered above. A positive family history is found in 30 per cent of cases. Several successive siblings may be affected, or unaffected siblings may intervene. Maximum incidence is at the ages of one to three years, but it can present between two weeks and ten years. No community or class is exempt, but in reported series Hindus are more frequently affected than Moslems, and the relatively wealthy Brahmins and Agarwal Baniyas make up a dis-proportionate percentage of cases compared with the frequency in the population at large (Sharma *et al.*, 1975). (The author is sceptical of the possible aetiological significance of this report, having observed that the children referred to his own unit with extrahepatic biliary atresia from outwith the hospital catchment area are most frequently from families of superior social class; the social class distribution of cases presenting within the catchment area mirrors that of the popu-lation of the area.) Neither quantitative nor qualitative malnutrition has been implicated. Aflatoxin has been suggested as a possible cause but this has not been supported by epidemiological or toxicological studies. The dermatoglyphics of affected children differ from controls with similar ethnic and racial background in having an increase in the total ridge count and an increased occurrence of whorls on the 4th and 5th fingers.

There is as yet no hypothesis which neatly explains these observations.

Treatment

There is no specific treatment. The complications of hepatitis and cirrhosis should be anticipated and treated.

BIBLIOGRAPHY AND REFERENCES

Chandra, R.K. (1974). Indian childhood cirrhosis – clinical biochemical, genealogical, histomorphological and immunological observations. *Med.chir.Dig.* **3**, 63

Chandra, R.K. (1975). Lymphocyte response to hepatitis B surface antigen. Findings in hepatitis and Indian childhood cirrhosis *Archs Dis.Childh.* **50**, 559

The Liver Disease Sub-Committee (1955). Infantile cirrhosis of the liver in India. *Indian J. med. Res.* **43**, 723

Nayak, N.C. and Ramalingaswami, V. (1975). Indian childhood cirrhosis. *Clin. Gastroent.* **4**, 333

Portmann, B., Tanner, M.S., Mowat, A.P. and Williams, R. (1978). Orcein positive liver deposits in Indian childhood cirrhosis. *Lancet* **1**, 1338

Sharma, U., Saxena, S., Mahta, J.B. and Sharma, M.L. (1975). Indian childhood cirrhosis. A clinico-pathological study of 50 cases. *Archs Chld Hlth, Calcutta* **17**, 56

CHAPTER 18

Disorders of the Portal and Hepatic Venous Systems

Anatomy of the portal vein

The portal venous system carries blood to the liver from the stomach, intestine, spleen, pancreas and gallbladder. The superior mesenteric and splenic veins join to form the portal vein. Within the liver it divides into two major trunks supplying the right and left lobes of the liver. These trunks undergo a series of divisions terminating in small branches which eventually pierce the limiting plate of the liver cells and enter adjacent sinusoids through short channels.

The main branches of the portal vein and tributaries are shown in *Figure 18.1*. The superior mesenteric vein is formed from vessels draining the small intestine, colon and stomach. The splenic vein carries blood from the spleen and the short gastric vessels.

PORTAL HYPERTENSION

Portal hypertension exists when the pressure in the portal venous system rises above 10–12 mmHg. The normal value depends on the mode of measurement but is generally around 7 mmHg. Portal hypertension may arise due to pre-hepatic, intrahepatic, or post-hepatic obstruction of blood flow to and through the liver.

The intrahepatic block may be pre-sinusoidal, para-sinusoidal, or post-sinusoidal. Rarely, portal hypertension results from increased blood flow to the liver from arteriovenous anastomosis. Sometimes only part of the portal system is affected.

The mode of presentation of each of these categories may be similar but the complications, naturally history and therapy can be very different. *Precise diagnosis is essential* if appropriate managment is to be offered. The possible causes include intrahepatic disorders such as chronic active hepatitis, and Wilson's disease, which can be arrested and the effects reversed by specific therapy; or they can be greatly

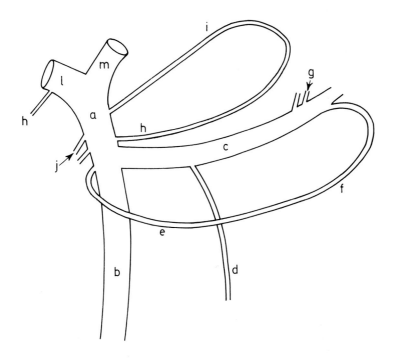

Figure 18.1. The portal vein and its tributaries.

(a)	portal vein	(h)	right gastric vein
(b)	superior mesenteric vein	(i)	left gastric vein
(c)	splenic vein	(j)	pancreatico-duodenal vein
(d)	inferior mesenteric vein	(k)	cystic vein
(e)	right gastro-epiploic vein	(l)	right branch of portal vein
(f)	left gastro-epiploic vein	(m)	left branch of portal vein
(g)	short gastric veins		

aggravated by inappropriate surgery. Intra-abdominal surgery must therefore be delayed until a complete anatomical and pathological diagnosis is established. Iatrogenic factors frequently contribute to the morbidity and mortality of this disorder.

Pathology

Because of reduced portal vein flow the liver becomes dependent on the hepatic artery for oxygen and nutrition. In extrahepatic block particularly, the total liver bulk and individual liver cells are reduced in size, especially if there is a large collateral circulation. The other hepatic changes in intrahepatic or post-hepatic causes are those of the primary disorder. The spleen becomes enlarged with a thickened capsule and increased reticulum around its dilated sinusoids. Histiocytes proliferate in the sinusoids. Erythrophagocytosis may be prominent. The splenic artery is enlarged and tortuous, and frequently there are aneurysms along its length or within the splenic substance. If the splenic vein and portal vein are patent they may also be enlarged, tortuous and occasionally calcified.

A major pathological effect is the development of collateral vessels which carry blood from the portal venous system to the systemic circulation, accounting for much of the symptoms and signs of this disorder. Collateral vessels develop: (a) where absorptive epithelium joins stratified epithelium in the oesophagus or anus; (b) in the falciform ligament; (c) on the posterior abdominal wall, draining into the inferior vena cava; (d) draining to the left kidney; and (e) rarely, into the pulmonary vein. In extrahepatic obstruction, there are, in addition, collaterals which attempt to carry blood around the blocked portal vein into the liver. They are also found in the suspensory ligaments of the liver and may include venae communicans of the portal vein and hepatic artery. Portal hypertension may be complicated by ascites and by considerable oedema of the mucosa of the small intestine, which may lead to malabsorption.

An important complication where there are large portosystemic shunts is hepatic encephalopathy. Septicaemia caused by Gram-negative intestinal organisms is an important cause of morbidity. A cause for failure to thrive may be by-passing of the liver by both absorbed food material and enteric hormones, such as insulin and glucagon which pass directly to the systemic circulation where the metabolic effects are quite different from those which would have occurred had they passed directly into the liver.

Clinical features

Portal hypertension may present with any of the features listed in *Table 18.1*. It may also present with features of the underlying hepatic disease, of which it is a complication. Clinical examination may show jaundice or the stigmata of cirrhosis, such as vascular spiders, palmar

TABLE 18.1
Clinical Features of Portal Hypertension

Splenomegaly	Internal haemorrhoids
Haematemesis	Small liver or hepatomegaly
Melaena	Hypersplenism
Oesophageal varices	Ascites
Cutaneous portosystemic shunts	Malabsorption
Caput medusae	Protein losing enteropathy
Venous hum above umbilicus	

erythema or xanthelasma. The patient may be anaemic, and there may be features of hepatic encephalopathy.

An important clinical sign is dilated cutaneous collateral vessels carrying blood from the portal to the systemic circulation. These are seen carrying blood away from the umbilicus towards the tributaries of the superior venacaval system.

EXTRAHEPATIC PORTAL HYPERTENSION

In this disorder the main portal vein or splenic vein is obstructed somewhere along its course, between the hilum of the spleen and the portohepatis. The portal vein may be replaced by a fibrous remnant, contain an organized blood clot, be compressed from outside, be obstructed by a web or diaphragm, or be replaced by a sheath of small channels usually described as cavernous transformation.

Aetiology

Many causes of extrahepatic portal hypertension are given in *Table 18.2*. In most series, over 50 per cent of cases have no evident cause. It has been inferred that a developmental defect may be responsible for some of the idiopathic cases. Congenital abnormalities in the heart, major blood vessels, biliary tree and renal system were found in 40 per cent of cases (Odievre, Pige and Alagille, 1977).

Clinical features

The patients usually present with asymptomatic splenomegaly or with alimentary haemorrhage from oesophageal varices. Less commonly, they may present with ascites or failure to thrive. Signs may be found at any time from birth to the age of 15 years. Where alimentary

TABLE 18.2
Extrahepatic Causes of Portal Hypertension

Obstruction of portal or splenic vein	
Idiopathic	Septicaemia
Congenital	Cholangitis
Structural lesions	Trauma
Oomphalitis	Duodenal ulcer
Umbilical vein catheterization	Pancreatitis
Portal pyelophlebitis	Malignant disease
Intra-abdominal sepsis	Lymph gland enlargement

Increased blood flow	
Arteriovenous fistulae	Tropical splenomegaly

bleeding is the presenting feature, this most commonly occurs by the age of seven years. Asymptomatic splenomegaly is more frequently a feature between the ages of 5 and 15 years.

Splenomegaly

Patients presenting with splenomegaly as the only feature are frequently well grown. There is no history of past liver disease although a history of umbilical infection, catheterization or intra-abdominal problems early in life may be elicited. On clinical examination there is

TABLE 18.3
Investigations in Suspected Portal Hypertension

Liver function tests:	Liver scan
Complete blood count	Endoscopy
Reticulocyte count	Barium swallow
Paul Bunnell test	Investigation for causes of
Prothrombin time	chronic liver disease
Ultrasonic echography of the	Liver biopsy
upper abdomen	

Investigations before surgery

(1) Venous phase of splanchnic angiogram
and/or splenic venogram or
umbilical portography
(2) Liver biopsy
(3) In some instances:
Hepatic vein pressures
Inferior vena cavagram
Retrograde hepatic venogram
Cardiac catheterization
Percutaneous transhepatic
portal venography

no jaundice or other evidence of chronic liver disease, generalized hyperplasia of the reticulo-endothelial system, bleeding diathesis, or intra-abdominal abnormality other than splenomegaly and, rarely, ascites.

A full history and clinical evaluation will often exclude the many infectious acquired causes of splenomegaly, such as infectious mononucleosis, respiratory tract infection or metabolic storage disorders such as Gaucher's disease. More detailed confirmatory investigations as shown in *Table 18.3* must be considered.

Alimentary bleeding

Extrahepatic portal hypertension may present with haematemesis or malaena. This typically occurs in a child who has previously been well, but complains of an acute onset of abdominal pain. Shortly thereafter, the child is notably pale and vomits blood and/or has a malaena. This may be a life-threatening complication leading to rapid exanguination and is said to be a contributory factor in early death in up to 12 per cent of patients. Upper respiratory tract infections, especially if treated with aspirin, are frequent antecedents. The alimentary bleeding usually stops spontaneously. Bleeding, however, recurs at irregular intervals but becomes less frequent if collaterals develop in areas other than those immediately below the alimentary mucosal endothelium. Often, this occurs between the ages of 12 and 18 years. Encephalopathy rarely complicates the alimentary bleeding.

On clinical evaluation, no cause for bleeding is found other than the splenomegaly, and even this may not be evident if there is marked blood loss and the spleen contracts. Collateral blood vessels also are often collapsed and inapparent at this stage. The diagnosis of the cause of the bleeding is best made by emergency endoscopy. Barium contrast studies may be negative because of the reduced vascular volume.

Ascites

Ascites may occur around the time of onset of the portal hypertension. It can also occur following brisk intestinal haemorrhage. It is thought that this causes a degree of hepatic decompensation since the serum albumin level frequently falls also at this time. If there is no further bleeding, ascites usually clears over the course of two to three weeks.

Dilated superficial portosystemic collaterals are very rarely seen in extrahepatic portal hypertension, partly because the thrombosis frequently involves vessels draining into the falciform ligament.

Rarely, *steatorrhoea and protein-losing enteropathy* may occur as part of the portal hypertension. Hepatic encephalopathy is distinctly uncommon. Minor features consistent with hepatic encephalopathy have been found in some patients following portal systemic shunts. Where the main portal vein has been blocked, some deterioration of hepatic parenchymal function does occur with increasing age and features of liver failure including encephalopathy may develop.

INTRAHEPATIC PORTAL HYPERTENSION

Cirrhosis

Cirrhosis from whatever cause, is almost inevitably followed by portal hypertension. In many instances, symptoms and signs of hepatic disease have been present for years before portal hypertension is manifest. In others, the portal hypertension is found to be present when symptoms and signs first appear, while in yet others all liver injury is asymptomatic and advanced liver disease may first become manifest as portal hypertension.

Physical examination of such patients may well show stigmata of chronic liver disease. In some, however, the patients still look extremely well, in spite of the presence of fairly severe cirrhosis. This is particularly likely to occur when cirrhosis complicates disorders such as Wilson's disease, Type IV glycogen storage disease, and can be a presentation of cystic fibrosis, and fructose intolerance. Other causes of intrahepatic portal hypertension are given in *Table 18.4*.

TABLE 18.4
Intrahepatic Causes of Portal Hypertension

Pre-sinusoidal	Cirrhosis
	Congenital hepatic fibrosis
	Schistosomiasis
	Portal tract infiltration
	Haematomata
	Hereditary telangiectasia (Rondu–Weber–Osler disease)
Parasinusoidal	Cirrhosis
	Acute hepatitis
	Fatty liver
Post-sinusoidal	Cirrhosis
	Metastatic malignancy
	Veno-occlusive disease
	Hepatic vein thrombosis

Clinical features

The clinical features are those of the underlying liver disease, together with features similar to those seen in extrahepatic portal hypertension. Hypersplenism with low haemoglobin concentrations, low total white count and thrombocytopenia are more frequently found.

When gastrointestinal bleeding occurs, there may be a rapid deterioration in hepatic function and features of hepatic encephalopathy frequently occur.

Intrahepatic portal hypertension due to congenital hepatic fibrosis

Parenchymal liver function is usually normal in such patients. The clinical features are very similar to those of extrahepatic portal hypertension. The child is healthy and well grown without stigmata of chronic liver disease. Splenomegaly, alimentary bleeding or ascites may all be the presenting features. There may be a family history of liver, renal or vascular disease. On examination, there are no features indicative of chronic liver disease. Kidneys may be enlarged and these are palpable if they are polycystic. The blood pressure may be elevated.

Investigations will show normal liver function tests other than the serum alkaline phosphatase which may be elevated. Serum urea and creatinin may be elevated. Intravenous pyelogram shows features consistent with polycystic disease (*see* page 205).

POST-HEPATIC PORTAL HYPERTENSION

Budd—Chiari syndrome (hepatic vein occlusion)

This syndrome is produced by obstruction of the hepatic vein occurring anywhere between the efferent hepatic veins and the entry of the inferior vena cava into the right atrium. Similar intrahepatic changes may occur complicating constrictive pericarditis or severe congestive cardiac failure.

Pathology

Thrombosis of the hepatic vein is almost invariably found at some point in the course. The thrombus may contain malignant cells or polymorphs depending on the initial cause. In chronic cases the hepatic vein wall may be thickened, while in some instances the hepatic vein lumen is completely occluded, or the vein replaced by a fibrous strand.

The liver is enlarged and smooth. There is marked venous congestion around the central vein with necrosis of hepatocytes in this area. Periportal areas are spared and the portal zones are normal. There is increased fibrosis in the central areas. Lymphatics may be dilated. Surviving liver cells are very similar to regenerating cells in cirrhosis. They often contain bile plugs. The caudate lobe may be spared if its hepatic veins, which often drain directly into the inferior vena cava, are not involved in the primary cause. Ascites is almost invariable and mild jaundice occurs in most patients. Rarely, cirrhosis occurs in chronic cases.

Aetiology

In the vast majority of cases, no cause can be found. It may be associated with thrombosis complicating polycythaemia, leukaemia, neoplasms (particularly hepatomas, and hypernephromas) paroxysmal nocturnal haemoglobinuria, infection and trauma. In adolescents it may complicate the use of oral contraceptives. It may arise secondary to a membranous obstruction in the inferior vena cava. We have seen one case in which it complicated intrahepatic haemangiomata.

Clinical features

In the acute form there is severe abdominal pain with vomiting, marked hepatomegaly and the rapid onset of ascites which may be blood-stained. There may be features of the underlying disorder. Diarrhoea is a frequent complication. If the hepatic vein occlusion is complete, death from hepatic failure may rapidly ensue.

In the more chronic form the patient presents with abdominal pain and ascites. The liver is enlarged and tender. Pressure over the liver fails to fill the jugular veins. Splenomegaly and oesophageal varices develop as the increased pressure within the liver is transmitted to the portal system.

If the inferior vena cava is affected, oedema of the legs occurs and distended superficial abdominal veins appear. There may be transient albuminuria.

Gradually a picture of chronic portal hypertension with hepatic damage may evolve.

Diagnosis

The diagnosis may be suspected on the typical clinical features. A helpful investigation is liver scan which shows decreased isotope uptake. If the venous drainage of the caudate lobe has been spared, however, uptake in this area is excellent. If a needle biopsy can be performed typical histological features will be seen, but confirmation of the diagnosis requires hepatic venography. An hepatic catheter cannot be

TABLE 18.5
Post-hepatic Causes of Portal Hypertension

Congestive cardiac failure
Constrictive pericarditis
Budd–Chiari syndrome
Polycythaemia
Neoplasm
Trauma
Inferior vena-caval webs

passed even a short distance along the hepatic vein wedging within a few centimetres from the diaphragm. It is impossible to obtain a normal wedged hepatic venogram. Inferior venocavography may be necessary to establish the patency of the inferior vena cava (*Table 18.5*). The hepatic segment of the vein may be compressed from side to side due to the enlarged liver. Right heart catheterization may be necessary to exclude constrictive pericarditis. Appropriate investigations may be necessary to exclude underlying diseases considered in aetiology.

Treatment

In the absence of a surgically treatable cause such as a web in the inferior vena cava or constrictive pericarditis, treatment is symptomatic. There is no evidence that anticoagulants, such as heparin, are helpful. Agents to lyse clots such as streptokinase have not been shown to modify the disorder.

VENO-OCCLUSIVE DISEASE OF THE LIVER

This is a particular form of hepatic vein obstruction which occurs more commonly in children than in other age-groups, and is the most frequent cause of hepatic vein obstruction in children. It was first recognized in Jamaica but subsequently has been shown to occur in other parts of the world such as South Africa, India, Dominica, Columbia, Venezuela and in Israel.

Pathology

The disorder starts in the endothelium of the small branches of the hepatic vein. The initial lesion is of endothelial oedema followed by marked fibroblastic proliferation, leading to phlebosclerosis with occlusion of the vessel lumen. There is secondary necrosis of hepatic cells leading to a progressive fibrosis and ultimately cirrhosis.

Aetiology

The condition is thought to arise from the ingestion of herbs infused as teas. The following plants have been implicated: *Senecio, Crotalaria, Borrago officinales, Cordia alba* and *Helitropicum indicum*. Similar pathological changes have followed irradiation injury to the liver.

Clinical features

The clinical features are those of the Budd–Chiari syndrome. The maximum age incidence is between one and six years. The syndrome starts with the sudden onset of abdominal distension and pain due to hepatomegaly. There may be associated ascites. Approximately 20 per cent of patients die in the acute stage, while 30 per cent develop chronic liver disease with cirrhosis and portal hypertension. Fifty per cent gradually recover over the course of four to six weeks. There is no specific treatment.

CHRONIC CONSTRICTIVE PERICARDITIS

Hepatic effects

Chronic constrictive pericarditis is an example of a disorder in which hepatic damage arises because of increased pressure within the hepatic veins secondary to increased pressure on the right heart.

Clinical features

Symptoms start insiduously. Fatigue, dyspnoea on effort but classically without orthopnoea, and massive abdominal swelling due to hepatomegaly, splenomegaly and ascites, develop often over the course of six to twelve months. There may be noticeable facial oedema. Weight-loss, failure to grow, and symptoms attributable to steatorrhoea and protein-losing enteropathy may also occur.

Diagnosis

The following cardiovascular abnormalities should suggest the diagnosis: persistently raised jugular venous pressure with absent hepatojugular reflux; poor pulse pressure with low blood pressure; and a quiet, inactive heart. On chest radiography pericardial calcification may be seen and on screening of the pericardium there is limited pulsation. The ECG classically shows flat or inverted 'T' waves and a QRS complex of reduced amplitude.

It must be noted, however, that many of the cardiac abnormalities may be minimal as indicated in the case history given in *Figure 18.2*.

The diagnosis may be suggested on the basis of ultrasonic examination of the liver showing distended hepatic veins. Liver biopsy will show loss of hepatocytes and collapse of the reticulin framework around the hepatic vein tributaries. This area will show dilated sinusoids with many red cells present. Confirmation of the diagnosis is by cardiac catheterization which confirms a high pressure in the right side of the heart with a characteristic appearance of the right atrial pulsewave, a steep Y descent being diagnostic.

Differential diagnosis

Difficulty may arise in distinguishing pericarditis from patients with chronic liver disease and much fluid retention.

Treatment

If the disorder is due to active tuberculosis it should be treated with anti-tuberculous drugs and corticosteroids. If the disease is inactive, or the disorder is idiopathic, pericardectomy should be undertaken. Provided the underlying myocardial damage is not severe, there will be a gradual return of cardiac efficiency during the subsequent 24 months. The hepatic lesion regresses similarly.

INVESTIGATION OF A PATIENT WITH SUSPECTED PORTAL HYPERTENSION

When portal hypertension is suspected as the cause of splenomegaly, alimentary haemorrhage, ascites or malabsorption, a systematic approach is required to confirm the presence of portal hypertension and to determine its cause.

Initial investigations

Simple non-invasive investigations are used initially.

A plain film of the abdomen may occasionally contribute by confirming the size of the liver and spleen and by showing the presence of abnormal calcification in the abdomen in the splenic or portal veins. It rarely adds to clinical evaluation. A liver scan using technetium 99 may be helpful in that in extrahepatic portal hypertension the liver will be small or normal in size with a homogenous uptake of isotope with a normal peak count rate, the spleen being enlarged in size but with a low uptake. In contrast, in intrahepatic disorders, the isotope distribution is likely to be mottled, the uptake reduced, and the splenic uptake increased. These investigations are non-invasive and provide, at best, only inferential evidence of portal hypertension. A barium study of the upper digestive tract is more helpful in that it may demonstrate sub-epithelial veins elevating the mucosa. These are characteristically serpiginous channels which change with respiration. They are usually best seen with barium sulphate suspension which coats the mucosa in the distal oesophagus. Varices may also be seen in the stomach or duodenum. Peptic ulceration should be excluded. Retroperitoneal oedema, a feature complicating extrahepatic portal hypertension, may cause distortion of the duodenum.

Endoscopy is the most reliable method for detecting sub-mucosal varices and has the additional advantage in the patient with alimentary bleeding of identifying its source. In children over the age of nine years it may be possible to perform this investigation with the help of diazepam but a general anaesthetic is required in younger children.

Hepatic state

Simultaneously with these relatively non-invasive investigations, simple tests should be carried out to assess the hepatic state. If liver function tests are abnormal, common causes of liver disease should be excluded. These are listed in *Tables 14.6* and *14.7*. A full blood count, including total differential white blood count and platelet count should be performed. Prothrombin time should be determined. A potentially useful investigation is ultrasonic scan of the upper abdomen to document the presence or absence of a normal patent portal vein. This technique has not yet been fully evaluated in children but in adults it has been shown to be a useful measure, confirming the presence of extrahepatic portal vein obstruction. These investigations are often sufficient to confirm the presence of portal hypertension and to indicate its likely cause. Liver biopsy, however, may be necessary to exclude certain disorders, for example, Wilson's disease.

Anatomical diagnosis

If surgical correction of the portal hypertension is to be considered, further investigations are necessary to define the portal venous anatomy.

Splanchnic angiography and/or splenic venography

The most useful investigation is a splanchnic angiogram performed by catheterizing the coeliac and superior mesenteric arteries, using catheters inserted percutaneously via the femoral arteries. Films taken during the venous phase outline the anatomy of portal venous system (*Figures 18.1* and *18.2*). The alternative is to perform a splenic venogram, which allows visualization of the splenic vein, portal vein and its intrahepatic branches if these are patent. If it is obstructed collateral vessels are shown as dilated, tortuous channels. There is poor hepatic sinusoidal filling. If cirrhosis is present, little blood may enter the portal vein due to stagnant or reversed blood flow.

The technique has the advantage over selective splanchnic angiograms in that it may more clearly show the splenic vein, and allow direct measurement of the intrasplenic pulp pressure, a measure of portal hypertension. Since intrasplenic pressure does not necessarily produce a reliable measure of portal hypertension and is unnecessary for clinical management, this investigation is rarely necessary. Further, its complications include subcapsular and intraperitoneal haemorrhage, sometimes leading to emergency splenectomy. While it provides very clear contrast of the collateral vessels running to the oesophagus, it may not demonstrate channels which may be utilized for surgery. Splenic venography should not be performed unless splenectomy can be undertaken without jeopardy. Splanchnic angiography does carry the risks of arterial puncture, occasionally including thrombosis of the

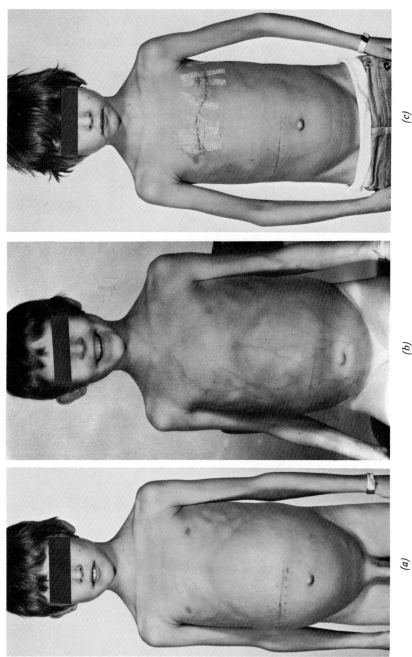

(a)　　　　　(b)　　　　　(c)

femoral artery, particularly if done in young infants. It gives less satis-factory radiological contrast in the splenic vein than splenic porto-graphy. It does demonstrate much more of the portal venous system. Occasionally, both investigations are necessary to give the surgeon optimum information on the venous system. Both require skilled personnel and appropriate radiological equipment.

Umbilical portography

Umbilical portography, in which contrast is injected into the portal vein or its tributaries following catheterization of the umbilical vein, demonstrates the portal vein, its intrahepatic branches and the hepatic sinusoids. It may be used to evaluate portal hypertension when the above studies are inconclusive or contra-indicated. In extrahepatic portal hypertension, in which the portal vein is usually involved, this technique rarely demonstrates the splenic vein. It will fail also if the umbilical vein has previously been transected at laparotomy or invaded by neoplasms. It does allow reliable measurement of portal venous pressure.

Hepatic vein pressure measurement

The free hepatic vein pressure is recorded with a catheter which lies in an unobstructed major hepatic vein branch. The pressures obtained must be considered in contrast with the pressure recorded in the inferior vena cava and in the right atrium. The hepatic vein pressure is

Figure 18.2. (a) Showing the trunk of a boy aged seven years who presented at another hospital with a 12-month history of abdominal distension and inter-mittent vomiting. For six months he had been anorexic and had vague epigastric pain. Clinical examination showed hepatomegaly, ascites, umbilical hernia and increased jugular venous pressure. (b) An infrared photograph showing distended veins over the abdomen carrying blood towards the diaphragm. Constrictive pericarditis was suspected but the diagnosis dismissed when no cardiac abnormality could be shown on clinical, radiological or electrocardiographic investigation. Laparotomy was considered to show cirrhosis. Liver biopsy showed hepatocyte loss around the central vein with some increased fibrosis and congested sinusoids in the central area, findings compatible with hepatic venous outflow obstruction. Cardiac catheterization showed the typical features of constrictive pericarditis. The hepatic vein and inferior vena cava were shown to be patent. At thoracotomy the pericardium was found to be densely fibrosed and constricting. Following resection, there was an immediate improvement in the clinical features (c). By six months the liver had returned to normal on clinical, laboratory and scintigraphic assessment

directly related to the measured portal vein pressure. A normal hepatic wedged pressure is about 5–6 mmHg. The values of approximately 20 mmHg are found in patients with sinusoidal or post-sinusoidal hypertension. In congenital hepatic fibrosis, schistiosomiasis and hepato-portal sclerosis the gradient is between ! and 10 mmHg. In extrahepatic portal vein block, both the wedged pressure and the free hepatic vein pressure are normal. Ascites can produce falsely high values. The main value of this investigation is in indicating the presence of significant intrahepatic disease when other more definitive tests are contra-indicated. In most instances, a percutaneous liver biopsy will give much more information at little extra risk.

Further investigations in selected patients

Investigations occasionally required include inferior venocavography to detect partial or complete obstruction to the inferior vena cava or its compression by tumour or enlarged cardiac lobe; retrograde hepatic venography to demonstrate the Budd–Chiari syndrome; cardiac catheterization to indicate constrictive pericarditis or cardiomyopathy; percutaneous transhepatic venography using a contrast medium injected directly into the portal or hepatic vein through the hepatic substance. This technique has been used largely in adults as an aid to a therapeutic measure in which a fine catheter is passed in a retrograde fashion along the portal vein into its coronary tributaries which are then occluded by fibrin plugs.

Liver biopsy

In intrahepatic disease the diagnosis and prognosis is largely dependent on the liver biopsy findings. These may be entirely morphological but on occasions biochemical studies will also be necessary. If congenital hepatic fibrosis is a possibility it is important to use the Trucut needle to obtain a diagnostic specimen of tissue.

TREATMENT OF PORTAL HYPERTENSION

Emergency treatment

Bleeding due to portal hypertension contributes to death in over 10 per cent of cases of extrahepatic portal hypertension, and causes even more mortality and morbidity where the cause is intrahepatic. It is vital therefore that blood-loss be arrested and significant blood-loss replaced. This necessitates admission to a hospital with facilities for blood transfusion in the first instance, and early transfer to a unit accustomed to dealing with the problems of portal hypertension irrespective of the cause. This should be arranged as soon as the patient is fit to travel and an adequate supply of cross-matched blood is available to accompany the patient to the central unit.

Following clinical assessment the haemoglobin, white blood count, platelet count, and standard liver function tests should be determined.

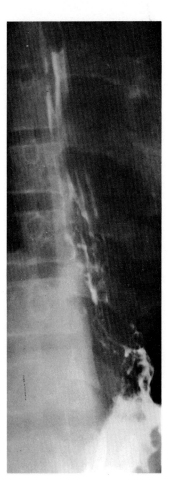

Figure 18.3. Barium swallow demonstrating oesophageal varices. These occupy the lower third of the oesophagus. The linear mucosal folds seen in the upper two-thirds are replaced by tortuous lines where the mucosa has been elevated by serpiginous subepithelial veins

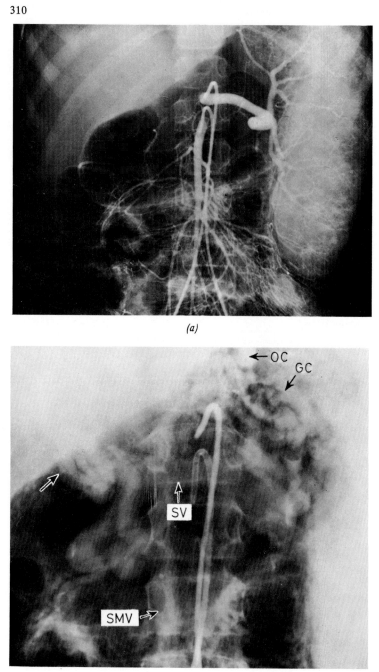

(a)

(b)

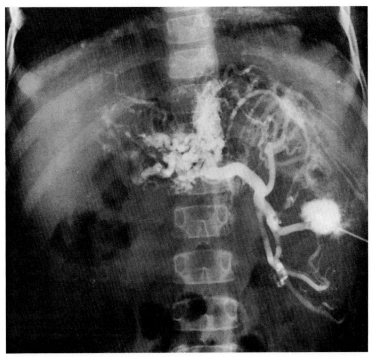

(c)

Figure 18.4. Arterial portogram of a patient with extrahepatic portal hypertension. This child developed umbilical sepsis in the neonatal period, followed by osteomyelitis and a parotid abscess. He was treated with vigorous antibiotic therapy. At the age of seven years he had a haematemesis which had recurred on three occasions. On each occasion these had been preceded by viral infections which were treated with aspirin. Severe anaemia resulted. Physical examination showed a healthy looking child with a markedly enlarged spleen but no features of chronic liver disease. Laboratory investigations were unremarkable, except that the total white count was 3,800 with a platelet count of 80,000/mm³. Liver function tests were normal and specific causes of liver disease in this age-group were negative. (a) Showing an arterio-portogram carried out by simultaneous selective catheterization of the coeliac and superior mesenteric arteries, 30 ml/ of 45 per cent Hypaque were injected into each catheter at a rate of 7.5 ml/ second. (b) The portal vein is thrombosed and replaced by numerous large collaterals (→) running alongside it taking the venous flow from the patent superior mesenteric (SMV) and splenic veins (SV). The diameter of the superior mesenteric vein was estimated at 1.0 cm, that of the splenic vein 0.8 cm. Gastric (GC) and lower oesophageal collaterals are visible. The patient was advised to avoid aspirin and in the 2 years since investigation, has not yet had further alimentary bleeding. (c) Splenic portogram in a girl aged ten years with idiopathic extrahepatic portal hypertension. Contrast medium flows through a dilated splenic vein but at the mid-line is replaced by numerous collateral vessels which drain towards the portalhepatis and to the gastric veins. These collaterals completely replace the portal vein

Regular monitoring of the pulse, blood pressure, urinary output, stool appearance, the recording of any haematemesis and haemoglobin concentration is necessary. The frequency with which these will have to be checked is indicated by the patient's clinical condition. To assess the possible continuance of alimentary bleeding, a fine naso-gastric tube should be passed to allow gastric aspiration.

Endoscopy

As soon as the patient's condition permits, arrangements should be made for endoscopy to ascertain the source of bleeding. This is important as the patients with portal hypertension may bleed from duodenal ulcers and gastric erosions, even if they do have oesophageal varices. In adults, such bleeding accounts for approximately 30 per cent of deaths. I know of no comparable figures for paediatric patients.

If bleeding is not profuse the patient is confined to bed, given some mild sedation, and antacids are precribed. Recently, the hydrogen-ion antagonist cimetidene has been introduced to try to prevent recurrence of haemorrhage. Its exact role in therapy has not been defined, but initial reports are encouraging. If a patient is suspected of having cirrhosis, purgation and neomycin by naso-gastric tube is recommended to prevent the development of hepatic encephalopathy.

Pitressin

If bleeding continues two further emergency measures must be considered. The first is the use of pitressin, 20 units/100 ml of 5 per cent dextrose, given intravenously over the course of 20–40 minutes. This often stops bleeding at least temporarily. An alternative is to use octapressin in a dose of 20 units given in a 20-minute period. The effect of this drug is also temporary. Intra-arterial pitressin, 0.2 units/ml per minute for 60 minutes directly into the hepatic or coeliac arteries is also effective in the short term but has a high complication rate.

Sengstaken–Blakemore tube

If the above measures fail to control bleeding, consideration must be given to the use of balloon tamponade with a paediatric Sengstaken–Blakemore tube. This a complex triple lumen tube, one tube of which communicates with the stomach. A second lumen connects with the stomach balloon, and this is filled with weak radioopaque solution and with gentle traction is positioned under radiological control well into the fundus of the stomach (*Figure 18.5*). A third lumen is connected with the oesophageal balloon which is inflated to a pressure of between 20 and 30 mmHg. This should compress oesophageal varices, while the stomach balloon may help to control varices in the fundus of the stomach. A fourth tube may be added to allow aspiration of the pharynx (*Figure 18.6*).

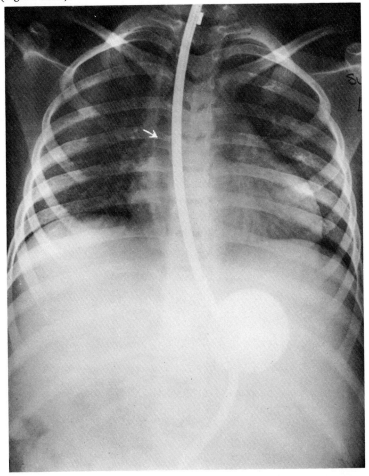

Figure 18.5. Radiograph of the chest and abdomen to show a Sengstaken–Blakemore tube in situ in a patient bleeding from oesophageal varices. The gastric balloon is well placed in the fundus of the stomach. The arrow indicates the air-filled oesophageal balloon.

These tubes are very successful in controlling bleeding from varices but they do have many complications and should only be used in preparation for more definitive surgical management if the patient's condition permits this. The complications of the tube include mal-positioning of the various balloons leading to asphyxia and aspiration of secretions into the lungs. Erosions at pressure points also occur. Considerable nursing skill is required to manage such complicated situations.

Direct obliteration of varices

In most instances, these measures will allow control of haemorrhage, at least sufficiently long to allow full investigation of the portal hyper-tension and its possible causes. In some instances, this may not be

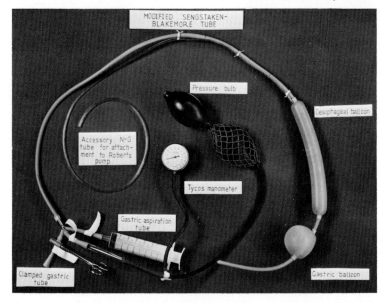

Figure 18.6. Modified Sengstaken–Blakemore tube and accessories. Note the naso-gastric tube which has been added to allow continuous aspiration of the pharynx

possible. Two measures should be considered. The first is direct injection of the oesophageal varices by sclerosing solutions. This has been used for many years but recently has been reintroduced with additional enthusiasm, particularly for the 'poor-risk' patient. The development in technique which gives more satisfactory results is one which allows one varix to prolapse through a hole in an oeso-phagoscope into the lumen of the instrument where it can then be injected. The instrument is then rotated and the injected varix moves outside the oesophagoscope and is compressed against the oesophageal wall. In the meantime, a further varix has prolapsed and can be injected. Occasionally, transthoracic oesophageal transection with direct ligation of the varices may be justified in the patient who continues to bleed and does not achieve sufficient homeostasis to allow complete investi-gation.

In adults, percutaneous transhepatic obliteration of varices has been performed with very satisfactory results in the short term. In this technique a catheter is threaded under fluoroscopic control via an intra-hepatic branch of the portal vein, along the portal vein and into the short gastric or lower oesophageal veins. Fibrin and gel foam is injected obliterating these vessels.

PORTOSYSTEMIC SURGICAL SHUNTS

Extrahepatic portal hypertension

It is important to completely exclude intrahepatic disease by liver biopsy and to demonstrate totally the patency and size of the portal, splenic and superior mesenteric veins. In addition, the state of the left renal vein and inferior vena cava should be determined because of the possibility of associated congenital anomalies of these vessels. The objective is to produce effective decompression of the portal venous system by means of an anastomosis with the systemic circulation. Since the portal vein is usually destroyed, considerable difficulty may be encountered in producing a shunt which remains patent. This usually involves fashioning a centrally placed *lieno-renal shunt*, often combined with splenectomy. At present the consensus view among paediatric surgeons is that surgery should be delayed until a shunt of 1cm in diameter can be guaranteed. It is rare for such surgery to be successful in children aged less than 10 years. The frequency of thrombosis of the lieno-renal shunt in such children varies in reported series from 50 to 82 per cent.

Splenectomy itself has possible disadvantages. It often deprives the patient of safe collaterals in the splanchnic bed, and if not associated with an effective shunt may lead to increased blood flow into the coronary-oesophageal venous system with more frequent and more severe alimentary haemorrhage following. Splenectomy is also fre-quently followed by thrombocythaemia with an increased tendency to vascular thrombosis. Such thrombosis, particularly, is likely to spread around a non-functioning shunt which has not entirely epithelialized.

For this reason, a more satisfactory alternative may be to create a *meso-caval shunt* in which the superior mesenteric vein is anastomosed to the inferior vena cava leaving the spleen *in situ*. This shunt can only be satisfactory for it decompresses the points that are bleeding. In the experience of most paediatric surgeons, both lieno-renal shunts and meso-caval shunts are frequently ineffective. Shunts fashioned between smaller vessels are even more likely to fail. All such intra-abdominal shunts are often associated with complications.

Variceal bleeding, however, does lead to repeated hospitalization, exposure to the risk of transfusion hepatitis as well as to occasional death. Thus, there is a case for considering active surgical management, especially if repeated bleeding occurs unprovoked by aspirin. Just what can be achieved is recorded in the paper of Bismuth and Franco (1976) who operated on 14 children with extrahepatic portal hypertension, all aged less than 6 years, performing 13 spleno-renal anastomoses and 1 meso-caval anastomosis. Only 3 of the spleno-renal shunts thrombosed, although the mean size of the shunt was 8.0 ± 0.6 mm, and the age of the patients 3.6 ± 1.6 years. These authors consider it of importance to confirm the patency of the shunt and the lack of mechanical compression or distortion of the anastomosis by intra-operative portography. They also attempted to prevent thrombosis by infusion of heparin in a dose of 1mg/kg per day into peripheral veins, as soon as the veins were clamped prior to anastomosis. The role of aspirin to decrease platelet stickiness following splenectomy has not been evaluated. These authors conclude that a permanent cure of portal hypertension by early portosystemic shunt can be achieved and may be the best management. Such a recommendation discounts the observation of almost all other authors that patients with portal vein thrombosis will frequently experience fewer and less severe bleeding episodes as they grow older. It takes no account of the possible harmful effects of splenectomy in infancy and early childhood in relation to their resistance to infection. It takes no account of the technical expertise which these authors have brought to bear in achieving such tremendous results.

Portosystemic shunting in cirrhosis

Controlled studies in adult patients have shown that a portocaval shunt is remarkably effective in preventing further haemorrhage from oesophageal varices, but it does not prolong life. Patients treated medically frequently died of bleeding but the surgically treated group died equally early of hepatic failure. Even if the patient does not develop rapid hepatic failure, there is a risk of progressive hepatic deterioration and encephalopathy. One of the main reasons for this is that portocaval shunting as well as decreasing the pressure in the portal venous system, decreases the blood flow to the liver.

In an effort to overcome this problem a selective decompression of the bleeding part of the portal venous system has been attempted. Studies using such technique have shown that distal spleno-renal shunt combined with coronary vein ligation, gastric devascularization and portal azygous disconnection results in a substantial decrease in the frequency and severity of alimentary heamorrhage without a corresponding increase in hepatic encephalopathy. Such reports require careful consideration when surgery is considered for children with intrahepatic disease. The underlying disease process may be very different from that seen in the adult with alcoholism or chronic hepatitis B infection or chronic active hepatitis. Dr Schuster's results in patients with cirrhosis complicating cystic fibrosis would seem to be a case in point where the patient appears to do well following effective shunting (*see* page 277). Unfortunately, in both adults and children, there is a great lack of long-term follow-up studies.

Surgery in portal hypertension due to congenital hepatic fibrosis

Effective portal decompression in this condition controls further alimentary bleeding and is unlikely to be followed by hepatic encephalopathy. Long-term follow-up studies have not been reported.

Schistosomiasis

Portocaval anastomosis for alimentary bleeding in this condition is said to be frequently followed by hepatic encephalopathy.

BIBLIOGRAPHY AND REFERENCES

Bismuth, H. and Franco, D. (1976). Portal diversion for portal hypertension in early childhood. *Ann.Surg.* **183**, 439

Britton, R.C. (1977). Clinical effectiveness of selective portal shunts. *Am.J. Surg.* **133**, 506

Datta, D.V., Saha, S., Sing, S.A.K., Gupta, D.B., Aikat, B.K., Chugh, K.F. and Chhuttani, P.M. (1972). Budd—Chiari syndrome due to obstruction of the intrahepatic portion of the inferior vena cava. *Gut* **13**, 372

Fonkalsrud, E.W., Myers, N.A. and Robinson, M.J. (1974). Management of extrahepatic portal hypertension in children. *Ann.Surg.* **180**, 487

Grases, P.J. (1972). Veno-occlusive disease of the liver *Am.J.Ped.* **53**, 511

Harshko, C. (1972). Hepatic vein thrombosis in children in the Near East. *Med. Chir.Dig.* **1**, 37

Odievre, M., Pige, G. and Alagille, D. (1977). Congenital abnormalities associated with extrahepatic portal hypertension. *Archs Dis.Childh.* **52**, 383

Resnick, R.H., Iber, F.L., Ishihara, A.M., Chalmers, T.C. and Zimmerman, H. (1974). A controlled study of the therapeutic portocaval shunt. *Gastroenterology* **67**, 843

Schuster, S.R., Shwachmann, H., Toyamane, W.M., Robino, A. and Taik-Khaw, K. (1977). The management of portal hypertension in cystic fibrosis. *J.Ped. Surg.* **12**, 201

Scott, J., Long, R.G., Dick, R. and Sherlock, S. (1976). Percutaneous transhepatic obliteration of gastro-oesophageal varices. *Lancet* **2** 53

Simcha, A. and Taylor, J.F.N. (1971). Constrictive pericarditis in childhood. *Archs Dis. Childh.* **46**, 508

Tavill, A.S., Wood, E.J., Kreol, L., Jones, E.A., Gregory, M. and Sherlock, S. (1975). The Budd–Chiari syndrome: Correlation between hepatic scintography and the clinical, radiological and pathological findings in 19 cases of hepatic venous outflow obstruction. *Gastroenterology* **68**, 509

Voorhees, A.B. and Christ, J.B. (1974). Extrahepatic portal hypertension. A retrospective analysis of 127 cases and associated clinical implications. *Archs Surg.* **108**, 338

CHAPTER 19

Liver Tumours

Introduction

Primary liver tumours are rare, accounting for between 0.5 and 2 per cent of paediatric malignancies, including leukaemia and lymphomas. They occur with approximately one-tenth of the frequency of nephroblastoma and neuroblastoma. Of the malignant tumours, hepatoblastoma and hepatocarcinoma, derived from hepatocytes, are the most frequent; rhabdomyosarcoma, sarcoma and mesenchymoma, derived from bile ductules or supportive structures, are very rare. The many benign hepatic tumours listed in *Table 19.1* are also rare.

HEPATOBLASTOMA

Hepatoblastomas are large single tumours which arise in and distort an otherwise normal liver. The majority are in the right lobe. Nodular extension of the tumour may occur. Characteristically they are supplied by large vessels and have many dilated sinusoidal channels. The cut surface is green, yellow or white. Direct spread occurs to adjacent tissues and lymph nodes or via the veins to the lungs, central nervous system and bone. Microscopically the tumour is characterized by

TABLE 19.1
Benign Hepatic Tumours in Childhood

Infantile haemangioendothelioma	Adenoma
Cavernous haemangioma	Lymphangioma
Mesenchymal hamartoma	Teratoma
Focal nodular hypoplasia	Cysts
	Abscess

epithelial cells resembling liver cells, but sometimes appear fetal, embryonal, or anaplastic in nature, usually arranged in cords but sometimes forming tubules or rosettes. In 50 per cent there is an admixture of mesenchymal tissue with ductular elements and even osteoid, cartilage or bone.

Clinical features

Over 75 per cent of cases occur before the age of 3 years, the majority by one year. The male to female ratio is 2:1. The commonest presentation is abdominal distension, with or without malaise, weight-loss and pallor. Rarely, there may be vomiting and abdominal pain. On clinical examination the liver is found to be enlarged and there may be a palpable mass. Splenomegaly is frequently found. A striking complication may be marked osteoporosis leading to pathological fracture, but this occurs only rarely. Precocious puberty is another rare and unusual complication.

Diagnosis

The main conditions to be considered in differential diagnosis are listed in *Table 19.2*. As soon as malignancy is suspected, distinction on clinical grounds should not be attempted because of the risk of

TABLE 19.2
Differential Diagnosis of Hepatoblastoma

Neuroblastoma	Rhabdomyosarcoma
Nephroblastoma	Gastrointestinal malignancy
Hepatocellular carcinoma	Benign lesion

causing dissemination of malignant cells. A scheme of investigation in which the least invasive investigations are listed first is given in *Table 19.3*. An intravenous pyelogram, to exclude a right-sided Wilm's tumour or neuroblastoma pushing the liver forward, is essential in nearly all cases. Liver function tests are usually normal unless jaundice is present. The serum alphafetoprotein is elevated in between 40 and 60 per cent of cases. A more precise figure cannot be given because there may be considerable variation from area to area and also the different techniques used by investigators have varying sensitivity. A liver scan showing a filling defect with technetium-99m is positive in 95 per cent of cases but in only approximately 50 per cent will the selenomethianine scan show filling of the defect. Hepato-arteriography

TABLE 19.3
Investigation of Liver Tumour

Radiology of the abdomen, chest and bones	Ultrasonic echography
Intravenous pyelography	Bone scan
Liver function tests	V.M.A. excretion
Serum alphafetoprotein	Hepatic arteriography
Full blood count, prothrombin time, blood group	Inferior venocavogram
	Liver biopsy ± laparoscopy
Hepatic scintiscanning	Laparotomy

will show displacement and dilatation of the supplying vessels and an abnormal increased sinusoidal circulation appearing as an amorphous blush on the radiograph. The radiological appearance may be mimicked by focal nodular hypoplasias. Hepatic arteriography and an inferior venocavogram is essential to determine whether resection is possible.

Percutaneous liver biopsy done blindly or directed at the filling defect on the scintiscan or at the tumour as shown on the arteriogram or at laparoscopy is necessary to distinguish between hepatoblastoma, hepatocellular carcinoma, malignant mesenchymoma and focal nodular

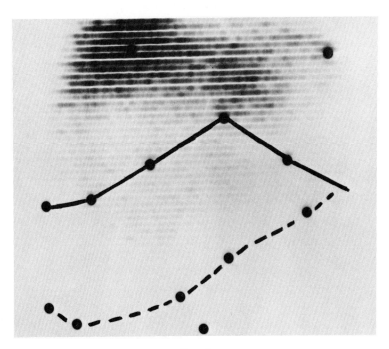

Scan 1

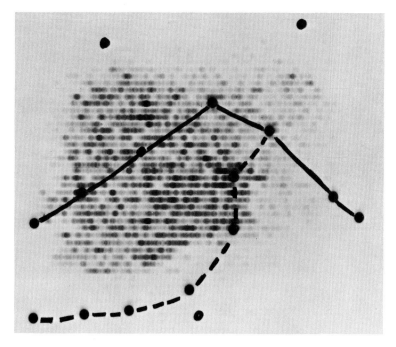

Scan 2

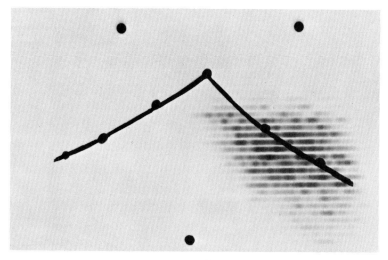

Scan 3

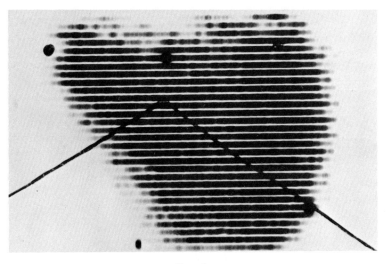

Scan 4

Figure 19.1. Photographs of serial liver scans from a child aged seven months who presented with abdominal distension and hepatomegaly due to a large hepatoblastoma involving the major part of the right lobe of the liver. Liver function tests were normal apart from a raised alkaline phosphatase. The serum alphafetoprotein was positive. The costal margin is indicated by a continuous line on the liver edge when palpable, on clinical examination by a broken line. The nipple and the umbilicus are marked with heavy black dots. Scan 1: Technetium-99m (^{99m}Tc) scan (50 microcuries) showing large filling defect in the lower part of the right lobe of the liver with maximal uptake in the right upper quadrant of the liver (peak count rate 68). Scan 2: L-selenomethionine (^{75}Se) scan on the same day showing uptake over the area of the filling defect on the technetium scan. Scan 3: $99m Tc$ scan (500 microcuries) 14 days after extended right hepatectomy with uptake limited to left lobe of liver or spleen (peak count rate 100). Scan 4: $99mTc$ scan (500 microcuries), 4 years 5 months after lobectomy (peak count rate 38). The serum alphafetoprotein has been persistently negative since laparotomy. The child is asymptomatic, fully active and growing normally, aged eight years

hyperplasia. Neuroblastoma is the most common form of metastatic liver disease in this age-group. Occasionally, diffuse hepatic enlargement or a focal metastasis may be the only feature because the primary is so small and inconspicuous. In these circumstances liver biopsy is essential to establish the correct diagnosis. Biopsy, however, may produce marked haemorrhage from a haemangiomatous lesion or cause dissemination of tumour both along the needle tract or more distally. These risks must be weighed against the advantages of establishing the correct histological diagnosis before operative exploration. Biopsy should only be undertaken after careful interpretation of other data and where it is considered its results could assist in planning surgical management. It is rarely necessary as a prelaparotomy investigation if the alpha-fetoprotein is positive.

Treatment

Total resection by hepatic lobectomy is the only effective treatment. The success rate with surgical removal is approximately 60 per cent but the operative mortality of between 10 and 25 per cent is still unacceptably high. This clearly is not a procedure for a tiro. It must be carefully planned following full study of the hepatic arteriogram and inferior venocavogram. Because of the localization of the tumour, in most instances a right lobectomy is performed, but it is sometimes necessary to remove also the medial segment of the left lobe. With

TABLE 19.4
Complications Following Hepatic Lobectomy

Complication	Mitigating action
Excessive blood loss during and immediately after surgery	Rapid blood replacement with central venous pressure determination via line inserted via upper limb
Air embolism	Control circulation
Ischaemic damage to remaining liver	Hypothermia during surgery
Post-operative Hepatic coma	Pre-operative neomycin orally
Hypoglycaemia	Intravenous glucose infusion
Hypo-albuminaemia	Intravenous albumin
Hypoprothrombinaemia	Intramuscular vitamin K
Hypofibrinogenaemia	Plasma infusions
Hypomagnesaemia	Oral magnesium supplements
Hepatic pain due to rapid regeneration of the liver	—

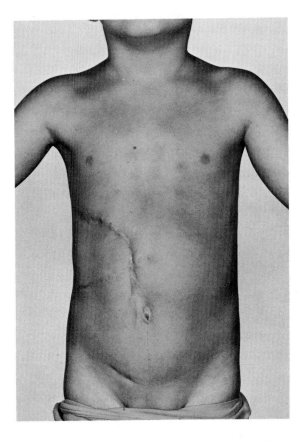

Figure 19.2. Clinical photograph of the patient referred to in Figure 19.1 at the age of 3½ years showing well healed abdominal scars

experienced, careful operators supported by good facilities, the proportion of cases which are operable should approach 80 per cent. In some instances resectability can only be assessed at laparotomy. The complications listed in *Table 19.4* must be anticipated by careful monitoring.

In some instances initial assessment of the patient will indicate that resection is impossible, but with radiotherapy and chemotherapeutic agents the tumour may be reduced in size to make subsequent surgery effective. If resection is not possible the outlook is bleak. Liver tumours are relatively resistant to radiotherapy, and chemotherapy for the vast majority is ineffective. Nevertheless, there are a number of individual case records where considerable reduction in tumour size will occur with radiation in a dose of 1,000/3,000 rads given over a two-week period with or without chemotherapeutic agents such as vincristine, actinomycin D, cyclophosphamide and doxorubicin hydrochloride. At present no established multi-drug regimen has yet been developed for this tumour, but preliminary reports of the use of doxorubicin hydrochloride (Adriamycin) are encouraging.

HEPATOCELLULAR CARCINOMA

Hepatocellular carcinoma is less common than hepatoblastoma. The peak incidence is also early in infancy but another peak occurs between the ages of 10 and 15.

Hepatocellular carcinoma frequently starts in a liver with underlying cirrhosis. The tumour is often multicentric. The tumour cells are polygomal, of varying size, with a hyperchromatic nucleus, and show frequent mitosis. Some secrete bile. They invade both hepatic and portal vein branches.

The clinical and biochemical features are similar to those of hepatoblastoma, except that they may reflect underlying primary disease process. Osteoporosis is rarely seen.

The investigation and management of hepatocellular carcinoma in childhood is as outlined for hepatoblastoma. Treatment is even less satisfactory. Hepatic resection is rarely possible and the survival rate is only about 30 per cent even when it is apparently complete. No effective chemotherapeutic regimens have been evolved but in individual cases there may be a dramatic improvement with radiation and chemotherapy.

RHABDOMYOSARCOMA

This very rare malignant tumour usually arises from the common bile duct but can occur in the common hepatic duct or even within the liver. The bile duct wall becomes thickened by a tumour which grows along it and encroaches on the lumen. The tumours commonly undergo necrosis and are the sites of bleeding. Bile duct rupture may occur. It may extend up into the liver or down to the pancreas. Histologically, the features are those of a sarcoma with, in some cells, cross-striations appearing.

The clinical features are fever, malaise, abdominal pain, jaundice, with an abdominal mass in most instances, but with intrahepatic tumours, there are no clinical differences between this and other hepatic malignancies.

The diagnosis may be suspected by cholangiography but it requires histological confirmation, usually at laparotomy. Treatment is by resection if possible, but considerable palliation is possible by radiotherapy and multiple drug chemotherapy.

MESENCHYMAL HAMARTOMA

These are usually multi-nucleated cystic lesions containing a variable amount of connective tissue and dysplastic bile ducts, liver cells in the surrounding solid structure. The cysts usually contain clear serous material. In most instances these present as a mass in the upper abdomen often without symptoms other than epigastric fullness. Selective hepatic arteriography is a most informative investigation showing an abnormal blood supply to the tumour but without the characteristic blush of a malignancy. Diagnosis requires biopsy. When the tumour is large resection is necessary.

ANGIOMATOUS MALFORMATION OF THE LIVER

Two main forms of these vascular tumours may be distinguished pathologically. The capillary haemangioma has small interconnecting vascular channels lined by epithelial cells several layers thick at the periphery of the lesion, but in the centre of the separation of vessels is less clear-cut. Cavernous haemangioma have larger blood-filled spaces lined by plump endothelial cells with a stroma of single plates of hepatocytes with or without varying amounts of fibrous tissue. Both types of tumour may undergo spontaneous regression by thrombosis and scarring, but in later infancy the latter form particularly may grow rapidly. Both tumours, if large, are supplied by wide blood vessels taking a large proportion of the cardiac output.

Clinical features

These tumours most commonly present in the first three months of life and rarely after the age of two years. Characteristically there is a hepatic mass over which a bruit may be heard. Liver scan will show a filling defect which may take up selenomethionine. Arteriography shows widely dilated supplying blood vessels leading to a very vascular tumour through which the radioopaque material passes very quickly. The most common complication is high output congestive cardiac failure but intraperitoneal haemorrhage and a haemorrhagic diathesis

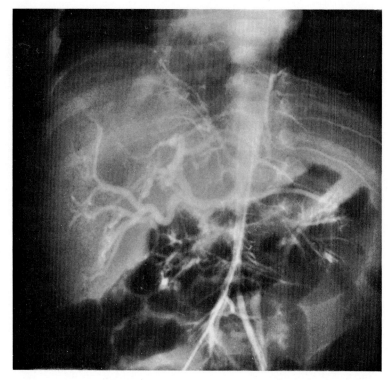

Figure 19.3. Aortic angiogram study in an infant aged three months who had
presented with congestive cardiac failure. Two superficial haemangiomas were
present on the trunk. A haemic murmur was heard over the liver. The angiogram
(a) shows that much of the contrast in the upper abdominal aorta passes into
large blood vessels supplying the liver (cont.)

with hypofibrinogenaemia or platelet sequestration in the tumour,
may also be life-threatening (*Table 19.5*).

Management

Since even large tumours may resolve spontaneously, if no complications
are present a period of observation is advocated. Steroids in some
instances speed regression and should certainly be given if complications
arise. Where indicated digoxin and diuretics control congestive cardiac
failure and vigorous replacement therapy for the bleeding diathesis is
necessary. If these measures fail, ligation of the hepatic artery or of

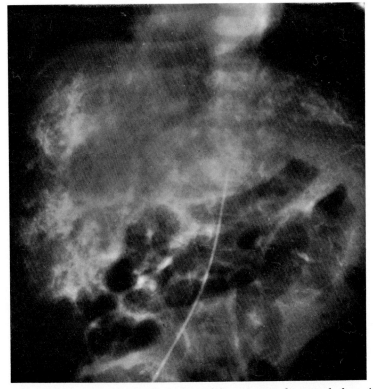

Figure 19.3 (cont.). (b) The capillary phase of the angiogram shows marked opacification of the hepatic parenchyma due to stasis of contrast material in angiomatous transformation within the liver. Following hepatic artery ligation the congestive cardiac failure was easily controlled with digoxin. This was withdrawn five months after surgery. The patient is now aged eight years and has no clinical or laboratory features of cardiovascular or hepatic disease. The haemangiomas on the skin regressed completely by the age of four years

its branch supplying a unilobular lesion, or hepatic lobectomy are necessary. Pre-operative hepatic angiography is essential.

FOCAL NODULAR HYPERPLASIA

This is a rare, slow growing, benign tumour of hepatic parenchyma, characterized pathologically by a central dense fibrous scar from which radiate septa containing proliferating bile ducts and blood vessels, often with medial and intimal hypertrophy. Between the septa there are normal hepatocytes. The exact nature of this well demarcated tumour is still debated.

TABLE 19.5
Syndromes Associated with Liver Tumours

Angiomas	Hypofibrinogenaemia
	Angiopathic haemolytic anaemia
	Thrombocytopenia
	Congestive cardiac failure
Liver tumours	Osteomalacia
	Polycythaemia
	Sexual precocity
	Cystathionuria
	Hypercalcaemia
	Hypoglycaemia
	Hyperlipidaemia

Clinical features and treatment

It presents as a hard hepatic mass which, in childhood, may be very large. There may be some abdominal discomfort but rarely other symptoms. Hepatocellular carcinoma or hepatoblastoma are the usual initial diagnoses until these have been excluded by biopsy. Small lesions require no treatment; in larger lesions resection has usually been advocated, but ligation of the supplying blood vessels should be considered rather than lobectomy which does carry a significant mortality.

VERY RARE TUMOURS

Hepatocellular adenoma, adenoma of the bile ducts, true teratomas and solitary non-parasitic cysts are all rare. Even less frequent are malignant mesodermal neoplasms such as mesenchymomas and sarcomas of the various structures within the liver.

BIBLIOGRAPHY

Edmondson, H.E. (1976). Benign epithelial tumours and tumour-like lesions of the liver. In *Hepatocellular Carcinoma*, p. 309. Ed. by Okuda, M. and Peters, R.L. New York: Wiley

Exelby, P.R., Filler, R.M. and Grosfield, J.L. (1975). Liver Tumours in Children. *J.Pediat.Surg.* 10, 329

Jones, P.G. and Campbell, P.E. (Eds) (1976). Tumours of the liver and bile ducts. In *Tumours of Infancy and Childhood*, p. 596. Oxford: Blackwell

Mowat, A.P., Gutjahr, P., Portmann, B., Dawson, J.L. and Williams, R. (1976). Focal nodular hyperplasia of the liver: a rational approach to treatment. *Gut* 17, 492

CHAPTER 20

Disorders of the Gallbladder and Biliary Tract

CONGENITAL ABNORMALITIES OF THE BILIARY TREE

Abnormalities may predispose to stasis, inflammation and cholelithiasis, but they are often asymptomatic and of no clinical importance. A knowledge of their occurrence is, however, important to the radiologist in interpreting cholecystograms and to the surgeon operating on the biliary system. Surgeons must recognize also that there is a wide variety of anomalies in the relationship of the hepatic artery — its right branch and the cystic artery to the common bile duct and cystic ducts — calling for careful surgical dissection in this area. When abnormalities occur they may do so in isolation, but they are often associated with other congenital lesions, such as polycystic disease and cardiac defects.

All the abnormalities are rare. Only those most frequently seen will be mentioned.

Absence of the gallbladder

This may occur as an isolated asymptomatic abnormality. It is often associated with other anomalies such as direct entry of the hepatic ducts into the duodenum with absence of the common bile duct. Failure of vacuolization of the gallbladder, which persists in its solid state, has been reported. This is usually associated with atresia of the extrahepatic ducts, giving a picture of biliary atresia. Whether this really does occur as a congenital abnormality or is an acquired condition, is considered elsewhere (page 79). It should be noted that the gallbladder may not be immediately obvious at operation if it is intrahepatic, buried in extensive fibrous tissue or atrophied because of previous cholecystitis. Such abnormalities are most commonly seen in childhood in association with cystic fibrosis.

Double gallbladder

Double gallbladders are usually recognized at cholecystography. The second gallbladder varies considerably in size and has an anomalous association with the biliary system; joining it within the hepatic substance, joining the common bile duct via its own cystic duct, or emptying directly into the duodenum. A double gallbladder may be confused with a bi-lobe gallbladder in which the gallbladder appears to form two distinct and separate fundi, having a common cystic duct.

Accessory bile ducts

An additional bile duct may leave the right lobe of the liver, draining directly to the common hepatic duct, to the cystic duct, the gallbladder or even the duodenum. In addition, accessory ducts may join the liver directly to the gallbladder.

CHOLEDOCHAL CYST

Definition

Choledochal cysts are dilatations of the biliary ducts. If unrecognized they cause progressive biliary obstruction leading to biliary cirrhosis and its complications. Four discrete varieties with distinct pathophysiological consequences are recognized.

(1) Spherical dilatation of the common bile duct with minimal dilatation of the hepatic duct and commonly a narrowing or obliteration of the distal common bile duct.
(2) A pedunculated diverticulum from the lateral wall of the common bile duct.
(3) Herniation of the terminal end of the common bile duct into the duodenum associated with the formation of the small cyst, usually termed a 'cholecystocele' (analagous to a ureterocele). There is little proximal bile duct dilatation, the cyst is small but it may obstruct the pancreatic duct causing pancreatitis.

(4) Multiple communicating dilatations of both intrahepatic and extrahepatic ducts. Rarely, single intrahepatic cysts coexist with single cysts of the common bile duct.

The complications of choledochal cyst are listed in *Table 20.1*.

TABLE 20.1
Complications of Coledochal Cyst

Recurrent ascending cholangitis	Portal vein thrombosis
Biliary cirrhosis	Hepatic abscess
Rupture with bile peritonitis	Carcinoma of cyst wall
Pancreatitis	Gallstones

Pathology

Histological examination of the cyst wall shows it to be up to 1.0cm thick and composed of dense fibrous tissue without muscle and with little or no epithelial lining. At the distal end where narrowing occurs there is commonly chronic inflammatory cell infiltrate, and scattered remnants of muscle are seen. The distal common bile duct may be narrowed or obliterated. In 14 instances adenocarcinoma has been seen to arise in the wall of the cyst (Kasai, Asakura and Taira, 1970). The cyst volume ranges from 5 ml to greater than 3,000 ml.

Secondary changes occur within the liver. The hepatic architecture is maintained but there are distinct histological changes, the earliest of which are minor cholestasis with inflammatory cell infiltrate in the portal tract with ever increasing fibrosis. In young infants, bile duct proliferation and bile plugging of canaliculi, similar to that seen in biliary atresia, may be observed. Such changes are reversible, but if obstruction persists and/or ascending cholangitis occurs, cirrhosis and its complications develop.

Incidence

Since the first cases were reported in 1852 (Douglas, 1852), over 700 cases have been documented (Saito and Ishida, 1974). An incidence of 1 in 13,000 live births has been calculated (Olbourne, 1975). Approximately 80 per cent of cases occur in females.

Aetiology

The aetiology is unknown; a congenital cause is commonly considered responsible, which seems likely in cases with an onset of features early

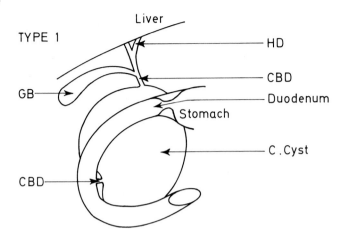

TYPE 1

Liver — HD — CBD — Duodenum — Stomach — C.Cyst — GB — CBD

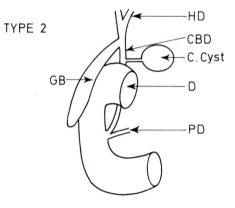

TYPE 2

HD — CBD — C.Cyst — D — PD — GB

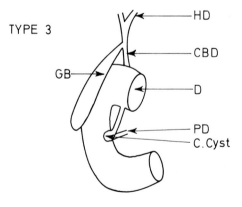

TYPE 3

HD — CBD — D — PD — C.Cyst — GB

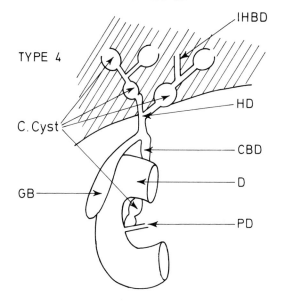

Figure 20.1. Choledochal cyst Types 1, 2, 3 and 4. Abbreviations: HD – hepatic duct; CBD – common bile duct; GB – gallbladder; D – duodenum; PD – pancreatic duct; IHBD – intrahepatic bile duct

in infancy or where there are other abnormalities in the biliary tree or gallbladder. This may also explain the localization of the lesion high in the common bile duct just distal to its point of formation. The aetiological mechanisms suggested include a congenital weakness of the muscle wall with a distal obstruction, congenital inflammation or valvular obstruction occurring in the ampulla of Vater or secondary to an angulated insertion of the common bile duct into the duodenal wall. A further hypothesis is that excessive proliferation of the epithelial cells of the primitive choledochus occurs leading to biliary dilatation when canalization or vacuolization occurs.

A further possibility is that pancreatic enzymes may regurgitate against the common bile duct causing tissue damage with subsequent inflammation, fibrosis and stenosis of the common bile duct at its distal end and proximal dilatation. In support of this hypothesis is the observation that the amylase content of the cyst is often high (Babbitt, 1969).

Clinical features

The classical triad of features suggesting the diagnosis of choledochal cyst is intermittent obstructive jaundice, abdominal pain and cystic abdominal mass. Unfortunately, these three features are rarely present early in the course and are found in less than 10 per cent of cases in recently reported series. The remaining cases may have one or two of these features but a proportion are asymptomatic. In most series, jaundice is reported to have occurred in between 60 and 90 per cent of cases. It is intermittent initially with pale stools and dark urine, but as progressive liver damage occurs and hepatocellular changes and fibrosis becomes marked, the jaundice may become persistent. The abdominal pain is often poorly defined and localized but it may be felt principally in the right upper quadrant and referred to the back. The mass, if palpable, is in the right hypochondrium. Typically it is smooth and appears continuous with the liver. Unfortunately, it may be palpable only intermittently. In infants, abdominal distension, fever and vomiting are commonly reported features.

In most cases, symptoms will have occurred for the first time between the ages of one and three years but, unfortunately, 75 per cent of the cases are unlikely to be diagnosed before the age of ten years, during which time progressive hepatocellular change leading to cirrhosis may have occurred.

Diagnosis

Laboratory investigations will confirm the presence of a conjugated hyperbilirubinaemia with markedly raised alkaline phosphatase and 5'nucleotidase. The cholesterol concentration may also be elevated to above the upper limit of normal for the age. Aspartate transaminase will show moderate elevation, usually to between two and five times normal. In long-standing cases where there is much evidence of hepatocellular dysfunction, the serum transaminases may be markedly elevated and the albumin depressed. In asymptomatic intervals all such investigations may be normal.

The diagnostic investigations are ultrasonic or radiological. The least invasive and most helpful is ultrasonic echography of the biliary tree which with appropriately sensitive apparatus ('grey scale') will show clearly a cystic mass in the course of the biliary tree. Where the lesion is large the barium meal is also helpful in showing the displacement of the duodenum forwards, downwards and to the left in the classical Type 1 case (*Figure 20.2*). If the patient is investigated in the non-jaundiced period, intravenous cholangiography – particularly if combined with tomography – is helpful. Pre-operative diagnosis may also be supported by the scintiscan findings following [131]I Rose Bengal injection. This dye is avidly taken up by the liver and excreted in the bile, but in the presence of choledochal cyst may be retained in the biliary tree.

If after these investigations the diagnosis is still in doubt, percutaneous liver biopsy may be helpful. Lesions will be found predominantly in the portal tract as described elsewhere. If the histological findings suggest biliary obstruction, pre-operative percutaneous cholan-

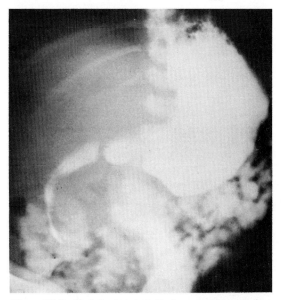

Figure 20.2. Choledochal cyst. Barium meal in an infant aged four months with conjugated hyperbilirubinaemia probably dating from the second week of life. The duodenum is compressed by a space-occupying lesion on its medial aspect. Laparotomy confirmed the presence of a choledochal cyst.

giography should be attempted. Endoscopy with inspection of the ampulla of Vater is helpful if a Type 3 lesion is present.

In some instances, the diagnosis has been suggested by the findings on selective angiography undertaken for the investigation of an abdominal mass which may have been malignant.

At laparotomy, an operative cholangiogram through the gallbladder is necessary to define other abnormalities in the biliary tree, both congenital and acquired, for example, cholelithiasis. Direct aspiration of the cyst must not be attempted.

Differential diagnosis

In infancy the main differential diagnosis lies between biliary atresia and the various forms of the hepatitis occurring in this age-group (Chapter 4). After exclusion of the recognized causes of the syndrome the most useful discriminatory investigations are ultrasonic echography and the barium meal. In this age-group hydronephrosis may also cause difficulties. In the older child the differential diagnosis will include chronic hepatitis and, if abdominal pain is marked, pancreatitis. The various intra-abdominal neoplasms must also be considered.

Treatment

The treatment is surgical. The best results are obtained if there is accurate pre-operative diagnosis; for example, no deaths occurred in a series of 97 such patients (Lee *et al.*, 1969). The exact technique which should be used is still controversial, the choice lying between an internal drainage procedure and excision.

Excision carries the risk of damage to the pancreatic duct, the hepatic artery and the portal vein. It requires a technically difficult anastomosis of the end of the proximal common bile duct to a Roux-en-Y loop of jejunum (Saito and Ishida, 1974). If the proximal bile duct is dilated an end-to-end anastomosis may be possible (Jones *et al.*, 1971). Excision has the advantage that the cyst with its propensity to dilate and form a focus for ascending cholangitis, or cholelithiasis, has been removed completely. Further, the risks of malignant change are averted.

The other procedure commonly used, a choledochocyst-jejunostomy to a Roux-en-Y loop, is technically much easier but leaves the problems mentioned above. Choledochocyst-jejunostomy or duodenostomy should not be performed as the risks of ascending cholangitis are unacceptable. Where the lesion is very high in the biliary tree, a hepatic porticoenterostomy will need to be fashioned (Kobayashi and Ohbe, 1977). Where a Type 2 cyst is found, excision is relatively simple and the biliary tree does not need to be disturbed.

The exact procedure adopted in any patient has to be tailored to the general condition of the patient, the thickness of the cyst wall, the exact anatomical abnormality in the biliary tree, as well as to the expertise of the surgeon.

Prognosis

The main hazards are the operative mortality, stricture formation, ascending cholangitis and the development of cirrhosis. The risks of carcinomatous change in the choledochal cyst appear to be at least five times that of the normal population. Without surgery 29 of 30 patients died in a series reported by Tsardakas and Robnett (1956). From the controversy regarding the best surgical procedure it is clear that none is ideal: 30–40 per cent of patients who have had chole-dococyst-jejunostomy performed will require further surgery within five years. The main problems are ascending cholangitis and pancreatitis; 65 per cent of all such patients will have recurrent features of hepato-biliary disease.

The overall mortality associated with cholecysto-jejunostomy is less than 10 per cent but up to 30 per cent of patients have continuing morbidity. In between 8 and 10 per cent of cases stromal stricture occurs.

If excision is performed the mortality is less than 10 per cent in ex-perienced hands (Saito and Ishida, 1974) but cholangitis still occurs in almost 10 per cent of cases and stricture in approximately 5 per cent. Although this would seem to be the procedure of choice in experienced hands, it does call for considerable technical expertise. Further, in most series, the mean period of follow-up is considerably less than ten years so that the quoted figures for complications are likely to be an underestimation.

SPONTANEOUS PERFORATION OF THE BILE DUCT IN INFANCY

In the first two years of life spontaneous bile peritonitis may develop due to a leakage of bile from the junction of the cystic duct and the common hepatic duct. It is commonest between the ages of one week and two months. Over 80 cases have been reported.

Pathology

Although the site of perforation is constant, its cause is unknown. Operative cholangiography frequently shows an obstruction to bile flow at the lower end of the common bile duct, but the nature of the obstruction is difficult to determine. This is an area which is not explored at surgery. Mucus plugs and gallstones have been responsible in individual cases. In other infants there is permanent obstruction with apparent fibrosis. Some of the affected children have normal common bile ducts.

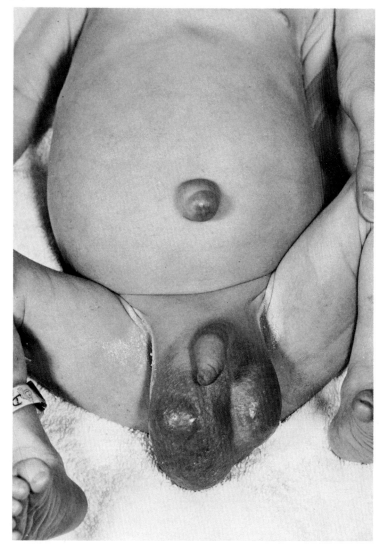

Figure 20.3. Strikingly bile-stained hydrocoeles and umbilicus in a child aged 7 weeks who had been jaundiced since the age of 14 days. The stools were acholic, weight-gain had been poor. At laparotomy there was clear bile-stained ascites and a large bile-containing cyst of the lower sac; the gallbladder was distended with bile. The liver was normal macroscopically, and subsequent histological examination showed no abnormality

The intrahepatic changes are minimal unless there is secondary ascending cholangitis. The bile initially causes little peritoneal reaction but later bacterial peritonitis may develop.

Clinical features

Birth and the immediate neonatal period is usually unremarkable and followed by a variable interval of apparently normal health. The initial features are of mild jaundice, failure to gain weight and, sometimes, vomiting. The stools are pale or acholic and the urine is usually dark due to bile. Progressive abdominal distension due to ascites develops. It is complicated by the development of hydrocoeles, or inguinal or umbilical hernia which typically are bile stained (*Figure 20.3*).

Laboratory investigations

The total serum bilirubin is usually less than 8 mg/100 ml (135 μmol/ litre) with between 40 and 90 per cent conjugated. The serum transaminase and alkaline phosphatase levels are usually normal. The prothrombin time may be prolonged but corrects immediately with parenteral vitamin K. Abdominal paracentesis confirms the presence of bile stained ascites.

The [131]I Rose Bengal faecal excretion test shows less than 10 per cent excretion in the stools in 72 hours. The ascitic fluid 36 hours after the injection of the isotope contains a much higher concentration of isotope than is found in the serum, thus confirming the presence of a bile leak.

Treatment

Laparotomy and operative cholangiography through the gallbladder should be undertaken. Cholangiography typically shows leakage of contrast medium from the junction of the cystic duct and the common hepatic duct (*Figure 20.4*). If there is free drainage of contrast medium through the common bile duct into the duodenum, the perforation should be sutured and the area of leakage drained. If there is obstruction to the common bile duct, a cholecyst-jejunostomy to a Roux-en-Y loop of jejunum should be constructed and the area drained. If the obstruction proves temporary, the cholecyst-jejunostomy will close spontaneously. Cholecyst-jejunostomy allows the biliary system to be decompressed, the perforation to heal and immediately corrects malabsorption caused by lack of bile.

The prognosis is good if ascending cholangitis does not occur.

GALLSTONES

Definition

Gallstones are amorphous or crystalline material which has precipitated in bile. Their pathological effects include obstruction of bile flow and the production of cholecystitis, cholangitis and, rarely, rupture of the biliary tree.

Types of gallstones

The most common type is a so-called mixed gallstone. It contains cholesterol, bile pigment, calcium and an organic or protein matrix. Such gallstones are usually multiple with faceted surfaces and contain enough calcium to be radioopaque.

Pure cholesterol stones are usually rounded single stones which are not radioopaque. However, when secondary infection occurs in the gallbladder a layer of radioopaque calcium is deposited, giving a radioopaque ring appearance on the radiograph.

Bile pigment stones are usually small, hard and amorphous. In addition to bile pigment they contain a variable amount of calcium and organic matter. They are rarely radioopaque.

Aetiology

Gallstones occur more commonly in adult life than in childhood. The pathogenesis of their formation has been the subject of extensive studies in the last decade. While many aspects of their aetiology remain unknown, the unusual physical chemical properties of bile, and the nature of the lipids in bile, are now recognized as being very important contributory factors. Approximately 8 per cent of the lipid in bile is in the form of cholesterol and between 15 and 20 per cent in the form of phospholipid. Both are virtually insoluble in water but are held in solution in bile by virtue of the detergent action of bile salts, which account for between 70 and 80 per cent of bile lipids. The cholesterol and phospholipid are kept in solution in micellar form. The bile salt micelle diagrammatically represented in *Figure 2.2* makes extremely efficient use of the detergent properties of bile salts to keep lecithin and cholesterol in solution. For a micellar solution to be stable, the relative concentrations of these substances are critical. The effect of

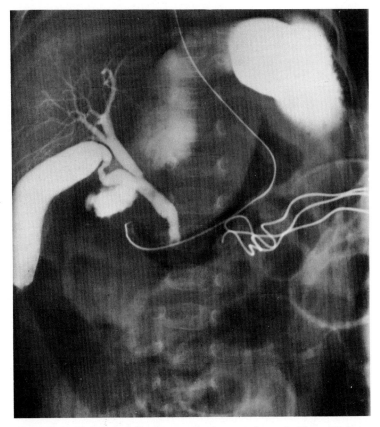

Figure 20.4. Operative cholangiogram (in the case shown in Figure 20.3) performed through the gallbladder showed normal intrahepatic biliary tree but with no flow from the distal common bile duct into the duodenum. Contrast medium leaked from the perforation at the junction of the cystic duct and common bile duct. The gallbladder was anastomosed to a Roux-en-Y loop of jejunum. Postoperative progress has been uneventful and at the age of two years the child is clinically well and liver function tests are normal

varying concentration of these substances on their solubility is shown diagrammatically in *Figure 2.2*. Only if their relative concentrations are within the micellar region will a stable solution occur. While some controversy still exists as to the exact critical levels in human bile, the basic physiological and chemical concept illustrated in *Figure 2.2* has not been challenged and, clearly, events which influence the relative concentrations of these substances may be of crucial importance in their solubility.

Micelles are thought to be formed in the bile canaliculi as bile is produced. In the gallbladder much liquid is absorbed from the bile causing an increase in micelle size. Initially it was considered that the abnormality causing gallstone formation lay in the gallbladder. More recent evidence suggests that the abnormality may be a primary abnormality in bile formation.

Thus, any condition causing *reduced bile acid excretion*, whether due to primary liver disease or from a reduced intrahepatic circulation of bile salts, may predispose to gallstone formation. Further evidence for the key role of bile acid metabolism in gallstone formation is the observation that in man oral administration of the bile salt chenodeoxycholic acid causes gradual dissolution of gallstones. Although it has been alleged that high cholesterol secretion predisposes to gallstones, this has not been confirmed. Indeed, subjects with gallstones frequently secrete low levels of lecithin.

Bacterial infection may also play a part in gallstone formation, by bacterial action on the components of micelles. Deconjugation of bile acids and diffusion of the free bile acids through the gallbladder wall may shift the concentration from the critical micellar phase. Similarly, the conversion of lecithin to lyso-lecithin and fatty acids may cause a precipitation of cholesterol.

Bacterial beta-glucuronidase may have a role in the production of bile pigment stones, causing the deconjugation of bilirubin glucuronide to insoluble bilirubin which may provide a pigment nucleus for gallstone formation. This mechanism may operate also in *haemolytic disorders* such as sickle cell anaemia, or acholuric jaundice, in which bilirubin excretion is excessive. It should be remembered, however, that such excretion is in a soluble form and therefore some additional factor is necessary to promote gallstone formation. It should also be noted that pigment gallstones occur in patients with idiopathic cirrhosis.

In *cystic fibrosis* the factors leading to gallstone formation are complex. It seems likely that in many instances, bile salt excretion in duodenal juice and in the stools may be reduced. The bile may contain abnormal mucin which provides a nucleus for gallstone formation.

The gallbladder is frequently small and the extrahepatic circulation of bile salts may be deranged. Finally, cirrhosis complicating the cystic fibrosis may produce secondary changes in bile salt secretion.

Pathological mechanisms predisposing to gallstone formation in children are shown in *Table 20.2*, while specific causes are listed in *Table 20.3*.

Clinical features

The vast majority of stones are found in the gallbladder, less than 6 per cent occluding the cystic duct or common bile duct. In many instances gallstones are asymptomatic, being discovered unexpectedly during investigation for problems seemingly unrelated to biliary tract disease. They may occur at any age, even in fetal life, but the majority are found at about the time of puberty. In early childhood the sex incidence is equal, but towards adolescence females predominate.

TABLE 20.2
Pathological Mechanisms in Cholelithiasis

Formation of abnormal bile due to primary liver disease
Ileal pathology causing reduced enterohepatic circulation of bile salts
Abnormality of gallbladder function:
    Impaired emptying causing reduction in bile salt recycling
    Excessive concentration of bile
    Hyperconcentration of bile at mucosal level
Abnormal bile constituents:
    Excess bilirubin in haemolytic disease
    Abnormal muco-protein in cystic fibrosis
    Bacteria
    Parasites, for example, Ascaris, *Clonorchis sinensis*
    Cell debris
Stasis due to obstruction of bile duct
Stasis due to abnormality of bile duct
Drugs or toxins causing cholestasis or bile salt depletion

TABLE 20.3
Contributory Factors in Cholelithiasis

Cholecystitis	Obesity
Liver disease	Intra-abdominal infection
Ileal disease or resection	Intra-abdominal surgery
Haemolytic disorders	Family history of liver or gallbladder
Cystic fibrosis	disease

Where symptoms occur they take the form of intermittent abdominal pain or mild or marked severity usually peri-umbilical in site, but occasionally localized to the right upper quadrant. In infants, the pain cannot be localized and irritability may be the most marked feature. Vomiting is a frequently reported complaint in all age-groups. On examination, mild jaundice may be observed together with tenderness localized to the right upper quadrant.

Laboratory investigations

Laboratory investigations are not particularly helpful, but a marked elevation of alkaline phosphatase, without similar elevation in bilirubin or aspartate aminotransferase, should suggest biliary tract disease. Plain radiographs of the gallbladder region may show calculi, but since the majority of calculi are not radioopaque, oral cholecystography is usually necessary to confirm the diagnosis. It may be necessary to repeat this investigation with a double dose of contrast medium if the gallbladder is not opacified.

Complications

Gallstones predispose to cholecystitis and biliary obstruction which can even lead to biliary cirrhosis. Perforation of the gallbladder has been reported. They may also predispose to carcinoma of the gallbladder in adult life.

Treatment

For the patient with symptoms or those with a non-functioning gallbladder, treatment is surgical with cholecystectomy and operative cholangiography, and exploration of the common bile duct where indicated. In uncomplicated cases the prognosis seems excellent, with common bile duct stenosis a very infrequent problem.

For the asymptomatic patient with normal liver function tests, the case for surgery is less clear-cut. Cholecystectomy may reasonably be carried out at the same time as splenectomy in a patient with microspherocytosis. For the patient with cystic fibrosis the hazards of general anaesthesia and the risks of exacerbation of respiratory infection in the post-operative period are such that cholecystectomy would be ill-advised. In yet less clear-cut circumstances, clinical judgment must be made assessing the risks of the procedure which in adults carries a mortality of 3.5 per cent against the risks of the complications which may arise and the overall prognosis related to the underlying disease.

If surgery is not undertaken, the patient should be told to report to the physician as soon as symptoms start so that cholecystectomy may be performed as early as possible to minimize the morbidity and mortality from acute cholecystitis (Arnold, 1970).

CALCULOUS CHOLECYSTITIS

Definition

Calculous cholecystitis is an acute or chronic inflammation of the gallbladder associated with the presence of gallstones in the gallbladder. In the acute form the cystic duct is commonly obstructed by the stone.

Pathogenesis

The pathological changes in acute cholecystitis range from small focal lesions that heal with little scarring, to widespread haemorrhagic necrosis with perforation and peritonitis. Increased pressure within the gallbladder causes vascular compression and subsequent hypoxic change, leading to infarction and gangrene. Except in rare instances bacteria appear to play no part in the initiation of the cholecystitis although within 24 hours of the onset of an attack, intestinal organisms such as *E.coli*, anaerobic streptococci, and lactobacilli are frequently recoverable from the gallbladder wall, gallbladder bile and in liver substance. It would thus seem that the initial inflammation is chemical in origin due to the action of bile, particularly of the bile salts on the mucosa. This may have initially been damaged by pressure from the gallstones or from the vascular effects mentioned above. Bacterial infection certainly contributes to the condition both by release of bacterial endotoxins and from the action of bacteria on bile salts which become deconjugated into more toxic forms.

In many instances chronic cholecystitis follows one or more attacks of acute cholecystitis,but it may also occur insidiously, presumably due to recurrent damage to the gallbladder mucosa produced by the gallstones. In addition, bile may have a direct toxic effect on areas of the gallbladder mucosa, such as the Rolitansky—Aschoff sinuses in which inspissated bile accumulates. However, these are rarely found in children.

Pathology

In acute disease the gallbladder is intensely inflamed with haemorrhage and oedema prominent. The wall may be thin, but more commonly it is somewhat thickened and often has a reddish-brown colour. The mucosa will show small areas of necrosis, and occasionally intramural abscesses are to be seen. Thrombi will be seen occluding some of the arterioles, leading in severe cases to a gangrenous cholecystitis. The exudate is rich in fibrin. The gallbladder content may appear frankly purulent; in most cases the content is not true pus but bile thickened by a mixture of inflammatory exudate and precipitated cholesterol and calcium carbonate.

In the second week of the illness the neutrophil infiltrate in the gallbladder wall increases, to be replaced in the third week by lymphocytes, plasma cells and macrophages, eventually leading to more or less extensive fibrosis of the wall of the gallbladder with destruction of its muscle coat. In chronic cholecystitis the mucosa is thin and flat and the wall contracted. There are commonly adhesions to adjacent structures. In the acute stages the related lymph glands are enlarged.

Clinical features

The majority of childhood cases have been reported in females, with a mean age of 12 years. An almost constant feature is the acute onset of a constant or colicky pain felt in the right upper quadrant. In the young child it may be difficult to localize. Occasionally, the pain may be felt in the epigastrium or peri-umbilical region. Rarely, it may be referred to the right scapula or shoulder. Vomiting occurs in about 75 per cent of cases. An equal percentage have nausea. Chills and rigors are not infrequent but fat intolerance is rarely reported.

Fever is common, 50 per cent of cases are jaundiced. The abdomen moves poorly with repiration. Palpation elicits tenderness and guarding in the right upper quadrant but a mass is rarely felt.

Appendicitis, acute pancreatitis, intussusception, and bowel perforation are the conditions which may be confused with acute cholecystitis. Rarely, right basal pneumonia with diaphragmatic involvement may cause diagnostic difficulties.

Laboratory investigations

The total white blood count may be normal initially but usually rises in the second or third day with a predominance of polymorphonuclear neutrophil leucytes. Serum bilirubin may be elevated, together with the alkaline phosphatase. The serum amylase may also be elevated. The finding of an extrarenal calcified area in the gallbladder region on antero-posterior or lateral radiographs of the abdomen should suggest the diagnosis. Oral cholecystograms are rarely helpful.

Treatment

Because of the rarity of the disorder and the difficulty in differential diagnosis, early laparotomy is usually undertaken at a time when cholecystectomy is a relatively simple procedure. If the child has fever tachycardia, poor peripheral circulation, hypotension or peritonitis a cholecystotomy should be performed and the patient treated vigorously with intravenous fluids, analgesics, and broad spectrum antibiotics. Ampicillin and gentamycin should be used until bacterial culture results are available. Insertion of a drainage tube through which cholangiography can be performed to exclude stones in the common bile duct is a necessary part of the procedure. Cholecystectomy should be performed 4–6 weeks later, provided signs of acute inflammation have settled and the liver function tests have returned to normal.

The prognosis following surgery is excellent except where there is significant underlying disease, such as cirrhosis.

NON-CALCULOUS CHOLECYSTITIS

Definition

Non-calculous cholecystitis is an acute inflammatory disease of the gallbladder in the absence of cholelithiasis.

Aetiology

Acute cholecystitis may occur as part of a systemic infection. It is reported in particular with bacterial enteric infections caused by *Salmonella typhi*, and in shigellosis and viral gastroenteritis. Parasitic infections with Giardia, Ascaris and, in the Orient, Clonorchis are rare causes. The liver fluke *Fasciola hepatica* does not survive in the gallbladder if bile is present.

Salmonella typhi and Clonorchis can both cause chronic cholecystitis. The other aetiological factors in non-calculous cholecystitis are congenital abnormalities of the gallbladder which result in bile stasis. This presumably causes the formation of inspissated bile with chemical injury to the gallbladder mucosa and subsequent cholecystitis.

Pathology

The pathological changes depend on the underlying cause. Many of the infections are self-limiting. The chronic ones have been referred to above. There is no acute distension of the gallbladder, so that the risks of perforation are less than in the calculous cholecystitis.

Clinical aspects

The clinical features, diagnosis and management are similar to that of calculous cholecystitis.

NON-CALCULOUS DISTENSION OF THE GALLBLADDER
(acute hydrops)

Definition

This is a rare, self-limiting disorder in which there is acute distension of the gallbladder in the absence of any mechnical obstruction to the cystic duct.

Aetiology and pathogenesis

The aetiology is unknown. In 13 of 25 cases (Chamberlain and Hung, 1970) there was a generalized mesenteric adenitis involving glands near the cystic duct. Although these lymph glands may be large there is no mechanical compression, although associated hyperaemia may cause mucosal oedema and thus obstruct the cystic duct lumen. No specific infectious agent has been incriminated as causing the adenitis, although a history of upper respiratory tract infection is frequently obtained. Some reports suggest that the hepatitis A virus may be implicated in that previous infectious hepatitis occurred in one patient, two were in contact with acute hepatitis and three were jaundiced, and a further three had abnormal liver function tests at the time of presentation. Other specific disorders which have been associated are scarlet fever and leptospirosis.

Pathology

There are few reports on excised gallbladders. These show either normal uncongested mucosa or oedematous mucosa with fibrous thickening of the gallbladder wall and cellular infiltration. One patient with cystic fibrosis had areas of infarction and fibrinoid necrosis in the arterioles. There are no reports of histological changes in the cystic duct.

The bile is reported to be green or yellow in the majority of cases. In a minority it is white, while small numbers have had turbid or brown bile. Where the bile has been examined it is often reported to be sterile, alkaline, with no protein and scanty leucocytes, but in 15 of 31 patients in which the bile was cultured a variety of pathogens were isolated.

Clinical features

A period of preceding illness is present in up to 60 per cent of cases. Age distribution ranges from one month to 15 years, the male-to-female ratio is 5:2. The principal feature is abdominal pain, most commonly severe and of sudden onset. Occasionally, it is intermittent, suggesting an intussusception. Fever is rare but anorexia, nausea and vomiting are prominent.

There is marked tenderness on palpation of the right upper quadrant but a mass is rarely palpable except under general anaesthesia. Jaundice is unusual but has been reported.

Diagnosis

Liver function tests are rarely recorded in case reports of this condition and laboratory investigations do not appear to have contributed to the diagnosis, which is most frequently made at laparotomy carried out to exclude intussusception or appendix abscess, although occasionally cholcystitis will be the pre-laparotomy diagnosis.

Treatment

Cholecystostomy is the treatment of choice. It is important to perform a post-operative cholangiogram to exclude an obstructive lesion in the biliary tree. Since the majority of patients can be expected to make a complete recovery with normal biliary tract function, cholecystectomy, which was often used as the initial therapy in earlier reported cases, should be reserved as a secondary procedure to be used only when indicated as a result of cholangiography.

The prognosis is excellent.

BIBLIOGRAPHY AND REFERENCES

Congenital abnormalities of the biliary tree

Flannery, M.G. and Caster, M.P. (1956). Congenital abnormalities of the gall-bladder; review of 101 cases. *Surg.Gynec.Obstet.* **103**, 439

Kassner, E.G. and Klotz, D.H. (1975). Cholecystitis and calculi in a diverticulum of the gallbladder. *J. pediat. Surg.* **10**, 967

Maingot, R. (1964). Anomolies of the gallbladder, bile ducts, and arteries. In *Surgery of the Gallbladder and Bile Ducts*, p. 12. Ed. by Smith, R. and Sherlock, S. London: Butterworths

Pinter, A., Pilaszanowich, I., Schaffer, J. and Weisenbach, J. (1975). Membranous obstruction of the common bile duct. *J. pediat. Surg.* **10**, 839

Choledochal cyst

Babbitt, D.P. (1969). Aetiology of congenital dilatation of biliary tree. *Ann. Radiol.* **12**, 231

Chen, W.J., Chang, C. and Hung, D.W. (1973). Congenital choledochal cyst with observation on rupture of the cyst and intrahepatic distal dilatation. *J. pediat. Surg.* **8**, 529

Douglas, A.H. (1852). Case of dilatation of the common bile duct. *Mon.J.med. Sci.(London)* **14**, 97

Jones, P.G., Smith, E.D., Clark, A.M. and Kent, M. (1971). Choledochal cyst: experience with radical excision. *J.pediat.Surg.* **6**, 112

Kasai, M., Asakura, Y. and Taira, Y. (1970). Surgical treatment of choledochal cyst. *Ann.Surg.* **172**, 844

Karjoo, M., Bishop, H.C., Borns, P. and Holtzapple, P.G. (1973). Choledochal cyst presenting as recurrent pancreatitis. *Pediatrics* **51**, 289

Klotz, D., Cohn, D.D. and Cottmeier, P.K. (1973). Choledochal cyst: diagnostic and therapeutic problems. *J.pediat.Surg.* **8**, 271

Kobayashi, A. and Ohbe, Y. (1977). Choledochal cyst in infancy and childhood: analysis of 16 cases. *Archs Dis.Childh.* **52**, 121

Lee, S.S., Min, P.C., Kim, G.W. and Hong, P.W. (1969). Choledochal cyst – a review of nine cases and review of the literature. *Archs Surg.* **99**, 19

Olbourne, N.A. (1975). Choledochal cysts. *Ann. R. Coll. Surg. Engl.* **56**, 26

Saito, S. and Ishida, M. (1974). Congenital choledochal cyst (cystic dilatation of the common bile duct). *Progr.ped.Surg.* **6**, 63

Tsardakas, E. and Robnett, A.H. (1956). Congenital cystic dilatation of the common bile duct. *Archs Surg.* **72**, 311

Volayer, J. and Alagille, D. (1975). Experience with choledochal cysts. *J.pediat. Surg.* **10**, 65

Gallstones

Admirand, W.H. and Small, D.M. (1968). The physiochemical basis of cholesterol gallstone formation in man. *J.clin.Invest.* **47**, 1043

Arnold, D.J. (1970). 28,621 cholecystectomies in Ohio. *Am. J. Surg.* **119**, 714

Bouchier, I.A.D. (1975). Gallstones. In *Topics of Gastroenterology*, p. 74. No. 3, Ed. by Truelove, S.C. and Trewell, J. Oxford: Blackwell

Pellerin, D., Pertin, P., Mihoul-Fekete, C.L. and Ricour, C. (1975). Cholelithiasis and ileal pathology in childhood, *J.pediat.Surg.* **10**, 35

Shrand, H. and Ackroyd, F.W. (1973). Gallstones in children. *Clin. Pediat.* **12**, 191

Strauss, R.G. (1969). Cholelithiasis in childhood. *Am.J.Dis.Child.* **117**, 689

Cholecystitis

Bass, H.N. (1970). Gallbladder disease in childhood: report of 4 cases, including one with 'milk of calcium bile'. *Clin.Pediat.* **9**, 229

Duttat, G.C., Shana, G.B. and Mesnakshi, T. (1975). Gallbladder disease in infancy and childhood. *Progr.pediat.Surg.* **8**, 109

Hanson, B.A., Mahour, G.H. and Woolley, N.M. (1971). Diseases of the gallbladder in infancy and childhood. *J. pediat. Surg.* **6**, 277

Marks, C., Espinosa, J. and Hyman, L.J. (1968). Acute acalculous cholecystitis in childhood. *J.pediat.Surg.* **3**, 608

Pieretti, R., Auldisu, A.W. and Stephens, C.A. (1975). Acute cholecystitis in children. *Surg. Gynec. Obstet.* **140**, 16

Stears, H., Golden, G.T. and Horsley, J.S. (1973). Cholecystitis in childhood and adolescence. *Archs Surg.* **106**, 651

Ternberg, J.L. and Keating, J.P. (1975). Acute acalculous cholecystitis. *Archs Surg.* **110**, 543

Non-calculous distension of the gallbladder

Chamberlain, J.W. and Hight, D.W. (1970). Acute hydrops of the gallbladder in childhood. *Surgery* **68**, 899

Loom, R.A.B. and Swain, V.A.J. (1966). Non-calculous distension of the gallbladder in childhood. *Archs Dis.Childh.* **41**, 503

CHAPTER 21

Laboratory Assessment of Hepatobiliary Disease

Laboratory investigations are frequently essential to establish or confirm a clinical diagnosis. They are of value in monitoring the progress of disease. They are also important in *excluding* hepatic disease, for example, in acute unexplained coma in childhood which might suggest a diagnosis of Reye's syndrome, or in the assessment of possible hepatotoxic effects of new drugs.

The relative importance of the available tests in the diagnosis of particular disorders is considered throughout the text. The most useful tests are those which identify specific aetiological factors, for example, alpha-1 antitrypsin deficiency Type PiZ or hepatitis B surface antigen and e antigen. Tests which give anatomical or histological information, for example, splenic angiography or liver biopsy, are often of considerable value in diagnosis. Radiology of the biliary system is considered in Chapter 22 (page 380). Routine tests of liver function are frequently influenced by many non-hepatic factors. Their value lies in screening and for monitoring progress.

LABORATORY TESTS OF LIVER FUNCTION

Aminotransferases

Aminotransferases (transaminases) are intracellular enzymes found in nearly all tissues. They are most active within the cells of the liver, heart, skeletal muscle, adipose tissue, brain and kidney. Plasma activity is believed to be due to the release of enzyme proteins as a result of cell turnover or injury. They are constantly being removed from the plasma. Two aminotransferase determinations are widely used clinically.

Aspartate aminotransferase (AsAT or AST, L-aspartate-2-oxaloglutarate aminotransferase, E.C.2.6.1.1, formerly serum glutamic-oxalo-acetic transaminase, SGOT)
catalyses the reaction:
Aspartate + 2-oxaloglutarate → oxaloacetate + glutamate

Alanine aminotransferase (AlAT or ALT, L-alanin -2-oxaloglutarate aminotransferase, E.C.2.6.1.2, formerly serum glutamic-pyruvic transaminase, SGPT).
catalyses the reaction:
Alanine + 2-oxaloglutarate → pyruvate + glutamate

There are a number of different techniques for measuring transferases. These can be influenced by the conditions under which the assay is performed. The clinician, therefore, must always be aware of the normal range of values relevant to the method used in the laboratory in which the test was done, as well as the composition of the 'normal' control population. Typical normal paediatric ranges for spectrophotometric units vary from 5 to 40 units/litre, while the range is from 3 to 16 for iu/litre. Values are frequently twice as high in the first month of life falling to normal paediatric levels by two years.

Serum aminotransferase activity is increased in minor cell injury making such determinations useful in the early detection of hepatitis due to infection or drugs. It is of value also in monitoring the course of the hepatitis. Persistently elevated transaminase levels are good evidence that the disease is still active and indicate that chronic active hepatitis be considered in the differential diagnosis.

In many other forms of hepatobiliary disease, such as biliary atresia, choledochal cyst, gallstones, cholecystitis and intrahepatic neoplasms, transaminases may be elevated. They are elevated also in such non-hepatic conditions as myocarditis, myopathies, pancreatitis and infarction of the kidney, brain or lung. Minor elevations may also occur in haemolytic anaemias.

Other enzyme activities which can be determined in serum and have been correlated with hepatocellular necrosis include sorbitol dehydrogenase, isocitrate dehydrogenase, lactic acid dehydrogenase, and leucine aminopeptidase. There seems little evidence that these add significantly to the information obtained from the more commonly measured transaminases.

Serum alkaline phosphatase

Isoenzymes of alkaline phosphatase (3.13.1, orthophosphoric monoester phosphohydrolase, AIP) are widely distributed in various organs of the body, including the liver, bone, kidney, intestines and placenta. In the liver they are located on both the sinusoidal and canalicular borders of the hepatocytes. Serum concentrations of the enzyme are increased in liver disease where there is interference with hepatic excretion.

The isoenzymes of alkaline phosphatase may be separated by electrophoresis or by heat inactivation. Placental alkaline phosphatase is resistant to incubation at $56°C$, liver enzymes somewhat less so, and bone enzyme loses much of its activity rapidly at this temperature. Neither method is particularly precise. Consideration of the clinical circumstances often allows assessment of the probable source of excessive activity.

Increased serum activity of alkaline phosphatase may occur with liver damage before the bilirubin rises, for example, in anicteric hepatitis or in congenital hepatic fibrosis or extrahepatic bile duct obstruction. The activity is frequently elevated in the presence of malignant and benign infiltrations of the liver, including liver abscess. In jaundiced patients, elevations occur both in chronic hepatitis and in bile duct obstruction. Alkaline phosphatase is commonly elevated in hepatitis in infancy and in extrahepatic biliary atresia. It is of no value in distinguishing between these two conditions.

Early in the course of hepatocellular jaundice in older children there is usually a more marked elevation of transaminases than of alkaline phosphatase. If jaundice results from bile duct obstruction, for example, due to choledochal cyst, the converse is found. If jaundice has been present for more than 2 weeks these differences may no longer be present.

In the first month of life, the alkaline phosphatase is usually raised to between 50 and 110 iu/litre, but by the age of 1 month the range is usually between 60 and 200 iu/litre. During puberty, levels of up to 240 iu/litre occur without disease being detected.

5'-nucleotidase

5'-nucleotidase (5 prime-ribonucleotide phosphohydrolase, EC, 3.1.3.5) is an enzyme which has a similar distribution within the hepatocytes as alkaline phosphatase, and may play a role in membrane mediated transport. Although present in bone, its concentration does not change with growth. It has been stated to be of value in differentiating between neonatal hepatitis and extrahepatic biliary atresia. It has been said that the level in extrahepatic biliary atresia is likely to be above 35 iu/litre while in hepatitis it is likely to be below this level. There are many methods for measuring 5'-nucleotidase and this may explain why in the cases in which I have seen this estimation made it has not distinguished these conditions.

Serum protein determination

Serum albumin is produced by the liver. Hypo-albuminaemia is frequently found in liver diseases. This may not necessarily be due to decreased synthesis or increased degradation, but may be due to increased plasma volume. Hypo-albuminaemia is most frequent in the presence of advanced chronic liver disease, particularly cirrhosis. It is a useful index of the severity of cellular dysfunction in such chronic liver disease and has been of value in adults in predicting the patient's response to portosystemic shunting or portal hypertension. In acute liver disease, its value is less striking, perhaps because of the long half-life of albumin (about 20 days).

Serum gammaglobulin is composed of immunoglobulins produced in the reticulo-endothelial system. High levels are found in chronic liver diseases.

Specific immunoglobulins are produced by T lymphocytes. Elevations of serum immunoglobulins A, G and M may be found in chronic liver disease. IgM is raised in viral hepatitis; IgG is commonly raised in chronic active hepatitis. Abnormally low levels, particularly of IgA, may be found in patients with chronic active hepatitis. Similarly, low levels may be found in their relatives. Some patients with chronic active hepatitis do, however, have raised IgA levels. In Wilson's disease the serum immoglobulins are normal, but in the early stages the IgM may be elevated.

Auto-antibodies to nuclei, smooth muscle, mitochondria, and microsomes

These are antibodies which are directed against subcellular organelles or soluble proteins. Their presence in serum may indicate an underlying genetic predisposition to immunological disorders. Persistently high titres may suggest particular disorders. High levels of anti-nuclear factor are commonly found in chronic active hepatitis. In adults high levels of anti-mitochondrial antibody are of value in the diagnosis of primary biliary cirrhosis.

Prothrombin time

The liver is the site of synthesis of many coagulation factors. The half-life of these varies from a few hours to four days. Thus, a decrease in hepatic synthesis due to liver damage is rapidly reflected in a decrease in the plasma levels of these factors (I,II,V,VII,IX and X). The one-stage prothrombin time is now considered to be largely dependent on factors II,V,VII,X and fibrinogen; these factors require vitamin K for synthesis. The test should be run in combination with a healthy control specimen and the result expressed in seconds. The test does not measure prothrombin concentration alone and the common method of expressing prothrombin results as a percentage prothrombin concentration should be abandoned.

Prolongation of the prothrombin time which is rapidly corrected following intramuscular injection of vitamin K, indicates obstructive biliary disease without marked hepatocellular impairment.

Vitamin K resistant prolongation of the prothrombin time indicates severe intrahepatic disease. Prolongation is commonly found in fulminant hepatic failure, in severe chronic active hepatitis and in decompensated cirrhosis. It is also found in metabolic liver injury in the newborn, for example, galactosaemia and fructosaemia.

Gammaglutamyl transpeptidase (GGPT)

This enzyme is found in hepatocytes, both in the cell membranes and in microzomes, as well as in the soluble fraction. It is not localized to the liver but has been found to be a sensitive screening enzyme assay for disorders of the hepatobiliary tract. It is elevated in patients who have no other abnormality of standard tests of liver function but who do have histological abnormalities within the liver. It may be elevated by drug injury to the liver, by cholestatic syndromes and by extrahepatic bile duct obstruction. By itself it is not a particularly useful parameter for the classification or characterization of liver disease or as a means of following its course. It may give additional information if used in conjunction with other enzymatic tests. The normal paediatric range is from 0 to 45 iu/litre.

Serum bilirubin and its metabolism

See Chapter 3.

Urine bilirubin

Bilirubin in the urine may be the first indication of hepatobiliary disease in patients who are not overtly jaundiced. In jaundiced patients it indicates the presence of conjugated bilirubin in the serum, a sign of hepatocellular parenchymal damage or bile duct obstruction. The commercially prepared Icto-test is the best available test. Urine that has been standing at room temperature for several hours may give a false-negative test. Beeturia and chlorpromazine metabolites in the urine may interfere with the test.

Serum cholesterol

The total serum cholesterol is low in newborn infants. It increases during the first year of life and thereafter slowly approaches adult levels. There is a wide range of normal values which, to some extent, are determined by dietary intake.

Although low serum values for cholesterol may be found in acute and chronic liver disease, the main abnormality is likely to be a high serum cholesterol in patients with chronic biliary obstruction or intra-hepatic cholestasis. In such patients values up to twice the upper limit of normal for adults are frequently found.

Normal cord serum cholesterol is between 50 and 150 mg/100 ml. This increases to from 90 to 200 mg/100 ml by the age of six weeks, and in children over the age of 1 year it is between 120 and 160 mg/100 ml. Adult values range from 120 to 250 mg/100 ml. Such normal values, however, may vary from community to community, depending on dietary habits.

Ammonia

The concentration of blood ammonia is primarily regulated by the liver. Endogenous ammonia is derived from the colon where it is produced mainly through the action of bacterial urease. Some is ela-borated in the kidney and small intestine. Exogenous sources include dietary protein and aminoacids.

No standard method has been generally accepted for the deter-mination of ammonia in blood. It is elevated in acute and chronic hepatic encephalopathy. In these circumstances diagnosis and moni-toring of the patient's progress can usually be determined in other ways. Perhaps the main role of blood ammonia determination is in the diagnosis and management of congenital hyperammonaemic states.

Serum bile salts

The major excretory function of the hepatocyte is the excretion of bile salts into bile. As this function is lost the peripheral plasma concentration of these compounds rises. This occurs whether the disease attacks primarily the liver or the biliary tract. Maximum values may be found following a meal. In chronic active hepatitis it has been found that this is a sensitive measure of disordered liver function when tests other than liver biopsy give normal results. The clinical value of serum bile salt determination is still undergoing evaluation. Contrary to an early report, it has not proven of value in the differentiation of hepatitis in infancy from extrahepatic biliary atresia.

Sulphobromophthalein sodium (BP) retention

Sulphobromophthalein sodium is a dye which is avidly taken up by the liver, and is actively excreted into the bile following conjugation with glutathione. Some reflux of conjugated sulphobromophthalein from the liver into the plasma occurs. The test is normally performed by injecting the dye as a 5 per cent aqueous solution into the vein in one arm. A dose of 5 mg/kg bodyweight is used. Blood is taken from the other arm 45 minutes later, and in healthy children less than 5 per cent is retained at that time. Abnormally high levels are found in a wide range of disorders; it is thus of little value in the differential diagnosis of liver disease but may indicate hepatic dysfunction which is not evident clinically. A wide range of non-hepatic disorders and drugs influence retention of the dye.

Sulphobromophthalein sodium may cause thrombophlebitis. It is intensely irritating when injected outside the vein. It can produce systemic allergic or anaphylactic reactions. It has in rare instances caused death. The test has at present no role in routine clinical practice.

SPECIFIC TESTS

Caeruloplasmin

Caeruloplasmin is a copper-binding protein which possesses copper oxidase enzymatic activity. In its purified state, as an alpha-2 globulin, it is blue.

Its concentration may be determined by immunoprecipitation techniques, or enzymatically by the oxidation of certain polyamines. The rate of oxidation is proportional to the plasma concentration of caeruloplasmin. The normal range is from 20 to 40mg/100 ml, much lower values are found in cord blood and in the first two months of life. In Wilson's disease caeruloplasmin may be absent or present in low concentrations in up to 95 per cent of cases. In most other forms of liver disease the caeruloplasmin concentration is high. In fulminant hepatic failure or subacute hepatic necrosis low levels may be found, returning to normal if the liver recovers.

Alpha-1 antitrypsin

Alpha-1 antitrypsin is a glycoprotein produced in the liver and found in the serum in association with the alpha-1 globulin fraction. Approximately 90 per cent of the alpha-1 globulin consists of alpha-1 antitrypsin. Alpha-1 antitrypsin is an acute phase protein. Its concentration rises in response to acute infection, surgical trauma, pregnancy and such drugs as oral contraceptives. Genetically determined very low levels have been associated with liver disease starting as a cholestatic syndrome in infancy or, rarely, with cirrhosis manifest in early childhood or young adult life, or with emphysema having its onset usually before the age of 40 years. More recently it has been associated with glomerulonephritis.

The serum concentration of alpha-1 antitrypsin is determined by more than 20 co-dominant genes. The alpha-1 antitrypsin produced by these can be identified by acid starch-gel electrophoresis and by immunoprecipitation techniques. These alleles are identified alphabetically depending on their rate of migration in an acid starch-gel electrophoretic system. The majority of the population have alpha-1 antitrypsin type MM which is usually identified as Pi (protease inhibitor) MM. Patients with severe liver and lung disease usually have the PiZZ phenotype but rarely have the PiZ nul phenotype. One family has been described in which 2 infants have cirrhosis with PiSZ phenotype. This latter association may be coincidental.

Alpha-1 antitrypsin deficiency may be suspected on visual examination of a routine serum protein electrophoretic strip by the detection of very low or absent alpha-1 globulin fraction. Alpha-1 antitrypsin may be determined semi-quantitatively by immunoprecipitation techniques. The serum concentration, however, is determined by the genetic make up of the individual as well as by stresses mentioned above. Immunoprecipitation techniques are therefore valuable only if they show a high level of alpha-1 antitrypsin. If the serum concentration is found by such techniques to be less than 200 mg/100 ml in a patient with liver disease, it is imperative to have the protease inhibitor phenotype determined by starch gel techniques. This is so because 'stress' of hepatic disease may in some instances increase the serum concentration of alpha-1 antitrypsin, even in a deficient individual, into the range commonly found in healthy individuals.

Alpha-1 antitrypsin deficiency may be suspected by the appearance in the liver biopsy of diastase-resistant, PAS-positive, magenta-coloured globules within the hepatic cells, particularly in the periportal zones.

This material is very difficult to find in deficient individuals before the age of 12 weeks and cannot be relied on to suggest the diagnosis. The material has been shown on electronmicroscopy to be localized to the lumens of the rough endoplasmic reticulum. It has been identified as alpha-1 antitrypsin by immunofluorescent techniques.

Alpha-1 antitrypsin deficiency itself does not cause liver disease. Clinically significant liver disease appears in approximately 15 per cent of such infants while up to 50 per cent have abnormal liver function tests in the first two years of life. Methods have been described for the detection of alpha-1 antitrypsin in amniotic fluid late in pregnancy, but as yet I am aware of no report on phenotyping of the fetus early in pregnancy.

Alpha-fetoprotein

Alpha-fetoprotein is normally synthesized by embryonic liver cells. In intrauterine life it is the major serum protein. It reaches its peak levels in serum between the ages of 13 and 20 weeks, after which it declines until birth. It is detectable in cord blood but is not normally detectable after the age of six to eight weeks.

Alphafetoprotein may be determined by immunoprecipitation techniques, counterimmune electrophoresis, and by radioimmunoassay. The latter has the greater sensitivity and allows accurate quantification.

High levels of alpha-fetoprotein concentrations are found in infants with intrahepatic cholestatic syndromes in the first 10–20 weeks of life. Patients with extrahepatic biliary atresia have levels which tend to be slightly lower but there is a large overlap between the values found in these two conditions, and alpha-fetoprotein determination cannot be recommended as a method for distinguishing the two conditions.

Elevated levels of alpha-fetoprotein are found in the serum of 50–70 per cent of children with hepatocellular carcinoma or hepatoblastoma. Where positive it is a useful test for assessing whether surgery has been completely effective. It may also have a role in monitoring the effects of chemotherapy. Approximately one-third of children with embryonal teratoblastoma have elevated alphafetoprotein in the blood. Yolk sac tumours also produce elevated levels.

It has been said that levels of greater than 100 ng/ml are associated with a good prognosis in fulminant hepatic failure. This has not yet been confirmed.

HEPATIC SCINTIGRAPHY

A gamma-emitting isotope such as technetium-99m or colloidal gold-198, is injected intravenously and the uptake of these isotopes by the reticulo-endothelial system is monitored using a rectilinear scinti-scanner or a gamma camera. The rectilinear scanner has the advantage that the gamma radiation from the liver may be represented by coloured dots which vary in colour with the intensity of radiation and thus indicate the spatial distribution and concentration of the isotope within the liver, as well as indicating liver shape and size. The gamma camera gives a more rapid picture but loses some definition. Technetium-99m is the radionuclide in most general use, giving a clear scan and having a short half-life.

The normal liver has a fairly even distribution of activity, the scan giving a good index of liver size and shape. Lesions that do not take up the isotope appear as filling defects. Primary or secondary tumours, cysts or abscesses may thus be localized. Other extrinsic lesions, such as a subphrenic abscess, may be suggested. Hepatic scintiscanning is valuable in the diagnosis of space-occupying lesions, particularly if larger than 2cm in diameter. The sensitivity of scanning also depends on the position of the lesion. Those placed anteriorally are more easily shown than posterior ones. Lateral scanning may help in localization.

Cirrhosis or any generalized hepatocellular disorder, such as acute hepatitis, is suggested by generalized decrease in uptake, an irregular pattern of isotope distribution and by uptake of technetium-99m by the spleen and bone marrow. In contrast, isotope uptake in extra-hepatic portal hypertension is not reduced and the pattern is homo-genous although there is marked increase in splenic size. The picture of severe hepatocellular disease is particularly useful when a bleeding tendency contra-indicates biopsy.

Obstruction to the hepatic veins will show reduced uptake through-out much of the liver but with good uptake in the caudate lobe. Serial scans are of value in following the course of lesions such as amoebic abscesses, or where precise determination of serial changes in hepatic size are necessary, as in the intravenous treatment of glycogen storage disease.

Radionuclides which are utilized in synthesizing protein, as opposed to being taken up by the reticulo-endothelial system, are of value in the further diagnosis of filling defects in the technetium-99m scan. For example, selenomethionine-75 is taken up by primary liver cell cancer and some secondary tumours but is not by cysts. It is often not taken up by haemangiomas but this is not invariable. Ultrasonic echography, serum alpha-fetoprotein determination, hepatic arteriography and tissue diagnosis must complement liver scanning in the management of patients with space-occupying lesions. In children the liver scan is of value in confirming the presence of liver disease when biochemical and clinical findings are equivocal, and points to the necessity for further more definitive investigations. There is considerable observer error in assessing scans.

Scintiscanning in biliary tract disease

Rose Bengal tagged with ^{131}I or with technetium-99m has been used to demonstrate the gallbladder. The main role has been in the identification of choledochal cysts. These appear as accumulations of isotope below the liver when scanning is repeated 12 hours following the intravenous injection. Recently, technetium-99m has been used to label such compounds such as pyridoxyline glutamate. This substance is rapidly taken up by the liver and excreted into the biliary system. It is concentrated in the gallbladder and thereafter discharged into the intestine. It can give valuable information about the gallbladder when the patient is jaundiced thereby precluding the use of oral cholecystography and intravenous cholangiography.

Ultrasonic scanning

Progressive development of ultrasonography, particularly the introduction of 'grey scale' sonography, has greatly enhanced the value of this technique. Initially, the main value was in distinguishing clearly between fluid-filled and solid lesions. Ultrasonography can now be used to determine accurately the size of the liver and spleen. It has also been shown to be of considerable value in demonstrating gallstones, dilatation of the biliary tree and mechanical obstruction of the biliary system by choledochal cysts and has also been of value in demonstrating the size of the main vessels supplying and draining the liver. The size and patency of the portal vein may be demonstrated. The technique is rapidly performed and involves no discomfort for the patient. It is thus a valuable initial investigation in suspected liver tumours, bile duct obstruction or portal hypertension.

Computerised axial tomography

By mathematically combining x-ray images made from numerous angles, a cross-sectional image of the biliary tract and liver may be constructed, visualized and photographed. Advances in computer technology and in display techniques have allowed this to be done with a total dose of x-ray approximately similar to that needed to make a single conventional radiograph of the abdomen. The equipment is expensive and unlikely to be available in many units. A further problem is that the patient must remain still during the period of the scan. This can make it difficult to use in infants and young children. In adults it has facilitated the early recognition of tumours, bile duct abnormality, cirrhosis and vascular lesions involving the liver and biliary tree. The value of this investigation, as opposed to the information gained from conventional radioisotope scanning and ultrasonic scanning, is still being assessed.

LABORATORY DIAGNOSIS OF INFECTIONS OF THE LIVER

Viral infections

Hepatitis A and B viruses and the yellow fever virus are the most important infectious causes of acute inflammation of the liver. Hepatitis has also been associated with cytomegalovirus (human herpes virus Type V,) and AB virus (human herpes virus Type IV). Other viruses which occasionally display increased hepatotrophism include rubella, various adenovirus serotypes, paramyxoviruses, herpes simplex virus, enteroviruses, various arbovirus serotypes and Marburg virus.

Hepatitis A virus

Tests for this virus are as yet only available in specialized referral centres. The virus may be identified in the stools as a spherical particle measuring 27 μm in diameter. It is detected by immune electron-microscopy.

Complement fixing specific antibody to viral hepatitis A can be demonstrated in serum soon after the onset of infection. Antibody can be detected by immune adherence within three to five weeks of infection and persists for many years. The hepatitis A antigen has been identified in serum in the early pre-clinical phases of the disease by immune adherence haemagglutination and radio-immunoassay.

Hepatitis B virus

There is now substantial evidence that hepatitis B virus is a 42 nm particle having an inner nucleocapsid core and an outer protein coat. In this protein coat the surface antigen is complex. There are at least four phenotypes, adw, adr, ayw, and ayr. The e antigen complex is distinct from the surface antigen. Its precise relationship to the virus has not been established. The extent of cross-immunity between the main sub-types is still undetermined. Antibody can be demonstrated to both the hepatitis B surface antigen and to the core. Core

TABLE 21.1
Laboratory Methods for Detecting Hepatitis B Surface Antigen

Method	Complexity	Specificity	Rapidity	Relative sensitivity
Immunodiffusion	Simple	+++		1
Counter-immuno-electrophoresis	Less simple	+++	++	X 4
Inert particle agglutination	Simple	+	+++	X 10
Reverse passive haemagglutination	Simple	+	+++	X 1,000
Complement fixation	Difficult	++		X 10
Passive haem-agglutination	Difficult	+	++	X 10
Radio-immunoassay	Complex	+		X 10,000
Electromicroscopy or immuno-electron microscopy	Complex	+++		

antibodies frequently persist in high concentrations in chronic carriers of the hepatitis B surface antigen. Antibody to the core has been measured by complement fixation and radioimmunoassay. It is not readily available as a laboratory investigation.

Immunofluorescent techniques have been used to study localization of the core and surface antigens in cells and tissue. There are many laboratory tests for the hepatitis B surface antigen. The principal tests are compared in *Table 21.1*.

Other viruses

Yellow fever may be suspected from the appearance of the characteristic bile-containing vacuoles in necrotic hepatocytes, the so-called 'councilman bodies'. The virus itself may be isolated by subcutaneous innoculation of susceptible non-human primates or into the brains of baby mice. Serological tests are difficult to assess since there are frequently cross-reactions with other Group B arboviruses.

Ebstein—Barr (EB) virus infections are best confirmed by demonstration of the specific antibody to EB virus. Monospot tests and the Paul—Bunnell test may only become positive if repeated. Cytomegalovirus commonly causes an inapparent infection. The highest infection rates occur in early infancy, in adolescents and young adults. Infection acquired in the first five years of life or *in utero*, is likely to be chronic, although sub-clinical. Association with liver disease is confirmed by the finding of inclusion bodies in the nuclei of hepatocytes and bile ductule cells.

Tests of value in other non-viral infections are listed in *Table 21.2*.

PERCUTANEOUS LIVER BIOPSY

Microscopic examination of liver tissue often provides invaluable information for the management of the child with liver disease, providing evidence which is not available by other means (*Table 21.3*). It can also provide material for bacterial and viral culture, analysis of enzymatic activity, chemical content as well as histochemical, immunofluorescent and electronmicroscopic studies. The technique does carry a slight but definite morbidity and even mortality. It can therefore only be justified when it is necessary to know the nature and severity of liver disease more precisely than can be assessed by less invasive techniques, and where the information sought may be crucial in modifying management. Certain contra-indications should be observed and complications anticipated.

The procedure should be performed by physicians who have had adequate instruction and supervision by others who have frequently performed this procedure. Except in intrahepatic biliary hypoplasia and in some rare metabolic disorders, percutaneous liver biopsy will provide sufficient material for full diagnosis. This is extremely surprising since it is likely that less than 1/20,000 of the liver is removed at biopsy. The smallness of the sample removed should be borne in mind since over-interpretation of minor changes in successive biopsies, particularly in chronic hepatitis, may be due more to sampling errors than the evolution of the disease.

TABLE 21.2
Diagnostic Investigations in Protozoal, Helminthic and Mitotic
Infections of the Liver

Disorder	Identification of organism	Antibody test
Amoebiasis	Active haemophagocytic tropho-zoite of *Entamoeba histo-lytica* in stool, rectal scrapings and liver aspirate	Specific of long duration
Leishmaniasis	*Leishmania donovani* parasites in reticulo-endothelial cells of lymph nodes, bone marrow, liver and spleen	Specific but not strain specific
Malaria	Parasite in thin or thick blood film stained with Giemsa stain	
Hydatid disease		Haemaglutination test 75 per cent positive Soluble flourescent antibody test 2 per cent *Echinococcus granulosus*-positive if titre greater than 1:40 Casoni intradermal test posi-tive in 70-80 per cent of cases but 10−15 per cent false-positives
Schistosomiasis	Ova in stool, rectal or liver biopsy	Specific complement fixation test (skin test, non-specific)
Clonorchiasis	Ova in stools	Tanned, red cell agglutination technique for antibody
Fascioliasis	Eggs in faeces or duodenum. Adult worm or eggs in dilated bile ducts on liver biopsy	−
Toxoplasmosis		Indirect fluorescent antibody test > 1/64 Complement fixation test > 1/4
Toxocara canis		Fluorescent antibody technique

Percutaneous liver biopsy may be done under local anaesthesia in young infants and in some children over the age of six years, depending on their personality. In most children between the age of six months and six years, a brief general anaesthetic is probably preferable to the very deep sedation necessary to ensure the child's compliance during the procedure. I have found intravenous Diazepam, in a dose of 0.25 mg/kg intravenously, the most satisfactory premedication, if sedation is required.

TABLE 21.3
Indications for Percutaneous Liver Biopsy

Differentation of conjugated hyperbilirubinaemia in infancy
Investigation of obscure hepatomegaly
Chronic hepatitis
Chronic or recurrent conjugated hyperbilirubinaemia
Investigation of portal hypertension
Diagnosis of Wilson's disease
Diagnosis of metabolic or storage disorders
Reye's syndrome
Drug, toxic or irradiation hepatitis
Pyrexia of uncertain origin
Staging of lymphoma

Consideration must also be given as to which type of liver biopsy should be performed. The aspiration biopsy, using the Menghini needle, is safer since the needle requires to be in the liver for only a very short time, and is thus less likely to tear the liver capsule if the patient breathes while the needle is in the liver. The fact that it by-passes fibrous structures, and is thus less likely to damage large intrahepatic blood vessels or bile ducts also makes it safer. This may, however, give a false estimate of the degree of hepatic fibrosis. For that reason,

TABLE 21.4
Contra-indications to Liver Biopsy

Purpura or a prothrombin time prolonged by more than three seconds compared with the control, or a platelet count of less than 40,000/mm^3
Extreme dyspnoea
Hydatid disease in the right lobe of the liver
A pyogenic abscess in the right lobe of the liver
Biliary tract infection
Infection of the peritoneum, right pleura or lung
Angiomatous malformation of the liver
Alphafetoprotein-positive suspected primary hepatic tumour
Suspected extrahepatic bile duct obstruction with possibly dilated biliary tree
    (ultrasonography or percutaneous cholangiography are better investigations)
Ascites

---

the Tru-cut needle which cuts a core of tissue from within the liver must be used if it is believed the liver has increased fibrosis.

Pre-operative preparation should include haematocrit blood count and platelet count, and the prothrombin time should be determined. The patient's blood group should be determined and a unit of blood cross-matched. In most circumstances a liver scan should have already been performed to exclude the possibility of filling defects within the right lobe of the liver. Careful consideration should be given to the possibility of there being any contra-indications such as those mentioned in *Table 21.4*.

Menghini technique

The Menghini needle is hollow, 40, 70, or 120 mm in length and 1.0, 1.2 or 1.4 mm in diameter. The tip is bevelled at 45 degrees and flat ground. A square 'nail' or obturator measuring 10 or 40mm and having a flattened head is inserted into the proximal end of the needle before assembly with the syringe. The obturator prevents aspiration of the specimen into the syringe.

The patient is placed in a supine position on a firm bed with the right flank exposed and the right arm drawn up beside the head. The point of entry of the needle into the liver is then selected. The upper limit of liver dullness is determined by percussion in the anterior axillary line. The site is one intercostal space below. It usually lies in the 7th and 8th intercostal space. The point of entry of the needle should be marked by applying tincture of iodine to the point or using an indelible marker.

The operator then prepares for the procedure by washing his hands and wearing surgical gloves. The area of the biopsy is prepared by using a chlorhexidine solution. The needle tract is anaesthetized down to the liver capsule with local anaesthetic. While this is taking effect, the Menghini needle, obturator and 20 ml syringe containing approximately 10 ml of sterile normal saline solution, is assembled. The system should be checked for leaks by occluding the biopsy needle opening with a gloved fingertip and retracting the plunger of the syringe. The connection of the needle and syringe must be adjusted until a 'leak-proof' system is achieved. A small nick is then made in the skin with a small-bladed scalpel, a trocar is then passed through the intercostal muscles to form a track for the biopsy needle. It should follow an imaginary line that will place the needle at right-angles in the liver surface. The Menghini needle on its syringe is then introduced as far as the inter-costal ligament which can often be felt to give way on penetration. A few drops of normal saline solution are then expressed through the needle to clear debris from the tip. With the patient's breath in expiration and the syringe barrel in full suction, the needle is rapidly advanced into the liver 2—5 cm and rapidly withdrawn. At all times the needle is directed at right-angles to the liver surface.

In young infants, the procedure should be done four hours after the last feed. The baby will normally be fractious during the preparation period, and can usually be soothed by means of a 'dummy' or comforter. This is withdrawn after the needle tip has been cleared of any debris. The infant will then usually cry vigorously and, during the expiratory cry, the biopsy can be performed safely.

Following the procedure, the patient should be advised to lie on his right side for four hours. The pulse and respiration should be monitored at quarter-hourly intervals for two hours, and thereafter at half-hourly intervals for a further six hours. The abdomen should be gently palpated six hours after the procedure for signs of peritoneal irritation.

Complications

Complications are likely to be minimal if careful consideration is given to the contra-indications listed and if the procedural details for performing the biopsy are followed. They appear to occur in less than 1:1,000 biopsies.

Important complications have been reported with this procedure. They include local pain and infection, subcapsular and intrahepatic haematomata, capsular bleeding, bile peritonitis, haemobilia, pleural pain, pneumothorax, penetration of other abdominal organs and arteriovenous fistula. Death has also occurred.

Problems are most likely to arise if the puncture is made low; the needle then transverses the thinnest part of the right lobe of the liver and may well impinge on the gallbladder and portohepatis structures.

Tru-cut liver biopsy

The Tru-cut needle (*Figure 21.1*) consists of a sharp, pointed needle with a 2 cm notch and cutting sleeve. The patient is prepared as for aspiration biopsy, including the injection of local anaesthetic down to the capsule of the liver. The skin is nicked. Respiration is arrested in expiration. The needle with the sleeve advanced is introduced just within the liver capsule. The needle alone is then advanced into the liver, the sleeve advanced to close over the notch, to cut and trap a cylinder of liver within the lumen of the needle, and the needle and sleeve are withdrawn together immediately. This technique is thus

372

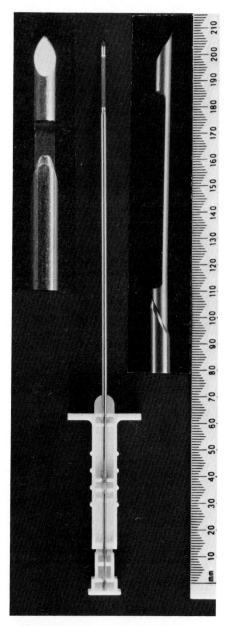

Figure 21.1. Composite photograph of Tru-cut liver biopsy needle with a magnified view of the end of the needle to show the notch

much more complicated than for a Menghini needle biopsy. It involves three distinct manoeuvres while the needle is within the liver. Inexperienced operators frequently pull the needle back within the liver, rather than advancing the sleeve. The author's technique is to introduce the needle and sleeve with the right hand, to advance the needle with the left hand, placing the 5th finger of the left hand on the surgical drape, to ensure that the left hand does not move, and then to advance the sleeve with the right hand. It is clearly important that this technique be perfected in the autopsy room.

Handling the tissue

The liver tissue is removed from the Menghini needle by expelling a little saline solution from the tip of the needle, or by dismantling the syringe and pushing the core of tissue out, using a fine trocar. The material should be transferred into the bedding or fixative material as quickly as possible. This is particularly important if enzymatic studies or electronmicroscopy is to be performed. It is important not to use forceps to manipulate the biopsy as these squeeze and distort the tissue. In general, it is best not to apply the tissue to filter paper or other mounting material provided one can guarantee to get the material to the laboratory without undue shaking and fragmentation of the tissue.

Transjugular liver biopsy

This technique has been used with adult patients as a method that avoids puncturing the peritoneum or liver capsule, where liver biopsy is indicated in patients with impaired coagulation, or with thrombocytopenia. These, of course, commonly occur in patients with severe liver disease. The liver biopsy is taken through the hepatic vein. This is entered by a catheter which is passed through the internal jugular vein into the right lobe of the liver. The catheter is introduced under fluoroscopic control. The technique has not to my knowledge been described in children. The size of the biopsy obtained from adults has sometimes been inadequate for diagnosis. Provided this technique is used by those experienced in catheterization and cannulation of the internal jugular vein, transjugular liver biopsy may be of value when percutaneous biopsy is hazardous, particularly also in instances where intracardiac and hepatic vein pressures are required.

SPLENOPORTOGRAPHY (PERCUTANEOUS TRANS-SPLENIC PORTAL VENOGRAPHY)

The injection of radioopaque dye into the pulp of the spleen is followed by the rapid uptake of the dye into the portal-venous system demonstrating it and its collateral vessels. Normally venous blood from the stomach and spleen flow into the splenic vein and on into the portal vein. Obstruction to portal blood flow, either due to intrahepatic or extrahepatic causes reverses this blood flow and causes the secondary development of collaterals, usually involving the gastric and oesophageal veins.

Contra-indications

Splenoportography is contra-indicated in the presence of allergy to contrast media. This should be tested by the intravenous injection of 1ml prior to the procedure. It is contra-indicated also if the prothrombin time is prolonged by more than three seconds, or if the platelet count is less than 50,000. The presence of an infectious cause for splenomegaly makes the spleen more liable to rupture. Deep jaundice, ascities or a non-palpable or small spleen are also contra-indications. The procedure should not be done unless removal of the spleen can safely be performed if the procedure causes splenic rupture. It should therefore rarely be undertaken below the age of eight years.

Indications

Splenic portography has been used as a means of establishing the localization of obstruction to blood flow in portal hypertension and the extent of collateral vessels. It also indicates whether blood is flowing to or from the liver along the portal vein. This may be of value in assessing the effects of sudden diversion of blood flow from the portal venous system. If there is already a reduction of blood flow to the liver, such a procedure may further compromise the liver and result in hepatic failure or encephalopathy. The procedure does indicate the size, position and patency of the portal and splenic veins. It may therefore be essential when considering an appropriate surgical approach should portal vein decompression become necessary.

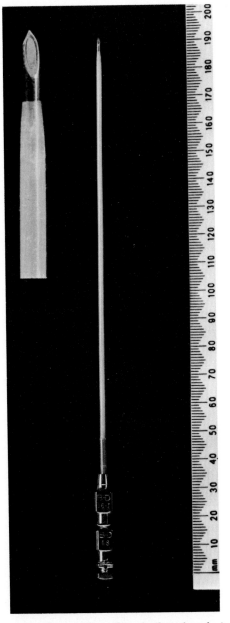

Figure 21.2. Teflon catheter with needle and stilette for splenic venography

Technique

This procedure should be performed under general anaesthesia in children aged less than ten years. In older children it may reasonably be performed with the patient under local anaesthesia. It is important to cross-match two units of blood before commencing the procedure, and a surgeon should be available should problems arise following the procedure. The technique is carried out in the radiological department on a table which allows image intensification, cineradiography, and a rapid film changer which will allow two films per second to be taken for the first two seconds and thereafter one film per second for 15 seconds. The patient is placed supine on the table. The point of maximum splenic dullness in the mid-axillary line (usually between the 8th and 9th intercostal space) is determined. A Teflon catheter with a needle and stilette (*Figure 21.2*) is inserted through a small skin incision in a horizontal and slightly cephaled direction. A distinct sensation can usually be felt as the needle pierces the capsule of the spleen, the needle should then be advanced for a further 2.5 cm. The stilette is then removed, blood should drop out at a rapid rate. The needle can then be removed leaving the flexible Teflon catheter. The correct position of the catheter is established by making a test injection of 5–10 ml 50 per cent of Hypaque. Rapid filling of the veins can then be established fluoroscopically. If the position is satisfactory, 20 ml of 20 per cent Hypaque is rapidly injected.

The cassette changer is programmed at the rate indicated above. It is often convenient to measure the splenic pressure between the test hand injection and the mechanical injection.

When the study is complete the cannula is withdrawn and the patient observed closely for signs of intraperitoneal bleeding or for pneumothorax.

BIBLIOGRAPHY

Aminotransferases

Leevy, C.M. (1974). *Evaluation of Liver Function in Clinical Practice*, 2nd Ed. Indianapolis: Lilly Research Laboratories

Mowat, A.P., Pscharopolous, H.T. and Williams, R. (1976). Extrahepatic biliary atresia versus neonatal hepatitis: a review of 137 prospectively investigated infants. *Archs Dis. Childh.* 51, 763

Wilkinson, J.H. *et al.* (1972). Standardization of clinical enzyme assays; a reference method for aspartate and alanine transaminases. *J.clin.Path.* 25, 940

Zimmerman, H.J. (1964). Serum enzymes in the diagnosis of hepatic disease. *Gastroenterology* 46, 613

Alkaline phosphatase

Boat, T.F., Doershuk, C.F., Stern, R.C. and Mathews, L.W. (1974). Serum alkaline phosphatase in cystic fibrosis. *Clin.Pediat.* **13**, 505

Kaplan, M.M. (1972). Alkaline phosphatase. *New Engl.J.Med.* **286**, 200

Kattwinklel, J., Taussig, L.M., Statland, B.E. and Verter, J.I. (1973). The effects of age on alkaline phosphatase and other serological liver function tests in normal subjects and patients with cystic fibrosis. *J.Pediat.* **82**, 243

5'Nucleotidase

Belfield, A. and Goldberg, D.M. (1971). Normal ranges and diagnostic value of serum 5'-nucleotidase and alkaline phosphatase activities in infancy. *Archs Dis.Childh.* **46**, 842

Yeung, C.Y. (1972). 5'Nucleotidase in neonatal hepatitis and biliary atresia; preliminary observations. *J.Pediat.* **50**, 812

Proteins, immunoglobulins and tissue auto-antibodies

Alper, C.A. (1974). Plasma protein measurements as a diagnostic aid. *New Engl. J.Med.* **291**, 287

Frommel, D. and Good, R.A. (1971). Immunological mechanisms and disorders. In *Recent Advances in Paediatrics*, p. 401. 4th ed. Ed. by Gardiner, D.M. and Hull, D. London: Churchill

Glynn, L.E. (1976). Immunopathology of liver disease. In *Progress in Liver Diseases*, p. 311. Ed. by Popper, H. and Schaffner, F. New York: Grune and Stratton

Sherlock, S. (1977). Immunological changes in liver disease. *Proc.R.Soc.Med.* **70**, 851

Prothrombin

Aledort, L.M. (1976). Blood clotting abnormalities in liver disease. In *Progress in Liver Diseases*, p. 350, Vol 5. Ed. by Popper, H. and Schaffner, F. New York: Grune and Stratton

Roberts, H.R. and Cederbaum, A.I. (1972). The liver and blood coagulation physiology and pathology. *Gastroenterology* **63**, 297

Smith, C.H. (1972). *Blood Diseases of Infancy and Childhood*, 3rd ed. St. Louis: Mosby

Gammaglutamyl transpeptidase

Gragosics, B., Ferenci, P., Pesendorfer, F. and Wewalka, F.G. (1976). Gamma glutamyl transpeptidase. Its relationship with other enzymes for diagnosis of liver disease. In *Progress in Liver Diseases*, p. 436, Vol. V. Ed. by Popper, H. and Schaffner, F. New York: Grune and Stratton

Cholesterol

Dietschy, J.M. and Wilson, J.D. (1970). Regulations of cholesterol metabolism. *New Engl.J.Med.* **282**, 1128

Tsang, R.C., Fellat, R.W. and Glueck, C.J. (1974). Cholesterol at birth, part 1: comparison of normal and hypercholesterolaemic neonates. *J.Pediat.* **53**, 458

Ammonia

Stahl, J. (1963). Studies of blood ammonia in liver disease: its diagnostic, prognostic and therapeutic significance. *Ann.intern.Med.* **58**, 1

Bile salts

Manthorpe, D. and Mowat, A.P. (1976). Serum bile acids in the neonatal hepatitis syndrome. In *Liver Diseases in Children, INSERM* (Colloquim, 23) **49**, 57

Hofmann, A.F., Korman, M.G. and Krugman, S. (1974). Sensitivity of serum bile acid assay for detection of liver damage in viral hepatitis Type B. *Am.J.dig. Dis.* **19**, 908

Caeruloplasmin

Aisen, P. *et al.* (1960). A rapid screening test for deficiency of plasma caeruloplasmin and its value in the diagnosis of Wilson's disease. *Am.J.Med.* **28**, 550

Ritland, S., Steinnes, E. and Skrede, S. (1977). Hepatic copper content, urinary copper excretion and serum caeruloplasmin in liver disease. *Scand.J.Gastroent.* **12**, 81

Alpha-1-antitrypsin

Arnaud, P., Chabuis-Cellier, C. and Creyssel, R. (1975). The Pi system: its study by means of thin-layer gel electrofocusing. In *Proceedings of the 22nd Colloquim on Protides.* Oxford: Pergamon Press

Fagerhol, M.K. (1976). The genetics of alpha-1-antitrypsin and its implications. In *Aspects of Genetics in Paediatrics*, p. 515. Ed. by Baltrop, D. London: Fellowship Postgrad. Med.

Alpha-fetoprotein

Johnston, D.I., Mowat, A.P., Orr, H. and Kohn, J. (1976). Serum alphafetoprotein levels in extrahepatic biliary atresia, idiopathic neonatal hepatitis and alpha-1 antitrypsin deficiency (PiZ). *Acta pediat.Scand.* **65**, 623

Silver, H.K.B. *et al.* (1974). Alpha-1 fetoprotein in chronic liver disease. *New Engl.J.Med.* **291**, 506

Scanning

Kreel, L. and Meire, H.B. (1977). The diagnostic process: a comparison of scanning techniques. *Br.med.J.* **2**, 809

Smith, A.L., Mowat, A.P. and Williams, R. (1977). Hepatic scintigraphy in the management of infants and children with liver disease. *Archs Dis. Childh.* **52**, 633

Infections of the liver

Apt, W. and Knierim, F. (1970). An evaluation of diagnostic tests for hydatid disease. *Am.J.trop.Med.Hyg.* **19**, 943

Jelliffe, D. (1971). *Diseases of Children in the Tropics and Sub-Tropics,* 2nd ed. London: Arnold

Krugman, S. and Ward, (1973). *Infectious Diseases of Children and Adults,* 5th ed. St. Louis: Mosby

Liver biopsy

Gilmore, I.T., Bradley, R.D. and Thompson, R.T.H. (1977). Transjugular liver biopsy. *Br. med. J.* **2**, 100

Menghini, G. (1970). One-second biopsy of the liver – problems in its clinical application. *Ind. J. Med.* **283**, 582

Rake, M.O., Ansell, I.B., Murray-Lyon, I.M. and Williams, R. (1969). Tru-cut biopsy of the liver. *Lancet* **2**, 1283

Roschlau, G. and Hinkel, G-K. (1974). Leber biopsie im Kindesalter, Jena: Fischer

Scheuer, P.J. (1973). *Liver Biopsy Interpretation,* 2nd ed. London: Bailliere Tindall

Splenoportography

Melham, R.E. and Rizk, G.K. (1970). Splenoportographic evaluation of portal hypertension in children. *J.pediat. Surg.* **5**, 522

Reynolds, T.B., Ito, S. and Iwaksuki, S. (1970). Measurement of portal pressure and its clinical applications. *Am.J.Med.* **49**, 649

CHAPTER 22

Investigation of Biliary Tract Disease

BIOCHEMICAL INVESTIGATIONS

Standard tests for liver function may be of value in distinguishing biliary tract disease from intrahepatic disease, particularly early in the course of the illness. In the former there is characteristically disproportionate elevation of alkaline phosphatase and $5'$-nucleotidase to values of between two and three times normal, while serum levels of enzymes which indicate hepatocellular damage such as aspartate aminotransferase, and gammaglutamyl-transpeptidase are elevated only by 20–25 per cent.

RADIOLOGICAL INVESTIGATIONS

Radiology of the abdomen and gallbladder region

Radiology will show radioopaque calculi both in the gallbladder and in the common bile duct and, more rarely, may show calculi within the hepatic bile duct. Gas in the biliary tree may be seen following spontaneous or post-operative biliary-bowel fistulae. A similar radiological appearance may be seen in cholecystitis and cholangitis if there are strictures in the bile duct.

Ultrasonic scanning of the biliary tree

With modern equipment it is possible to demonstrate cavities with diameters as little as 0.5 cm by ultrasonic echography. Thus, it is possible to demonstrate a normal gallbladder and to show its size and contraction following a fatty meal. Distension of the common bile duct or intrahepatic ducts can also be shown with this non-invasive technique.

Oral cholecystography

The main value of this investigation is in demonstrating gallstones and in detecting gallbladder disease by assessing the ability of the gallbladder to concentrate the radioopaque medium and to contract following a fatty meal. Most commonly, oral cholecystography will show the cystic duct and common bile duct.

The contrast media used are actively absorbed in the gastrointestinal tract, and in the presence of normal hepatic function are taken from the blood into the hepatocytes, excreted in bile and concentrated in the gallbladder. Thus, failure to opacify the gallbladder may occur due to alimentary causes such as vomiting, gastric stasis, diarrhoea or malabsorption, or may be due to defective hepatic excretion. The last-named is particularly likely to occur if the serum bilirubin is greater than 34 mmol/litre (2 mg/100 ml). It may also occur because of inability of the gallbladder to absorb water and concentrate the dye.

If the gallbladder is normal the contrast medium is usually sufficiently concentrated within 10 hours to produce a radioopaque shadow, but the more typical homogenous ovoid shadow is usually seen at 12 hours. It frequently bears a concavity on its medial aspect due to pressure from the duodenum. One and a half hours after a fatty meal the gallbladder should have contracted to half or less its previous size and at this stage the bile ducts may even be visualized. Attention to detail is important if satisfactory results are to be obtained. A laxative should be taken for one or two days before the examination and a control film of the gallbladder area taken. A fatty meal about mid-day on the day preceding the investigations is recommended. The oral cholecystogram agent is taken on the evening following a light meal. This should be fat-free. No further fat should be ingested until the examination is complete. Fluids are permitted. Radiographs of the gallbladder area are taken some 10–12 hours after ingestion of the medium. Prone oblique films together with erect anteroposterior or oblique films are necessary to demonstrate mobile translucencies within the gallbladder.

If visualization is not obtained, tomography may be helpful as may a repeat film taken two or three hours later.

Examination is completed 30 minutes to two hours later following ingestion of the fatty meal. Contra-indications are listed in *Table 22.1*. Abnormalities to be anticipated are shown in *Table 22.2*.

TABLE 22.1
Contra-indications to Cholcystography or Cholangiography

Iodine sensitivity
Serum bilirubin of greater than 34 μmol/litre (2 mg/100 ml)
Intestinal obstruction
Severe impairment of hepatic or renal function
Thyrotoxicosis

TABLE 22.2
Abnormalities on Cholecystography

Non-opacification
    Non-functioning gallbladder
    Cholecystitis
    Hepatic disease
    Inadequate dosage
    Failure of absorption
    Absence of gallbladder

Demonstration of radiotranslucent gallstones

Failure of contraction due to chronic cholecystitis

Abnormal gallbladder anatomy

TABLE 22.3
Cholecystography –Cholecystangiography Agents

Agent	Age or weight	Dose	Route
Calcium ipodate	Newborn and infants	0.4 g of powder/kg	Oral
(Solu-Biloptin)	<4 years or 20 kg	0.3 g ” ” ”	”
	>4 years or 20 kg	0.15 g ” ”	”
Iopanoic acid	<13 kg	0.15g/kg	”
(Telepaque)	13–23 kg	2.0 g	”
	>23 kg	3.0 g	”
Meglumine			
iodipamide	<2 years	0.8 ml/kg	Intravenous
(0.3g/ml	2–6 years	0.6 ” ”	”
Biligrafin)	>6 years	0.4 ” ”	”
Meglumine	0–2 years	0.8 ” ”	”
ioglycamate	3–8 years	0.6 ” ”	”
35 per cent	>8 years	0.45 ” ”	”
(Biligram)			

Intravenous cholangiography

This technique is used to demonstrate the extrahepatic biliary tree and occasionally the gallbladder. A radioopaque dye, which is avidly taken up by the hepatocytes and excreted in the bile, is given intravenously either as a slow infusion over 10–15 minutes, or by a continuous infusion given over some hours.

Again, technical details are important in obtaining good results. It is important that the abdomen be as free from gas as possible. Physical activity and a low residue diet appear to promote this. A fat-containing meal should be given on the evening before the investigation. The patient should then fast for 10–12 hours but should not be deprived of fluids.

Dosage regimens are given in *Table 22.3*. Tomography is essential if good definition is to be obtained.

This investigation is contra-indicated in the presence of renal failure. It should be avoided also in patients with bronchial asthma. It is unlikely to be successful if the serum bilirubin is greater than 34 μmol/litre (2 mg/100 ml).

Percutaneous transhepatic cholangiography

This investigation is used to differentiate intracellular from obstructive jaundice when the clinical and biochemical findings are equivocal and where a high serum bilirubin precludes oral or intravenous cholangiography. The investigation is undertaken as a pre-operative procedure to demonstrate the site of extrahepatic obstruction of the biliary tree or obstruction to the bile ducts within the liver. The procedure has three major complications: bile leakage, haemorrhage from the liver substance, and bacteraemia or septicaemia sometimes complicated by shock if the bile ducts are infected. The procedure should only be undertaken by skilled personnel in circumstances where such complications can be anticipated and dealt with effectively.

In adult patients with dilated intrahepatic ducts transhepatic cholangiography using a fine polyethylene tubing drawn over a needle 12 cm in length and with a bore of 1.0 mm, is used. It is inserted under fluoroscopic control towards the main left and right hepatic ducts. The needle is withdrawn leaving the polyethylene cannula *in situ*. This is slowly withdrawn as suction is applied, until bile enters the syringe. Aspiration is continued until no further bile is obtained, then between 20 and 30 ml of 16 per cent Urographin is slowly injected under fluoroscopic control. After successful catheterization, the tube is left *in situ* and bile drainage continues until laparotomy is performed.

If no bile duct is entered on two attempts it is suggestive of intrahepatic choiestasis and laparotomy is not indicated. If obstruction has been prolonged, that is, more than six months, there may be so much sclerosis around the needle that it is unable to penetrate the thickened duct wall. This procedure, although important in adult hepatology, has rarely been reported of value in children. Even in adults its use has been largely replaced by the two techniques described below.

'Skinny needle'

The Okuda needle, made of fine flexible steel, 15 cm in length and with an outer diameter of 0.7 mm and an internal diameter of 0.5 mm through which dye can be injected while at transverse with the liver, has brought two major advantages. Bile leakage is much less frequent but more importantly, intrahepatic bile ducts which show no dilatation may be demonstrated in up to 67 per cent of adult patients with jaundice due to intrahepatic disease. We have used this technique in infants and children to demonstrate normal hepatic ducts, dilated hepatic ducts due to extrahepatic biliary obstruction and fine abnormal intrahepatic ducts in patients with biliary atresia.

The patient is anaesthetized, respiration is stopped, and with the patient lying supine the needle with a stilette is introduced just anterior to the right maxillary line in the 7th or 8th intercostal space and advanced under fluoroscopic control parallel to the surface of the liver to a point midway between the diaphragm and the upper border of the first part of the duodenum, to a point just above the junction of the right and left hepatic ducts. The stilette is removed and the needle connected to a syringe containing contrast medium. The needle is slowly withdrawn while gentle pressure is applied to the syringe plunger. If a needle enters a blood vessel the contrast is fleetingly seen. If dye enters the hepatic parenchyma it stays for up to two hours, but if it enters a bile duct it flows slowly towards the junction of the main hepatic ducts (*Figure 22.1*). The needle is too fine to allow aspiration of bile. The investigation is contra-indicated if there is a bleeding diathesis or ascites. The procedure should not be carried out unless there are facilities for laparotomy immediately if this is indicated.

Endoscopic retrograde choledochopancreatography

The development of fibre optic endoscopy, and the equipment and techniques for cannulating the ampulla of Vater, has led to the widespread use of endoscopic retrograde choledochopancreatography (ERCP) in the diagnosis and management of biliary and pancreatic disease in adults. In obstructive jaundice it is useful in demonstrating conditions such as sclerosing cholangitis, gallstones, carcinoma of the bile ducts, bile duct stricture and bile duct dilatation. It is thus of value in allowing precise pre-operative diagnosis in these disorders but also in avoiding surgery in such conditions as primary biliary cirrhosis. The technique must be considered in circumstances where oral cholecystography or intravenous cholangiography is unsuccessful

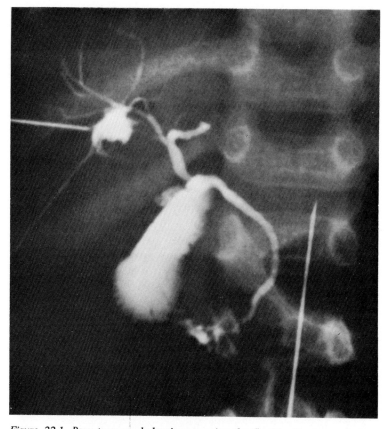

Figure 22.1. Percutaneous cholangiogram using the flexible Okuda needle in a child aged 21 months. The child had had three episodes of jaundice, had persistent pruritus and rickets. Liver biopsy findings did not exclude bile duct obstruction. The tip of the Okuda needle is obscured by a pool of contrast medium within the hepatic parenchyma. Contrast medium has entered fine normal distal bile ducts in the right lobe of the liver and opacified the main right and left hepatic ducts. The common hepatic duct, cystic duct, gallbladder and common hepatic bile duct are normal in calibre. Contrast is seen in the duodenum, excluding obstruction

or contra-indicated. It avoids the complications of percutaneous cholangiography. The procedure produces raised concentrations of serum in between 20 and 70 per cent of cases, and symptomatic acute pancreatitis in between 1 and 17 per cent of cases. As yet, no cannulating endoscope suitable for children has been marketed. With the present instruments a skilled operator may be successful in performing ERCP in children aged 7–8 years and upwards. It should be stressed, however, that this investigation requires considerable skill and expertise on the part of the operator, it is time-consuming and requires expensive endoscopic and radiographic equipment.

RADIOACTIVE TAGGED ROSE BENGAL FAECAL EXCRETION TEST

Principle

The dye, Rose Bengal, if given intravenously is avidly taken up by hepatocytes and, if the liver is normal, is excreted in the bile within a few hours. Since in man absorption from the gut is thought not to occur, the faecal excretion of the dye is related to the amount of bile reaching the duodenum. To avoid the unpleasant task of extracting the dye from the stool and subsequent chemical analysis, it is administered bound to a radioactive isotope such as ^{131}I or ^{125}I.

Problems

An important problem with the test, which causes considerable difficulties when it is applied to young children, is that in jaundice with reduced bile flow much of the radioactive material is excreted in the urine. If such urine contaminates the faeces a falsely high excretion will be reported. For that reason it is absolutely essential that faeces be collected uncontaminated with urine.

To avoid that necessity of meticulous quantitative stool collections many modifications of this test have been advocated. These have, in general, utilized serial counts of radioactivity over the liver and left iliac fossa at intervals up to 48 hours after the intravenous injection of the radioisotope. If no significant obstruction of the biliary tract is present, radioactivity is usually recognizable in the gut within the first three hours, and by 24 hours there is almost complete clearance of radioactivity from the liver, the majority being present in the colon. In total obstruction of the biliary tract there is prolonged retention of the radioisotope in the liver, considerable amounts localized to the kidney and bladder even after 24 hours with no activity appearing in the gut even if counting is done at 48 hours. Unfortunately, there is as yet no published evidence confirming that such techniques are as helpful in discriminating extrahepatic biliary atresia from idiopathic neonatal hepatitis as quantitative stool collection. A further problem is that the dose of radioisotope necessary to allow counting is usually between 20 and 50 times that necessary for the quantitative test.

Method

Although no unbound radioactive labelled iodine should be present in preparations used for this test (source: Radiochemical Centre, White Lion Road, Amersham, Bucks.) the patient is given Lugol's iodine, three drops per day for three days, to block thyroid uptake of any unbound radioactive contaminant. An accurately measured amount of radioactive labelled Rose Bengal is given intravenously by determining the amount of isotope in the syringe before and after injection. It is not necessary to use more than approximately 1 μCi/kg to obtain radioisotope counts significantly greater than background in the collected stool specimen.

Stools uncontaminated by urine are collected for a 72 hour period. In male infants the urine may easily be diverted by tubing attached to the penis or a sterile disposable urine collecting bag which is emptied as soon as micturition occurs. This latter technique is usually successful in female infants provided they are immobilized, but occasionally catheterization is required. It is worth emphasizing that the validity of the test is dependent on the reliability of stool collection. It is thus essential that every nurse involved in the care of the infant understands the necessity for complete stool collection while the test is being performed, including the collection of stools possibly contaminated with urine. Two large polythene bags in bins labelled 'stools uncontaminated with urine' and the second 'stools possibly contaminated with urine' should be provided. It is important to make this available since it is often impossible to avoid all urinary contamination, and indeed it may on occasions be difficult to decide whether slight contamination has occurred. Contamination does not necessarily invalidate the test result provided it has been recognized. If the total excretion from both samples is low, complete cholestasis is present, while if the excretion from the uncontaminated incomplete sample is high, biliary atresia is unlikely.

Evaluation

Where this test has been used in normal infants, the range of excretion in 72 hours has varied between 22 and 71 per cent of the administered dose. (The number of such control cases reported is mercifully low.) In infants with neonatal cholestatic hepatitis, indistinguishable clinically from biliary atresia, the range of excretion reported has varied from 4 to 73 per cent. In biliary atresia, the range reported is from 0 to 23 per cent. The wide range of values reported in the two conditions and the considerable overlap has resulted in this test falling into disrepute.

Where studies have been performed carefully, however, it has become evident that an excretion of less than 10 per cent is indicative of complete bile stasis compatible with biliary atresia. Sass-Kortsak (1974) reported 45 patients with biliary atresia in whom 44 gave an excretion of less than 10 per cent, the remaining patient 11 per cent. In a series of 34 consecutive infants with biliary atresia investigated in our own unit, all had an excretion of less than 10 per cent.

Unfortunately, in intrahepatic causes of cholestasis excretion may also be less than 10 per cent. Sass-Kortsak (1974) found 4 of 41 infants with low excretion, while in our own experience we have recorded it in 5 of 18 infants with intrahepatic causes of cholestasis.

It had been suggested that in such circumstances the infant should be given cholestyramine for 15—20 days and the test repeated towards the end of this period, in that in intrahepatic disease an increased excretion would then be found. We have certainly confirmed that in biliary atresia this measure produces no increase in excretion but, unfortunately, in two of the five cases of intrahepatic cholestasis referred to above, no increase in excretion occurred. With these limitations I consider that this test is a useful investigation to distinguish infants with idiopathic severe neonatal hepatitis with much cholestasis from infants with extrahepatic biliary atresia.

^{131}I ROSE BENGAL ABDOMINAL SCAN

This scan has been referred to above. One situation where it does appear to be helpful is in the patient with choledochal cyst in which it may be possible to demonstrate clearance of the radioisotope from the liver and its accumulation in the cyst lying immediately below the liver. The dose of isotope used in this test, however, is often greater than 100 μCi and cysts detectable in this fashion are likely to be detectable by ultrasonic echography or by barium meal.

BIBLIOGRAPHY

General

Cotton, E.B. (1972). Cannulation of the papilla of Vater by endoscopy and retrograde cholangiopancreatography (ERCP). *Gut* 13, 1014

Chaumont, P., Kalifa, C. and Fontaine, Y. (1974). Slow drip infusion cholangiography in children. *Ann.Radiol.* 17, 441

Fortier-Beaulieu, M. and Rymer, R. (1973). Radiological diagnosis of cholelithiasis in infancy and childhood. *Ann.Radiol.* 16, 167

Okuda, K. *et al.* (14 others) (1974). Non-surgical, percutaneous transhepatic cholangiography – diagnostic significance in medical problems of the liver. *Am. J. dig. Dis.* 19, 21

Rosenfald, N. and Griscom, N.T. (1975). Choledochus cyst – rontgenographic techniques. *Radiology* 114, 113

Rose Bengal faecal excretion test

Brent, R.L. and Geppert, L.J. (1959). The use of radioactive Rose Bengal in the evaluation of infantile jaundice. *Am.J.Dis.Child.* 98, 720

Maksoud, J.D., Thom, A.F., Kieffer, J. and Pinto, B.A.C. (1971). Faecal excretion of Rose Bengal ^{131}I in the diagnosis of obstructive jaundice in infancy, with special reference to biliary atresia. *J.Pediat.* 48, 966

Mowat, A.P., Psacharopolous, H. and Williams, R. (1976). Extrahepatic biliary atresia versus neonatal hepatitis: review of 137 prospectively investigated infants. *Archs Dis.Childh.* 51, 763

Poley, J.R., Smith, E.I., Boon, D.J., Bhatia, M., Smith, C.W. and Thompson, J.B. (1972). Lipoprotein-X and the double [131]I Rose Bengal test in the diagnosis of prolonged infantile jaundice. *J. pediat. Surg.* 7, 660

Sass-Kortsak, A. (1974). Management of young infants presenting with direct reacting hyperbilirubinaemia. *Pediat.Clin.N.Am.* 21, 777

Wicksman, R.S., Adcock, D.F., Bream, C.A. and Scatliff, J.H. (1975). [131]I Rose Bengal liver scanning in the differential diagnosis of neonatal jaundice. *South. med. J.* 68, 599

Index

Abdomen, radiology of, 380
Abscess, pyogenic, 112
Acid base disturbances in liver failure,
   131
Acid esterase deficiency, (See
   Wolman's disease)
Acidosis in glycogen storage diseases,
   166, 168
Acrodermatitis in hepatitis, 107
Actinomycin D, 326
Acute hydrops of gallbladder, 350
Adolescence, hepatic lesions of cystic
   fibrosis in, 273
Aflatoxins, 290
   Reye's syndrome and, 143
Age (See also under specific periods,
   Newborn, Infants etc)
   A-beta lipoproteinaemia and, 177
   alkaline phosphatase levels and, 356
   alphafetoprotein and, 362
   angiomatous malformations, in, 327
   bile acid levels and, 11
   choledochal cyst and, 336
   cholesterol levels and, 11
   chronic hepatitis and, 223
   cirrhosis in cystic fibrosis and, 270
   cystic fibrosis and, 269, 270, 271,
      273, 275
   distribution of hepatitis type A
      antibody and, 96
   diuretic dosage and, 262
   drug metabolism and, 12
   Dubin–Johnson syndrome and, 44

Age (*cont.*)
   gallbladder lesions in cystic fibrosis
      and, 271
   Gilbert's syndrome and, 30
   hepatic fibrosis and, 209
   hepatitis type A and, 96, 98
   hepatoblastoma and, 320
   Indian childhood cirrhosis and, 290
   intrahepatic biliary hypoplasia and,
      70
   jaundice and, 28
   liver cells and, 8
   management of cystic fibrosis and,
      275
   polycystic disease and, 203
   porphyria and, 189
   portal hypertension and, 295
   post-hepatitis syndrome and, 100
   prognosis of cystic fibrosis and, 269
   protein synthesis and, 12
   red cell life and, 32
   Reye's syndrome and, 140
   schistosomiasis and, 120
   sinusoids and, 5
   sodium restriction and, 261
   spleen palpation and, 2
   spontaneous perforation of
      gallbladder and, 339
   symptoms of Gaucher's disease and,
      174
   treatment of liver failure and, 136
   ulcerative colitis and, 121
   veno-occlusive disease and, 302